# PEDIATRIC

## CONTINUING EDUCATION
## REVIEW

By

GLORIA C. ESSOKA, R.N., M.S.

JOSEPHINE C. KIRSCH, R.N., M.A.

FELIX T. KROWINSKI, R.N., M.A.

DONNA L. WONG, R.N., B.S., M.N.

### 530 ESSAY QUESTIONS
### AND REFERENCED ANSWERS

MEDICAL EXAMINATION PUBLISHING COMPANY, INC.

65-36 Fresh Meadow Lane

Flushing, N.Y. 11365

# PREFACE

The questions presented in this volume have been specifically selected to bring the working nurse up-to-date with the latest scientific knowledge and procedures in pediatric nursing. Although this book was written primarily with the nursing practitioner in mind, it will prove to be of value to the educator and administrator as well.

The answers contain complete information, and present major ideas as well as comprehensive background information. They have been referenced to recent nursing journals and textbooks, providing original sources to which the reader may turn for further study and review.

It is hoped that this book, covering the many aspects of pediatrics which require the understanding and awareness of nurses involved in the care of children, will offer interesting and diverse reading for everyone in the field of pediatric nursing.

## ABOUT THE AUTHORS

GLORIA C. ESSOKA, R.N., M.S., teaches maternal-newborn nursing at Seton Hall University, South Orange, New Jersey, and is completing her doctoral studies at New York University. She is a graduate of Thomas Jefferson Hospital School of Nursing in Philadelphia, and later received B.S. and M.S. degrees in Nursing at the University of Pennsylvania. Mrs. Essoka is a co-author of *Obstetrical Nursing Continuing Education Review.*

JOSEPHINE COMITO KIRSCH, R.N., M.A., is Assistant Professor of Nursing, and teaches Maternal and Child Nursing at Hunter College, New York City. She received her B.S. degree in Nursing from Adelphi University, Garden City, New York, and her M.A. degree from New York University, New York.

FELIX T. KROWINSKI, R.N., M.A., teaches psychiatric-mental health nursing at The School of Health Sciences, Hunter College - Bellevue School of Nursing, New York City. Having graduated from Buffalo State Hospital School of Nursing in Buffalo, New York, he attended Black Mountain College in North Carolina. He then received his B.S. in Nursing from Teacher's College, Columbia University and an M.A. in psychiatric-mental health nursing at New York University. Prior to his present office, he held various staff and administrative positions with organizations in different parts of the world, ranging from Greenland to Sumatra, Indonesia. He was nurse-crew member aboard an oceanographic research vessel which discovered the Seamount Chain in the Atlantic Ocean. Currently, he is continuing his studies at New York University.

DONNA LEE WONG, R.N., B.S., M.N., teaches maternal and child nursing at Seton Hall College of Nursing in New Jersey. Prior to this, she was a pediatric clinical specialist, working with children who were terminally ill. She received her Bachelor of Science degree from Rutgers College of Nursing in Newark, New Jersey, and her Masters of Nursing degree from the University of California School of Nursing in Los Angeles.

PEDIATRIC NURSING
CONTINUING EDUCATION REVIEW

TABLE OF CONTENTS

Table of Contents (Continued)

# I. GROWTH AND DEVELOPMENT OF CHILDREN

1. Q. What are some developmental milestones of early childhood?

   A. The infant is born with several reflexes such as suck, swallow, blink, gag, startle, tonic neck and others. As he matures many of these primitive reflexes, such as the startle and tonic neck, disappear and other learned skills emerge. Although there are variations along the time scale for each skill to appear, normalcy seems to follow this rough schedule:

a) 1 month - follows an object to midline, regards a face, makes a face, makes a fist, coos and gurgles
b) 2 months - smiles at social gestures, follows an object 180 degrees
c) 3 months - turns head
d) 4 months - holds head up, reaches for objects
e) 5 months - rolls over
f) 6 months - transfers objects from either hand, has raking grasp
g) 7 months - sits briefly, unsupported
h) 8 months - creeps, sits alone steady, good hand-eye coordination
i) 9 months - pulls himself up with help, shows preference for using one hand instead of the other, can purposely release an object
j) 10 months - pincer grasp, walks holding on, stands alone
k) 12 to 14 months - walks unsupported, says 2 to 3 words
l) 18 months - builds 2 to 3 cube tower, scribbles with crayon, knows ten words
m) 24 months - builds tower of 5 or more blocks, runs well, has vocabulary of about 200 words, uses phrases or short sentences of 2 to 4 words

REF. Marlow D.: Textbook of Pediatric Nursing. W. B. Saunders Company, Philadelphia, 1973.

2. Q. What are the principles of basic learning and developmental processes of all children?

   A. The following chart lists the principal basic learning and development processes of children. Adapted from "The Visually Impaired Child. Growth Learning Development - Infancy to School Age (Halliday, 1970)".

| | |
|---|---|
| (1) More body movement | Less body involvement |
| (2) Large muscle usage | Small muscle usage |
| (3) The familiar | The unfamiliar |
| (4) Simple tasks | Harder tasks |
| (5) Immediate concerns | Remote concerns |
| (6) Short attention span | Increased attention span |
| (7) One concern | Several concerns |
| (8) Thinking of himself as the center of his world | Thinking of others |

7

|  |  |
|---|---|
| ( 9) Things "lived" | Things thought |
| (10) Using words as labels | Using words as organizers and enablers of thought |
| (11) One word sentences | Expressed thoughts, ideas |
| (12) Doing | Sensing, symbolizing |
| (13) Field dependence | Field independence |
| (14) Analysis | Synthesis |
| (15) Physically taking apart or undoing | Physically putting together or fastening |
| (16) Outlines | Details |
| (17) Identifying | Comparing |
| (18) Recognizing differences | Recognizing likenesses |
| (19) Recognizing | Reproducing |
| (20) Recognizing opposites | Determining varying kinds of relationships |
| (21) Random ordering | Dimension ordering |
| (22) Categorizing | Establishing hierarchies |
| (23) Perceiving objects through the senses | Noting their use; naming them and their uses |

REF. Zimmerman LD, Calvovini G.: Toys as Learning Materials for Preschool Children. Exceptional Children 37:9, 642-654, 1971.

3. Q. What are Erik Erikson's stages of development?

A. Erikson's stages of development encompass the life span, but his first five stages involve infancy, childhood and adolescence.

Stage I - Acquiring a Sense of Basic Trust:
    The first year involves the satisfaction of physical needs; during first half of year, the oral route affords the most pleasure, while later the relationship with the mother becomes very important.
Stage II - Acquiring a Sense of Autonomy:
    The second year (roughly 18 months to 3 years) marks a time of increasing motor ability and separation of the self from mother.
Stage III - Acquiring a Sense of Initiative:
    During the preschool years child begins to explore feelings of discomfort and guilt; it is also a time of energetic learning and accomplishment.
Stage IV - Acquiring a Sense of Industry:
    The school age child's theme is to master tasks set before him; he concentrates on his capacity to relate to and to communicate with those individuals most significant to him.
Stage V - Acquiring a Sense of Identity:
    An adolescent's major task is answering the question "Who am I?", while looking for acceptance and belonging among his peers and other significant individuals.

The last three stages of adulthood are acquiring a sense of intimacy, generativity, and integrity.
REF. Maier H.: Three Theories of Child Development. Harper and Row Publishers, New York, 1969.

4. Q. What is Piaget's theory of a child's cognitive development?

A. Jean Piaget's theories of learning and intelligence incorporate a developmental point of view, that is, learning is a function of development. Each phase of this development occurs in a specific order based on steps previously learned. To understand his theory, several principles must be understood. According to his theory, intellectual behavior is characterized by function and structure. Function remains stable throughout life, and the two main functions, organization and adaptation operate from infancy. Organization is the process of giving pattern and consistency to every act. Adaptation is the striving for equilibrium between the self and the environment. Adaptation involves the processes of assimilation and accommodation.

Assimilation involves a person's adaptation and use of something in the environment to incorporate it in himself. Accommodation is the converse of assimilation and represents the impact of the actual environment. For example, the visual perception of fire is assimilated as a perceptual idea. If the person touches the fire he has acquired another input and through the process of accommodation he has other perceptions of what fire is. Thus, these two properties always work together to achieve a balance. Although his stages of development are not clearly defined, they can be stated as:

(1) sensorimotor phase, 0 to 2 years
(2) preconceptual phase, 2 to 4 years
(3) phase of intuitive thought, 4 to 7 years
(4) phase of concrete operations, 7 to 11 years
(5) phase of formal operations, 11 to 15 years

REF. Maier H.: Three Theories of Child Development. Harper and Row, New York, 1969.

5. Q. What developmental stages are involved in feeding behavior?

A. At birth, the infant is born with a strong suck reflex and strong suck demands. By about one month, he is able to take solid food from a spoon, although he will thrust food back out of the mouth due to the extrusion reflex. Between 5 to 6 months, his swallowing becomes more mature, his preference for different tastes emerges, and he sucks on finger foods, such as toast or zwiebach. By 8 or 9 months, he is beginning to hold his own bottle during feeding and to manipulate a spoon to feed himself. Finger feeding also is gaining importance at this time. By about one year, he begins to drink from a cup, with spilling from the edges of his mouth. He feeds himself quite well, and refuses attempts to be fed. By 15 months, he is usually able to drink from a cup with little spilling.

REF. Chinn P.: Child Health Maintenance. C. V. Mosby Company, St. Louis, 1974, p. 197.

6. Q. Can infants recognize a human face?

A. One hundred and twenty subjects ranging in age from 12 weeks to 57 weeks were studied in order to observe age differences in response to facial stimuli. Four different face stimuli were presented to each subject. The stimuli shown were a male's photograph, a cyclops face, a line drawing of a face with features in their normal position and a line drawing of a face with all features misplaced.

The observers found that the male's photograph elicited the most fixation, smiling, vocalization, fretting and crying. By contrast, the face with all features misplaced elicited the least. The fact that the infants smiled more often at the normal face indicates that the infant is able to discriminate.
REF. Lewis M.: Infants' Responses to Facial Stimuli During the First Year of Life. Developmental Psychology 1:75-86, 1969.

7. Q. Does home environment influence infant intelligence?

A. In order to investigate the effect of environment upon intellectual growth 102 infants at five different age levels (7, 11, 15, 18 or 22 months of age) were studied. Half the infants in each age group were disadvantaged and half were middle-class. The development of each infant was assessed. In addition, learning and foresight tasks were given as well as other measures of development. The home environment as it related to the child was assessed.

At eleven months of age, the disadvantaged infants required more trials to achieve success than the middle-class infants. Also, middle-class infants in the 15 to 22 months categories used a larger number of words and a larger number of appropriate words than the disadvantaged infants.

The investigators conclude that the results of the study indicate that deficiencies in intellectual performance are appearing at a very early age. In pragmatic terms, perhaps Head Start should begin during the first year of life for disadvantaged children.
REF. Wachs TD, et al.: Cognitive Development in Infants of Different Age Levels and from Different Environmental Backgrounds: An Exploratory Investigation. Merrill-Palmer Quarterly 17:283-317, 1971.

8. Q. What are the basic needs of all preschool children?

A. Some children have specific needs depending on their particular endowments. Each child is a unique individual who learns and develops according to his own physical, mental, and emotional endowments, his own cultural and environmental experiences, and at his own rate. The basic needs are:

(1) An enriched, stimulating environment in which he can move
(2) Time to explore, discover, and organize information gleaned from his excursions

( 3) Motivating materials to encourage active involvement in the
learning process and to help him understand his environment
( 4) Success in a hurry
( 5) Play-self absorbed, socializing, imaginative, role playing
( 6) Respect - acceptance for what he is and approval
( 7) Responsible direction and challenge to do his best
( 8) Free choice - giving form and substance to his capabilities, and
practice in decision making
( 9) Help in determining his own behavior; building on privileges
(10) A place he can call his own; secret places into which he can curl
REF. Zimmerman L, Calvovini G.: Toys as Learning Materials for
Preschool Children. Exceptional Children 37:9, 642-654, 1971.

9. Q. Does paternal absence affect boys' sex role development?

A. A study was done of differences in behavior of seventeen boys
whose fathers did not live home and seventeen boys whose fathers
lived at home. The father-absent boys displayed greater sex role
orientation, but their manifest sex role development was less than
that of father-present boys. It appears that this phenomena is related to the degree to which mothers encourage masculine behavior.
The findings suggest that mothers of father-absent boys encourage
less masculine behavior than the mothers of father-present boys.
In father-absent homes the maternal encouragement seems more
important than in father-present homes where masculine behavior
is encouraged, observed and emulated. The mother of a father-absent boy is of critical importance in sex role behavior because of
the degree to which she encourages or discourages behavior in the
absence of a male role model.
REF. Biller HB.: Father Absence, Maternal Encouragement and
Sex Role Development in Kindergarten Age Boys. Child Development 40:539-545, 1969.

10. Q. Are there early differences in play between boys and girls?

A. A recent study of thirty-two boys and thirty-two girls, thirteen months of age, suggests that sex differences in play do occur
as early as the first year of life. The behavior of the subjects was
observed in a free play situation. In general, girls showed less exploratory behavior, and their play behavior was quieter. Boys, on
the other hand, were independent, showed more exploratory behavior and were more vigorous and aggressive. These investigators
believe that these behaviors approximate those of later life. Most
of the behaviors suggest that they have been reinforced by the mother, based upon her perception of sex-appropriate behavior for the
child. The authors conclude that because sex differences in behavior occur in the first year of life, it should be considered a variable
in every study.
REF. Goldberg S, Lewis M.: Play Behavior in the Year-Old Infant:
Early Sex Differences. Child Development 40:21-31, 1969.

11. Q. What is the background for the selection of toys as learning
materials for the preschool child?

A. Some consideration should be given to:

(1) Preschool environments: whether classroom, church basement, the environment should be attractive, inviting, and should encourage exploration. The autotelic, responsive controlled environment is one in which the child is free to explore, self initiate, self pace and self control his activities. It encourages him to make a series of discoveries and gives him immediate response to his success. Outdoor space should be included for big muscle play. Physically handicapped children need adaptively designed playground equipment.

(2) Curricula have been defined as the sum total of experiences to which a child is exposed. Most children follow the sequential developmental patterns of all human beings, each does so at his own pace. Curricula should be developed around input, integration, output, and feedback.

a) Self awareness: the child's total self concept and feelings of self worth will be a combination of his physical, kinesthetic, and psychological selves - his own body image concepts, awareness of himself in relation to movement and space, and awareness of his own identity.
b) Sensory-motor-perceptual development: as physical development progresses the child moves from large to small muscle usage and from identifying to comparing, recognizing differences, and recognizing likenesses.
c) Language, communication, cognition processes provides the child with the elements for intellectual development.
d) Social and emotional development: in time the self centered infant learns to play with someone, take turns, control his feelings, and take pride in his accomplishments.

REF. Zimmerman LD, Calvovini G.: Toys as Learning Materials for Preschool Children. Exceptional Children 37:9, 642-654, 1971.

12. Q. What kinds of play are most suited to the toddler and preschool child?

A. Play during this time is in a transition from parallel play toward cooperative play. Episodic play of infancy now gives rise to dramatic play, where themes emerge, especially the newly acquired concept of "I" during the stage of autonomy (Erikson). The toddler is especially interested in motor activity that uses large muscle groups, rather than fine muscles. Riding tricycles, pushing and pulling small wagons, jumping and running are examples of vigorous activity. This is also the time for discovery, and the toddler is curiously seeking every hidden corner, making him vulnerable for accidents.

The preschooler, although still enjoying the feel of clay, now likes to shape and mold it. Simple carpentry and building blocks provide hours of fun. Waterplay, sandbox activities and finger painting are special interests of this age group. This is also an age when acting out feelings is easier than verbalizing them. Puppets, miniature dolls, and dress-up clothes help the child through imaginative play to act out fears and anxieties that can build up inside him to cause problems later in life. Florence Erickson found that intrusive procedures (other than via the oral route) presented the greatest threat to this age group.

REF. Juenker D.: Play as a Tool of the Nurse. Care of the Child with Long-Term Illness. In Steele, 2nd Ed. Appleton-Century-Crofts, New York, 1971, pp. 40-46.

13. Q. When should certain toys be introduced as learning material for the preschool child?

A. Toys for any developmental age should be challenging since this challenge gives the child motivation to move to the next functional level. Problem children may need specific toys which provide practice at that particular developmental level.

REF. Zimmerman LD, Calvovini G.: Toys as Learning Materials for Preschool Children. Exceptional Children 37:9, 642-654, 1971.

14. Q. What is a toy and what are the qualities of a good toy as learning materials for the preschool child?

A. Any toy which stimulates children to discover relationships, stimulates curiosity and imagination, and lets him discover that which it was expected he would learn. A child understands through his toy certain aspects of the physical world.

A good toy is attractive and inviting, well constructed and durable, safe, nontoxic, challenging, and fun. Self correcting toys, those that go together in one way only, allow a child to proceed at his own pace and in his own way without supervision.

REF. Zimmerman LD, Calvovini G.: Toys as Learning Materials for Preschool Children. Exceptional Children 37:9, 642-654, 1971.

15. Q. Why should a specific toy be used as a learning material for the preschool child?

A. A toy should be selected on the basis of the developmental level of a child. Because of physical, mental, emotional, or environmental deprivations and disabilities, some children function at a lower developmental level than other children of the same chronological age. In depth ongoing diagnostic evaluations should be a part of each child's record. Evaluations should be made not only by specialists but can and should include observations by knowledgeable teachers (nurses). It is imperative to know the functioning level of the child in order to determine the use of appropriate materials.

REF. Zimmerman LD, Calvovini G.: Toys as Learning Materials for Preschool Children. Exceptional Children 37:9, 642-654, 1971.

16. Q. What is developmental day care?

A. Recent research has indicated that the early years are crucial periods during which the child develops many skills invaluable for future learning and functioning. In response to these findings, day care has changed from a purely custodial function to a supportive environment with activities designed to foster the child's overall development. Thus, the concept of developmental day care.

Developmental day care attempts to meet the physical, emotional, social and intellectual needs of each child. A key factor is a warm, affectionate staff who function as teachers and parent-substitutes. A variety of stimulating activities which foster curiosity and exploration should be planned. Opportunities to play, which is the child's work, should be provided.

Such day care can support and stimulate the child's development. On the other hand, day care not based upon the child's needs can negatively influence development.
REF. Caldwell BM.: Children Today 1:6-11, Jan.-Feb. 1972.

17. Q. What are the effects of day care on children under three?

A. Studies of children three years of age or younger were conducted in research-based day care projects. Their prime objective was to investigate the impact of day care upon development.

It was found that infants in day care do not suffer cognitive damage. Some demonstrated an increase in I.Q. while others showed no increase. However, none of the children demonstrated deterioration in cognitive ability.

No significant differences in attachment of the infant to its mother were found between day care and home-reared infants. Since day care infants had interaction with more people than the home-reared infants, they tended to develop more attachments. Illness among day care children was not significantly greater than among home-reared children.
REF. Klein JW.: Educational Component of Day Care. Children Today 1:2-5, Jan.-Feb. 1972.

18. Q. What is "PRESS"?

A. The "Preschool Readiness Experimental Reading Test" (PRESS) is a pre-school reading test that can be administered during a routine health check. Five areas of knowledge are tested: knowledge of colors, numbers, general knowledge, drawing coordination, and performance and maturity. The test is appropriate for children 4 years and 9 months through 5 years and 7 months. Interpretation of the test should be limited to white, middle-class children because no research has been done with other ethnic groups.

This test was designed to identify children with future learning problems.

REF. Rogers WB, Rogers RA.: A New Simplified Preschool Readiness Experimental Screening Scale (The PRESS). Clinical Pediatrics 11:558-562, Oct. 1972.

19. Q. Can children benefit from a preschool enrichment program?

A. Attempts have been made to intervene in the environment of low income children with the aim of boosting their usually lagging cognitive growth rates.

Project Headstart and Follow-Through programs for primary school children in low income areas found that gains often dissipate when children move on to primary school. Attempts have been made at intervention more comprehensive than school enrichment alone, recruiting practitioners in medicine, dentistry, and social work, as well as with attention to the children's living conditions and to a closer involvement of parents, particularly mothers. This study shows that an erosion of gains made at school are not unexpected since low income children tend to be exposed to nonconsolidating experiences before and after school, while they are attending the enrichment program and most of the time after they leave. It appears then that substantial and permanent cognitive gains are likely only after a modification of total life experience. This indicates a need for change on a broad front:

(1) Improvement in living conditions
(2) Preschool educational enrichment
(3) Follow through programs at primary school
(4) Fostering of intense parental involvement in the process of education

This study shows that a comprehensive broad front and not only the continuing refinement of pre-school enrichment programs is needed. REF. DeLacey PR, et al.: Effects of Enrichment Preschooling: An Australian Followup Study. Exceptional Children 40:3, 171-176, 1973.

20. Q. Does preschool enrichment have an effect on a child's intellectual performance?

A. Children whose early learning experiences have been impoverished enter public school restricted psychologically, socially, and intellectually, according to Deutsch (1964), Reissman (1961), and others. They have poor verbal skills, knowledge of cultural patterns generally known to other children is limited, and they have few abstract concepts. Lacking the fundamental cognitive skills commonly held by 5 year olds, they must quickly develop the new concepts upon which communication and classroom learning are based before they can progress normally in the primary and elementary grades. The school situation is unfamiliar, so these children must be given more individual attention and help in building self trust and confidence in the learning process.

A 3-1/2 year study of the intellectual performance of preschool Appalachian children, subjected to an enriched day care program, revealed marked improvement in the children who received enrichment. Significant gains in IQ scores during the 3-year period of enriched day care programming were shown for the 4 and 5 year old learning disadvantaged children. A control group showed an average loss of 6.45 IQ points during the year prior to public school entry. No further decrement or increment was noted during 2 years of public school education for these subjects. The overall results of the study support the use of preschool enrichment programming for disadvantaged children on a longitudinal basis.
REF. Kodman Jr. F.: Effects of Preschool Enrichment on Intellectual Performance of Appalachian Children. Exceptional Children 36:7, 503-507, 1970.

21. Q. What are some current concepts and changes in immunization?

A. The combination of diphtheria and tetanus toxoids, and pertussis vaccine (DPT) is still highly recommended for infants and young children. The Committee on Infectious Diseases of the American Academy of Pediatrics (1971) recommends that DPT and trivalent oral polio virus vaccine be given at 2, 4, and 6 months of age. Adult-type combination of tetanus-diphtheria toxoid (Td) is recommended after the age of six years, because of the risk of encephalitis and convulsions from the pertussis vaccine. One outstanding change has been in the schedule for Td. It is now recommended that a booster dose of Td be given every 10 years, or after five years for a contaminated wound.

One of the present problems about immunization is decreasing use of the vaccinations. For example, polio immunizations have been decreasing even though epidemic outbreaks haven't occurred. Such is not the case with rubeola. Present epidemic rates have been increasing even though the vaccine confirms at least 95% efficacy in prevention.

Much controversy is present concerning the rubella vaccine. This vaccine is given to prevent pregnant women from contracting the disease during the first trimester, which can cause severe anomalies in the fetus. The illness itself, however, is quite mild. Some of the present questions are whether or not the vaccine presents a hazard to pregnant contacts, will vaccine-induced immunity in young girls last until childbearing years, and who should be vaccinated to eliminate this threat to pregnant mothers?

A single dose of live mumps virus seems to provide durable immunity and causes fewer reactions than measles or rubella vaccines. It is now present in a combination measles-mumps-rubella preparation.

Two other changes in public health regulations are the discontinuance of routine smallpox vaccination for children and travelers to most

other countries and the discontinued requirement for cholera vaccination as a condition for entering the U. S. Although smallpox has
been discontinued routinely because of the hazard of vaccination and
the decreasing risk of infection, health personnel, military members
and travelers to special countries should still be immunized.
REF. Francis B.: Current Concepts in Immunization. American
Journal of Nursing 73:4, 646-649, April 1973.

22. Q. How effective is combined measles-mumps-rubella vaccine?

A. One hundred eighty-eight Chilean children, ages six months
to eleven years, were given combined measles-mumps-rubella vaccine. By six to thirteen weeks after administration of the vaccine,
96-100% of the children had formed antibodies against all three diseases. There were few complaints of clinical symptoms.

The combined measles-mumps-rubella vaccine has been recommend-
ed for use by the Committee on Infectious Diseases of the American
Academy of Pediatrics.
REF. Borgono M, et al.: A Field Trial of Combined Measles-
Mumps-Rubella Vaccine. Clinical Pediatrics 12:170-172, March
1973.

23. Q. Does the Sabin vaccine confirm long-term immunization for
polioviruses?

A. Ten years have elapsed since the oral Sabin vaccine was introduced during a mass immunization program. The oral polio vaccine stimulates natural poliovirus infection, producing circulating
antibodies and local resistance to reinfection of the intestines. However, little is known about expected serum antibody titers to the vaccine ten years after primary vaccination. A study was done on forty-
five young adults who had received the series of trivalent poliovirus
vaccines ten years previous. Results showed that 75% of the subjects had antibody titers to all three types of poliovirus at a dilution
of 1:4 or greater, and the rest had lower levels of circulating antibodies. Although the study was done on a small sample and definitive conclusions cannot be derived, it does seem that the majority
of the population does maintain circulating antibodies for as long as
ten years, although it may be at a very low level.
REF. Sanders D, Cramblett H.: Antibody Titers to Poliovirus in
Patients Ten Years after Immunization with Sabin Vaccine. Journal
of Pediatrics 84:3, 406-408, March 1974.

24. Q. Why has smallpox vaccination been eradicated in the U. S. ?

A. The United States has been free of smallpox since 1949.
However, since that time several deaths have occurred from complications of smallpox vaccination. In the 21 years since the last
case of smallpox disease in this country, about 160 vaccine associated deaths have occurred. Besides a mortality rate, a morbidity
rate of approximately 8000 cases of severe complications exists
each year. Fatal complications could have been prevented in sever-

al of the cases if three simple precautions were followed: (1) vaccination after age one year, (2) no vaccination for individuals with an altered immune state, and (3) no vaccination in individuals with eczema. However, despite these clear and simple recommendations, 40% of all infant deaths were in infants under one year of age.

Several facts about the variola virus contribute to its possible eradication as a disease: (1) it is a highly visible disease because of its dermal lesions; (2) there is no human carrier state; (3) there is no nonhuman reservoir; and (4) smallpox is not highly contagious.

Although routine primary vaccination is not recommended for the general public, three major groups still remain at risk: (1) travellers to endemic smallpox areas, (2) personnel in military service, and (3) hospital employees.

REF. Karzon D.: Smallpox Vaccination in the United States: The End of an Era. Journal of Pediatrics 1:3, 600-607, Sept. 1972.

25. Q. What is the "small-for-date" infant?

A. Regardless of the duration of pregnancy, an infant can be small-for-date. This includes infants who are postmature: 42 weeks or greater; term: 37-42 weeks; premature: under 37 weeks; or immature: under 28 weeks. Infants born after 37 weeks, who were once regarded as "premature" babies, are now classified as small-for-date babies by comparing birth weight with gestational age. Factors such as weight; length; head circumference; color; texture, kind, and number of skin creases; the presence of vernix and lanugo; ear cartilages, nails, breasts, genitalia and muscle tone; position and neurological reflexes, all are significant in diagnosing the small-for-date infant. These babies need to be identified in order to meet their special needs, since they represent a large proportion of perinatal mortality and morbidity and contribute largely to those children who develop cerebral palsy and mental retardation, as well as other defects.

REF. Andrews B, M.D., et al.: Small-For-Date Babies. Pediatric Clinics of North America 17:1, 185-198, 1970.

26. Q. Do infants who are small-for-date have normal physical growth and development?

A. Ninety-six full term infants were studied from birth to at least 4 years of age. These children were all products of gestations of 38 weeks or more and were at least 30% under expected normal weight. The results were that growth was found to be retarded in all aspects. The average weight and height at 4-6 years was between the 10th and the 25th percentile of the Stuart graphs. Thirty-five percent were below the third percentile and only 8% above the 50th percentile. Siblings and parents were of normal height distribution. Later growth cannot be predicted by the degree of weight retardation, but does bear some relationship to the rate of growth in the first six months. Some small-for-date infants have a growth rate which is

above normal for the first 6 months of life, and this allows the child
to eventually reach a satisfactory growth level.
REF. Fitzhardinge PM, Steven EM.: The Small-For-Date Infant
1. Later Growth Patterns. Pediatrics 49:5, 671-681, 1972.

27. Q. How do infants of low birthweight respond to cold stress?

A. Premature infants defend their body temperature by controlling skin blood flow and regulating heat production within hours of
birth, small babies easily become hypothermic in the first few weeks
of life. The tendency to hypothermia is generally attributed to lack
of tissue insulation and to the high surface area to body weight ratio.

Another factor, low birthweight, together with low incubator temperature in the first few days of life at a time when calorie intake was
low, might be implicated in the observed temporary loss of metabolic response to a cold stress of 29º C. (89.2º F.) for 20 minutes.
The defect in temperature regulation was only temporary, and could
have resulted from depletion of the fat stores available to the babies
calorigenic brown adipose tissues.
REF. Hey EN, Katz G.: Temporary Loss of a Metabolic Response
to Cold Stress in Infants of Low Birthweight. Archives of Disease
in Childhood 44:235, 323-329, 1969.

28. Q. What are the implications of environmental control for babies
that are 3-10 days old and weighing less than 2-3kg.?

A. In these babies, a cot may no longer provide optimum warmth
unless heating is provided below the mattress or the room temperature is maintained well above 25º C. (77º F.). This can be uncom-
fortable for nursing personnel unless they wear light clothing when
working in the nursery. There may be a case for returning to the
practice of nursing some tiny 1 kg. babies lightly clothed in an incubator at a little over 31º C. (87.8º F.) when they are no longer under continuous observation, since the clothing helps to minimize the
effect of any fluctuation in environmental temperature.
REF. Hey EN, O'Connell B.: Oxygen Consumption and Heat Balance
in the Cot-Nursed Baby. Archives of Disease in Childhood 45:241,
335-343, 1970.

29. Q. What is the difference between the environment provided for
a naked baby weighing 2-3kg., between 3-10 days old, in an incubator and that provided for a clothed baby in a cot?

A. Should the temperature within an incubator fall 2º C. (4º F.),
heat production would need to increase more than 35% for there to
be no fall in deep body temperature; should it rise 2º C., the baby
would become pyrexial even if it sweated more than average.

Similar fluctuations in room temperature would have a negligible
effect on a clothed baby in a cot; room temperature would have to
fall to 19º C. (66.2º F.) or rise to 31º C. (87.8º F.) to have a comparable effect on a clothed baby under blankets in a cot. To nurse

such a baby naked in an incubator with an operative temperature close to 32° C. (90° F.), it is important to keep the child under continuous observation. Close control needs to be maintained over incubator temperature because changes of as little as 1° C. (2° F.) will have a marked effect on thermal balance.

Where the baby is not under continuous observation, constant warmth can probably be more easily, cheaply, and safely provided by nursing the baby clothed and lightly wrapped in a warm room at a little over 24° C. (75° F.).
REF. Hey EN, O'Connel B.: Oxygen Consumption and Heat Balance in the Cot-Nursed Baby. Archives of Disease in Childhood 45:241, 335-343, 1970.

30. Q. What adoption resources are available for black children?

A. Although the supply of white infants available for adoption is small, there exists a large number of children in need of adoptive parents. These include minority and racially-mixed children, older children, emotionally or physically handicapped children and children from the same family. Most of the children who do not have homes are black or black and white.

In order to place these children, adoption agencies have established more flexible requirements than in the past. Families or persons who would have been rejected in the past as adoptive parents are now considered. Single persons, older persons, working mothers and low-income families may now adopt children.

In addition, subsidies are available in some states, after adoption, to families with limited financial resources. Foster parents may now become adoptive parents. A more recent trend has been transracial adoption. Also, many organizations concerned with finding homes for "hard-to-place" children have been formed. The paramount focus of these changes in policy is the child and his welfare.
REF. Gallagher U.: Adoption Resources for Black Children. Children 18:49-53, March - April 1971.

31. Q. What is the present status of one-parent adoptions?

A. Although it is generally believed that the two-parent family is best for the adoptable child, it is recognized that such a family cannot be found for every child. This is especially true when the adoptable child is from a racial minority, racially mixed, older or handicapped. Thus, children have been adopted by single men or women, divorcees and widows.

A study of 36 case records conducted in Los Angeles demonstrates that "many persons without marital partners have a great deal to offer children and do so when given an opportunity". When two-parent families are unavailable, the one-parent family is an alternative for placing "hard-to-place" children, so that their needs can be met.

REF. Branham E.: One parent Adoptions. Children 17:103-107, May - June 1970.

32. Q. What is the present status of school health services?

A. The rise in drug use among the young has forced schools to "take action" and provide drug education. Usually the presentation is singular, provides some information about drugs but is not effective.

Although the "crash program" approach has not been fruitful, health professionals continue to agree that drug education is the best way to prevent drug use. Rather than an exclusive focus upon drugs, however, health education should be part of a comprehensive health curriculum that begins in primary school and ends at the end of high school.

Within this health education structure, early school years should teach about the variables involved in health. Middle years should build on and reinforce earlier learning. During the adolescent years, drug use and abuse, including the responsibilities of the young person as a citizen and parent, should be the primary emphasis.
REF. Hester BB.: A New Approach to Teaching About Drugs. Clinical Pediatrics 10:632-636, Nov. 1971.

33. Q. What are some preliminary proposals of the 1971 White House Conference on Children?

A. Preliminary reports were developed by 24 pre-conference forums of experts and laymen from all facets of society. The proposals called for:

(1) The development of a network of experimental elementary schools free of all current regulations where obstacles to education could be overcome, and the best known education methods applied
(2) A system of model elementary schools be established based on democratic principles where students are the decision-makers
(3) Improved research to identify the components of literacy
(4) The priorities of the nation be re-ordered so that the child and family are of prime importance
(5) Parents be trained for the role of parenthood
(6) There be a system of advocacy for children
(7) A system be established to safeguard the health of all children
In general, the proposals emphasize that the United States must vastly change its attitudes and priorities that greatly contribute to the neglect of the needs of children and their families.
REF. Epstein N.: Priorities for Change - Some Preliminary Proposals from the White House Conference on Children. Children 18:2-7, Jan. - Feb. 1971.

34. Q. Should the American educational system be changed to accomodate the needs of multicultural children?

A. This change cannot come soon enough; it should reflect the growing recognition of the value of the many cultural groups in our society.

The special education classroom teacher and the culturally different child both have important contributions to make in molding this new educational system. There is a special need for teachers to realize that there will be cultural conflicts between themselves and some of their students, to try to understand different cultures, and to use these differences to enrich the education of their students.

A special need is that many of these children can and should be made politically aware and politically sophisticated. Along with basic skills and knowledge, children should be given the tools for social change. Many culturally different children want to succeed and they have high aspirations. These children are often thwarted, and the special education teacher must help them achieve as much as they possibly can.

REF. Jaramilli ML.: Cultural Conflict Curriculum and the Exceptional Child. Exceptional Children 40:8, 585-587, 1974.

35. Q. Does the self-concept of black children become more negative with age?

A. Forty 1st grade and forty 5th grade children were the subjects. One-half of each group was white; one-half, black. The self-concept of all children was measured. It was found that the self-concepts of all girls, particularly black girls, were more negative than those of boys, particularly black boys.

The authors suggest that the black mother may be a significant factor in fostering the girls' self-concept.

REF. Carpenter T, Busse TV.: Development of Self Concept in Negro and White Welfare Children. Child Development 40:935-939, 1969.

36. Q. How can parents be helped to answer their children's questions about sex?

A. Curiosity about sexual knowledge and exploration of one's body is normal developmental needs of children. Studies (by John Money and others) have shown that gender role is well established by about two years of age. Whether or not parents provide formal sex education, they do teach the child attitudes about sex through their own behavior and relationships. Because this information is usually supplied unknowingly, the child lacks a set of symbols to identify the sex organs and their functions, and in an attempt to understand, he uses fantasy and magical thinking.

The most important aspect of sex education is preparing a child to receive this information, often a most difficult task to accomplish. This preparation is the attitude of the informer. Nurses often have the opportunity of reeducating a mother to become more at ease while talking about sex, and helping her answer the child's questions. Sex information should be given in exactly the same manner as answers to questions about nature, a toy, etc. Questions should be answered simply, based on the child's level of understanding. For example, children between three and six years often ask, "Where do babies come from"? A truthful answer is "They grow inside their mothers". In answering questions, it is best to use words that avoid confusion with other bodily functions, for example, "The baby grows inside the mommy's abdomen", because "tummy" is often associated with eating.

As children enter school, their curiosity deepens and answers usually need to be more specific, such as a simple explanation of the reproductive system. Discussions of sex should be carried out in private to convey to the child that he should also do these things only in private. Along with sexual knowledge, children should know that love, pleasure, respect and concern are all part of sexuality.
REF. Wilbur C, Aug R.: Sex Education. American Journal of Nursing 73:1, 88-91, Jan. 1973.

37. Q. How useful are routine catheter examinations of the newborn?

A. Between 1965 and 1970, 6,119 term and premature infants were routinely given a catheter examination. This procedure consisted of gently introducing a soft catheter through the nostrils, esophagus, and rectum of every newborn infant. The objective was to immediately recognize some non-obnoxious gastrointestinal obstructions.

Of the 6,119 subjects examined, eight had anomalies such as tracheoesophageal fistula, duodenal atresia and annular pancreas. Nineteen infants had oral bleeding, vomited blood or both; five had rectal bleeding.

Whether or not to risk the danger of causing traumatic bleeding or other complications makes this "routine" procedure questionable.
REF. Quinn N.: Diagnostic Catheter Examinations of the Newborn. Clinical Pediatrics 10:251-253, May 1971.

38. Q. Does newborn behavior influence caretaker responses?

A. Newborn characteristics can influence the emotional and social responses of the adult caretaker. In turn, these characteristics are the variables that provide the caretaker with their perception of the infant's behavior and unique personality.

Of all infant behaviors, wide, bright eyes with search movements is most compelling. Alert eyes are seen as a sign of intelligence and curiosity. Mouth movements may appear to be greeting responses by the caretaker. The caretaker may often play with the infant by mimicking its mouth movements. Activity level also influences the way an infant is perceived.

The main importance of newborn behavior may be its effect upon the caretaker. Social responses perceived as positive will facilitate reciprocal interaction between infant and caretaker. As a result of this mutual interchange, personality, style and temperament can develop.
REF. Bennett S.: Infant Caretaker Interactions. Journal of Child Psychiatry 10:321-335, 1971.

39. Q. Is there a characteristic behavior pattern in a mother's first contact with her newborn baby?

A. The behavior of 12 mothers of full term babies and 9 mothers of premature babies was studied at first postnatal contact. Mothers of full term infants demonstrated a predictable and orderly pattern of behavior when presented with their nude newborns shortly after birth. Starting with fingertip touch on the infants extremities, they proceeded in 4-8 minutes to massaging, encompassing and palm contact on the trunk. The rapid progression from fingertip to palm contact does not agree with the findings of Rubin, who noted that this progression takes several days to occur. Early mother-infant eye-to-eye contact appears to be a significant interaction during the development of maternal affectional ties. Mothers in both groups expressed great interest in the infants opening their eyes and spent increasing time in the "en face" position, i. e. a position in which the mother's face is rotated so that her eyes and the infant's meet fully in the same vertical plane. In mothers of premature babies, this sequence was altered in that the progression from fingertip to palm contact did not occur for the first 3 contacts. Instead, fingertip contact increased. A comparison of immediate postnatal behavior with that observed in non-human species, suggests that this is a sensitive period in the development of close affectional maternal ties.
REF. Klaus M, et al.: Human Maternal Behavior at the First Contact with Her Young. Pediatrics 46:2, 187-192, 1970.

40. Q. What effect does maternal handling have upon the infant?

A. When a mother picks her infant up in order to soothe him, she will inadvertently provide him with visual experiences. Thus, one type of sensory stimulation provided by maternal care is visual experience. The infant who is picked up and soothed will have more opportunities to explore both his mother's and his environments. By contrast, when an infant is not picked up, he is not only deprived of soothing but also deprived of an opportunity to get acquainted with his environment.
REF. Korner AF, Thoman EB.: Visual Alertness in Neonates as Evoked by Maternal Care. Journal of Experimental Child Psychology 10:67-78, 1970.

41. Q. Does a father-absent-home influence emotional development of the child?

A. The life style of one hundred and five children from fatherless homes was studied. They were divided into two groups: (1) "Transitional" fatherless - those without fathers for two years or less (2) "Hard Core" fatherless -- those living with their mothers and apart from an adult male for more than two years. Fifty children were in a fathered control group.

The study found that fatherless children felt ostracized by their peers and were characterized as "loners". The Hard Core children had more intellectual and emotional problems than the other groups. Among this group, the mothers had few contacts with the children. In addition, mother-child interaction was impaired. The authors suggested that critical influences on parent-child interaction are:

(1) the style of the household
(2) different economic conditions
(3) households broken by divorce and desertion rather than death
(4) households which socioculturally differ a great deal from white middle-class norms

REF. Kogecschatz JL, et al.: Family Styles of Fatherless Household. Journal of Child Psychiatry 11:365-382, 1972.

42. Q. What behaviors are the signs of a toddler's separation anxiety?

A. One of the clues that can alert a nurse to the severity of separation anxiety in a toddler is the closeness of the mother-child relationship. For example, a child with a physical deformity may have been loved, but overly protected by the parents. Hospitalization and separation may represent a crisis to child and parent.

Bowlby has described the three (3) stages of separation as protest, despair, and detachment. Protest can be manifested by regressive behavior such as wetting or soiling, kicking, refusal to cooperate, constant crying. The violence and aggression are a child's way of attempting to recapture his mother. Despair occurs when the outbursts stop, and behavior of abandonment sets in. The child is passive, sits alone sucking his thumb or clutching a favorite toy or blanket, moans to himself, and refuses comfort from anyone even the parents. Detachment may appear as if the child has recovered from his loneliness, but actually he has resigned himself to the loss of his mother and will accept anyone, without a trusting relationship with a particular individual.

Nurses can help a child through the first and second stage, and prevent the third stage by explaining to the mother what is happening, that the child's behavior and rejection of the mother is the only understanding the child has about separation or desertion (in his eyes). Mothers need to be encouraged to stay with the child and participate in his care. If the mother is unable to stay all the time, one nurse should try to be the substitute mother, providing care as closely to the way the mother does it, using articles that are familiar to the child.

REF. Stephens K.: A Toddler's Separation Anxiety. American Journal of Nursing 73:9, 1553-1555, Sept. 1973.

43. Q. How can a nurse help a mother retain a symbiotic relationship with her infant, when they are separated because of hospitalization?

A. Many authors have talked about the close, symbiotic relationship that begins between mother and baby as early as conception. Rubin has described the initial phases of touch in the mothering process. But birth and consequent physical separation of mother and child can break this developing closeness. It is even more of a crisis when the newborn is deformed, and besides developing mothering, the mother is desperately trying to deal with her own anxieties, fear of her inadequacy and of her doubts of love for this child.

A nurse can help the mother and child reestablish and maintain a symbiotic relationship by gradually relinquishing much of the infant's care to the mother. When the mother cares for her child with nurse's support, the mother can see another person openly accepting her infant. Nurses and medical staff need to convey knowledge of the deformity in simple language and to discuss treatment and future implications for care.

The author of this article found that not only hospitalization but also a great distance, separated mother and child. In her effort to reestablish their relationship, the nurse used the telephone as communication media. Their conversations frequently were about the infant's progress, the nurse's care of him, and his growth in both physical and developmental terms. When the child returned home, the mother had been continuously growing with her child through the nurse.

REF. Penfold KM.: Supporting Mother Love. American Journal of Nursing 74:3, 464-466, March 1974.

44. Q. What is the nursing intervention in depression and recovery of a 9-week-old infant?

A. An infant is generally not injured by disruption of the infant-mother bond before 12 weeks of age. John Bowlby (Attachment and Loss, Vol. 1 Attachment. London: Hogarth Press, 1969), says that until 8 weeks, and more usually 12 weeks of age, the infant's ability to discriminate one person from another is either absent or extremely limited. Differential responsiveness to auditory stimuli may be observed after 4 weeks of age, and to visual stimuli, after 10 weeks. Robertson, J. (Mother-infant interaction from birth to twelve months: two case studies. In: Determinants of Infant Behavior, ed. B.M. Foss. London: Methuen, 1965, 3:111-127), describes an infant of 8 weeks who became depressed and retarded in psychomotor development upon his mother's withdrawal from a very warm responsive relationship with him.

In the case cited, a 9-week-old breast-fed baby was given minimal care by the mother while she attended to an older sibling's stay in a hospital. Care was left to the father, and, when not available, to a housekeeper. At 10 weeks of age, the nurse-author's examination of the baby showed him to be pale and listless, fontanel depressed, skin inelastic, expression lethargic; he looked cold. The mother stated he looked like a waif and was constantly sucking, which was unrelated to hunger. The nurse felt the infant had good mothering but was reacting much more strongly to deprivation than one who has never known care. A non-threatening expression was utilized, "weaning shock", which the mother accepted.

The nurse suggested that she feed him in a warm room so she could give him direct skin contact with herself; that she cuddle him, sing to him, rock him, encourage response from him, and in every possible way, indicate to him that she was there. The mother decided to do this, rather than subject the infant to hospitalization and various tests. The result at 28 weeks of age, on next examination, showed the infant's physical and motor development to be within normal limits.

REF. Taylor RW.: Depression and Recovery at 9 Weeks of Age. The American Academy Journal of Child Psychiatry 12:3, 506-510, 1973.

45. Q. What are maternal attitudes toward toilet training?

A. The present study was designed to elicit maternal expectations and attitudes regarding toilet training and to identify possible differences between the opinions of inner-city mothers versus middle-class suburban mothers. Some of the conclusions were:

(1) The majority of clinic mothers indicated that family members were the most common source of information regarding advice to toilet training. Middle-class mothers relied mostly on books and their own common sense. Neither group considered the physician (or other health personnel) to be an important source of information.
(2) Clinic mothers (63%) saw the ideal age for starting toilet training to be by 16 months of age for girls or boys. Only 17% of private practice mothers held this belief; most of them saw 17 to 24 months as more appropriate.
(3) Maternal expectation concerning the ideal age for completion of toilet training also varied. Approximately 50% of clinic mothers stated 2 years as completion age, whereas only 16% of the other group agreed. They saw 2 1/2 to 3 years as a proper time.
(4) Both groups responded almost equally to accidents of soiling. Approximately half of the mothers in each group answered that they would offer encouragement. No mother from the private group felt the child should be spanked, while 15% of the other mothers felt spanking was appropriate.

This understanding of parental attitudes is important for health workers who can detect conflicts regarding the parents' readiness versus

the child's readiness for toilet training, thereby preventing possible behavior problems. Some authorities believe that the child is physically and mentally mature enough by ages 18 to 30 months for training to begin.
REF. Carlson S, Asnes R.: Maternal Expectations and Attitudes toward Toilet Training: A Comparison between clinic mothers and private practice mothers. Journal of Pediatrics 84:1, 148-151, Jan. 1974.

46. Q. Should "Mothering" be taught to young boys and girls?

A. "Mothering" and motherliness is thought to be instinctive and universal. Very little is taught about "mothering" - a definition of "mothering" as meaning sensitive, generous, and individualistic approach to the young child by a very tender mother or father prepared to give promptly and predictably whatever the baby needs in the way of individual attention, food, and comfort.

Perhaps 20% of all young mothers have serious problems in mothering, sufficient to require a great deal of support on the part of husbands, health visitors, and physicians. One in five in this group does not know how to turn "mothering" on. Functions of mothering are often taken on by other people in the family, or else the child will receive insufficient mothering and be damaged for life. We must learn to "titrate" the amount of supplemental mothering a given child needs.
REF. Kempe HC.: Pediatric Implications of the Battered Baby Syndrome. Archives of Disease in Childhood 46:245, 28-37, 1971.

47. Q. How may parental over-protection affect the handicapped child?

A. The benevolent actions of the parents of a handicapped child may cause further handicaps by making the child unable to cooperate with others (physicians, nurses, therapists, teachers) as they try to help him overcome his basic handicap. In addition, the child may become emotionally disturbed, express a lack of self-esteem, initiative and self-control. Also, the child may develop some degree of mental retardation or aggravation of present retardation because of a poverty of experiences.

The principal parental (or family) actions which can precipitate this type of behavior are over-protection, permissiveness and excessive helping of the child. Basic guilt feelings, anxiety, love and compassion are usually the motivating factors.

Counselling by health professionals may be beneficial to parents. The main focus should usually be on parental feelings, parental actions and their effect upon the handicapped child. Parent counselling should begin immediately after the child's diagnosis is made; follow-up is essential.
REF. Boone DR, Hartman BH.: The Benevolent Over-Reaction. Clinical Pediatrics 11:268-271, May 1972.

48. Q. Does social class influence mother-infant interaction?

A. In an investigation of social class differences in mother-infant interaction, 30 middle-class and 26 working-class mothers and their firstborn female infants were studied. The major differences found were that middle-class mothers had more verbal interactions with their infants and provided infant stimulation more often than the working-class mothers. On interview, working-class mothers revealed that they felt it was futile to interact with infants. They perceived the infant as unable to express emotions or communicate with other people. Some mothers felt that the infant should be spoken to when he had the ability to verbalize. Many mothers felt they could do nothing to influence the infants' development.
REF. Tulkin SR, Kagan J.: Mother-Child Interaction in the First Year of Life. Child Development 43:31-41, 1972.

49. Q. What are the normal events which occur at puberty?

A. In boys, the first perceptible sign of puberty is the growth of the testes and scrotum. This is frequently unnoticed and is followed approximately one year later by the appearance of pubic hair and enlargement of the penis. In girls, breast development and the appearance of pubic hair usually precede menarche by more than one year. There is a typical adolescent growth spurt which, in boys, begins one year after the onset of testicular growth and about simultaneously with enlargement of the penis. In girls, the beginning of the growth spurt is closely related to the onset of breast development; the peak of growth has usually passed when menarche occurs.
REF. Illig R, M.D.: Delayed Adolescence. Pediatric Annals. 3:7, 17-29, 1974.

50. Q. What are the hormonal factors involved in the onset of puberty?

A. Some of the essentials of normal sexual maturation are as follows:

(1) Pubertal physical development, i.e., growth spurt, increase in muscle size, development of breasts and pubic hair, as well as menarche, are affected by increasing levels of sex steroid hormones in the blood.
(2) The increased production of estrogens and androgens in the gonads and the adrenal gland is caused by increasing levels of gonadotropins, which are protein hormones produced by the anterior lobe of the pituitary gland.
(3) This increase in gonadotropin production is due to enhanced stimulation of the gonadotropin-producing cells by gonadotropin releasing hormones. This gonadotropin-releasing hormone reaches the pituitary gland from the hypothalamus via special portal vessels along the stalk of the pituitary gland.

(4) It is not known why, at a certain stage of maturation, an increase in the production of hypothalamic gonadotropin hormones occurs; research in this area is being done.
REF. Blunck W, M.D.: Sexual Precocity. Pediatric Annals 3:7, 30-46, 1974.

51. Q. What are the stages of puberty in males?

A. Adolescent sexual development in American males begins somewhere between 11.5 and 11.8 years. The testes and scrotum begin to enlarge, with pigmentation and thinning of the scrotal sac. The penis follows with growth in length and circumference. Male pubic hair growth appears between 11.8 and 12.2 years. It begins at the base of the penis, progressing from straight, coarse hair to more profuse curly hair. Eventually it forms a triangle extending to umbilicus and linea alba. Full hair distribution usually is completed in the middle of the third decade. Axillary hair growth follows pubic hair growth. Facial and body hair appear during late adolescence, around 16 years.

Marked growth spurt in maximum height increment occurs about the time pubic hair first develops and decelerates by the time the hair growth is established. Peak height velocity was attained by an average of 14.06 years in this study.

During middle adolescence (13 to 16 years) the prostate and seminal vesicles mature but produce inadequate numbers of spermatozoa. Seminal emission contains an adequate number of motile sperm for fertility around 16 to 18 years. Muscle growth (increase in size and number of cells) occurs in males between 5 and 16 years with the peak increase at 10.5 years. Under the influence of the androgens, the size of the muscle cell continues to enlarge until the end of the third decade.
REF. Root A.: Endocrinology of Puberty. Journal of Pediatrics 83:1, 1-19, July 1973.

52. Q. What are the stages of puberty in females?

A. The characteristic physical changes of puberty progress sequentially until adult sexual characteristics have been attained. The physiologic and endocrinologic changes relate more significantly to the physical stages of sexual maturation than to chronological age. However, there is some uniformity in appearance of physical characteristics. Breast growth usually begins with budding, widening of the areola, and elevation of the mound of subareolar tissue. There is subareola, followed by the areola and papilla, projecting above the plane of the enlarging breast. The average age for the initiation of breast development in American females is 10.8 years.

Most females begin breast development before pubic hair growth, which usually begins at 11.0 years. The first stage is appearance of long, pigmented hair over the mons veneris or labia majora. Dark, coarse curly hair then grows over the mons veneris until an adult type distribution to the medial aspect of the thigh is present. Axillary hair begins to grow after pubic hair.

Menarche is best correlated with bone age and seems to appear between 12.6 to 12.9 years in American girls. Generally, menarche follows breast development and pubic hair growth. A marked growth spurt with maximum height increment may occur about 18 months before menarche.
REF. Root A.: Endocrinology of Puberty. Journal of Pediatrics 83:1, 1-19, July 1973.

53. Q. What is meant by the term delayed adolescence?

A. Delayed adolescence is a benign form of maturational retardation. Medical advice in cases of delayed sexual maturation is most frequently sought for boys between 14 and 16 years of age, but rarely for girls. One of the main complaints of these boys is small stature. The onset of puberty in 95% of boys is between 9 1/2 and 13 1/2 years of age. Five % of boys fall outside this normal range, in 2.5% puberty is more than two years late, therefore occurring in 25 of 1,000 children. The diagnosis is based on the simultaneous retardation of sexual maturation, bone age and linear growth in otherwise healthy boys or girls. Frequently there is a familial history of the occurrence of delayed adolescence. It may be necessary to make growth hormone determinations to differentiate between delayed puberty and severe growth retardation and growth hormone deficiency. In most cases, reassurance that growth will proceed and normal adult size will be reached, helps overcome the problem. In some cases, mainly with boys, psychological problems may necessitate the use of testosterone to induce puberty.
REF. Illig R, M.D.: Delayed Adolescence. Pediatric Annals 3:7, 17-29, 1974.

54. Q. Are there any new developments in the treatment of teenage acne vulgaris?

A. Significant improvements in the current therapy of acne await better understanding of the precise pathogenesis of this disease. However, understanding of the current status of knowledge about the pathogenesis of acne enables utilization of available methods of therapy for the maximum benefit of the affected adolescent. Rational selection of treatment modalities can be improved by considering acne as falling into 2 categories:

(1) Non-inflammatory acne, characterized by closed and open comedones (whiteheads and blackheads).
(2) Inflammatory acne, characterized by inflammation and appearing as papules, pustules and nodulocystic lesions with a propensity for scarring.

Treatment for non-inflammatory acne includes acne surgery, the mechanical removal of blackheads and whiteheads with an instrument known as a comedo extractor. Peeling agents are also used; these include cleansing agents, astringents, acne creams, lotions and gels, cryolush therapy (the application of carbon-dioxide slush to produce erythema and desquamation), natural and artificial ultraviolet light and topical vitamin A.

Inflammatory acne requires treatment which differs from that of non-inflammatory acne, although acne surgery may be used to some extent. The most significant advance in the management of the more severe pustulo-nodulo-cystic type of acne has been the use of long term, broad spectrum antibiotics. The tetracyclines are the most widely used and appear to be the safest for long-term use. Intralesional corticosteroid is a valuable modality in hastening involution of lesions and reducing scarring. Systemic corticosteroids may be used in selected severe cases, for short duration only, because of the hazard of side effects.

REF. Reisner R, M.D.: Acne Vulgaris. Pediatric Clinics of North America 20:4, 851-863, Nov. 1973.

55. Q. Does diet play a role in the treatment of acne?

A. At the present time, it appears that dietary restriction has little or no role in the management of acne, as is true of oral vitamin A administration. Appropriate use of cosmetics may be of great help in reducing the emotional impact of disfigurement produced by acne. Awareness of the physical and psychological scarring which acne can produce, coupled with a well thought out program of topical and systemic therapy can result in significant improvement in most cases.

REF. Reisner R, M.D.: Acne Vulgaris. Pediatric Clinics of North America 20:4, 851-863, Nov. 1973.

56. Q. What are the indications and methods for the treatment of acne with antibiotics?

A. The indication for the treatment of acne with antibiotics is the presence of inflammatory lesions. Little or no improvement can be expected with non-inflammatory lesions or comedones. Tetracycline is the antibiotic most frequently used. Numerous studies have attested to its effectiveness and it is also relatively inexpensive, an important consideration in a drug for long-term use. Therapy is usually begun with doses of from 500mg to 1000mg daily and adjusted downward to the optimal level for each patient. Some patients can be maintained on doses as low as 250mg every other day. Antibiotic therapy does not appear to affect existing lesions, but rather to prevent the formation and reduce the severity of newly formed or forming lesions. Response to treatment requires time and immediate improvement may be the result of coincidental remission or placebo effect. Some patients do not respond to antibiotic therapy, for unknown reasons. Treatment with antibiotics is suppressive rather than curative. Reports of serious toxicity to tetracycline are rare, but occasional side effects, such as G.I. symptoms or candidiasis may appear.

REF. Committee on Drugs: The Treatment of Acne with Antibiotics. Pediatric 48:4, 663-665, 1971.

57. Q. Have specific nutritional needs of adolescents been identified?

A. Because adolescence is a period of rapid growth, nutritional intake is of critical significance. Although many surveys of "teenagers" have been done, their precise meaning in relation to growth, development and reproductive maturation have not been clearly defined. However, some nutritional requirements have been identified as having especial importance during adolescence. They are:

1) Calories - these requirements are related to the stage of physiologic development, growth velocity and genital maturation. In addition, caloric requirements vary greatly with the adolescents' rate of growth and energy requirements. In general, at 16 years of age, boys consumed 3,600 calories daily as compared to 2,300 calories for girls.
2) Calcium - although there is little evidence of calcium deficiency in American adolescents, calcium requirements are not firmly established. However, it is known that calcium retention among adolescents increases and then decreases by age 20.
3) Iron - in response to the menarche, iron requirements for girls increase. Increased muscle and soft tissue growth increases the need in both sexes.

REF. American Journal of Public Health -Supplement, 63:53, Nov. 1973.

58. Q. What differences are there between obese and nonobese adolescents?

A. This study attempted to evaluate the physical, behavioral and psychosocial characteristics of obese teenagers as compared to a group of nonobese adolescents. Some of the results included:

(1) Obese girls were characterized by an earlier onset of puberty and menarche (11.3 years as compared to 12.8 years for the control group), by an accelerated skeletal maturation and by advanced height age. Physical development varied more in the obese boys than in the obese girls.
(2) Endocrinological studies for appropriate hormones were generally within normal limits for most of the obese subjects.
(3) Feeding patterns were prevalent in the obese adolescent's family since birth, such as increased infant feeding problems, food intolerances, earlier introduction of solid foods, and use of sweets as reward for good behavior. During adolescence, the total daily caloric intake and eating patterns were not statistically different between obese and nonobese, but the obese engaged in less physically exerting activities.

(4) Defective body image, low self-esteem, depression and social isolation were much more prevalent among the obese adolescents, particularly the females. The degree to which these character-istics were present seemed to correlate with the success or fail-ure of reducing plans.
(5) The obese adolescents seemed to be a focus of parental conflict, a source of embarrassment, and a scapegoat for their siblings. The parents seemed to defer treatment of the obesity until psy-chosocial problems were obvious, although the obesity had been apparent since early life. They viewed prognosis for weight loss as hopeless and offered minimal support to the adolescent.

REF. Hammar S, et al.: An Interdisciplinary Study of Adolescent Obesity. Journal of Pediatrics 80:3, 373-383, March 1972.

59. Q. What variables can be used to assess adolescent behavior?

A. Adolescent behavior is usually not understood by many with whom there is interaction. It ranges within a broad continuum from normality to abnormality. In order to assess the meaning of the be-havior, it must be viewed for what it is and what it is for. Adoles-cent behavior can be judged, organized and understood utilizing the concept of developmental tasks. The four "basic developmental tasks" represent milestones in development thoroughly which the adolescent must pass in order to become a psychologically normal adult. The tasks to be completed are:

(1) To become emancipated from parents and other adults
(2) To acquire skills for future economic independence
(3) To learn to function in an adult heterosexual role
(4) To establish a stable, realistic positive adult self-identity

Assessment of adolescent behavior should include an exploration of how he functions with family, peers, and in school and whether or not the behavior is age-appropriate. In situations where the behav-ior is not within the range of normality, family counselling may be necessary.

REF. Fine LL.: What's a Normal Adolescent? Clinical Pediatrics 12:1-5, Jan. 1973.

60. Q. What factors cause school failure in adolescent males?

A. Many factors interfere with learning. In the adolescent male, experiencing school failure may be due to resistance to a-chieving adulthood and separation- individuation from their parents. Because of the conflictual attachment to the mother and the inability to identify with the father, there is difficulty achieving adult auton-omy. Thus all demands to "grow up" are met with passive behavior.

With no desire to reach adult development, total passivity toward school and socialization develops. Development is arrested at the

oedipal stage, the conflicts continue to exist. Treatment is aimed at the development of more age-appropriate ego function and to rectify defective development early in life.
REF. Berman S.: A Type of Academic Failure Among Male Adolescents. 10:418-443, 1971.

61. Q. How does the adolescent respond to hospitalization?

A. During adolescence the major task is the establishment of identity. Erikson has identified seven task areas the adolescent must successfully master in order to achieve identity. These are:

(1) A sense of certainty as a person in his own right
(2) A sense of appropriate timing
(3) A sense of sexual adequacy
(4) A sense of social competence
(5) A sense of workmanship
(6) A sense of authority integration
(7) A sense of forming ideology

When the adolescent is hospitalized, his level of anxiety is increased. As a result, he finds task mastery even more difficult than usual. The nurse who cares for the adolescent must understand adolescent development and help him cope with his feelings.

As part of nursing interaction and intervention the nurse should help contribute to the adolescent's self development. That is, she must help him deal with his anxieties and fears related to hospitalization, illness and interruption of his normal life. The adolescent's dependency needs should be attended to by providing support and care when necessary. The nurse should involve the adolescent in his treatment. This will help him feel secure as he strives for independence.

At times, adolescent anxiety is acted out. This may be manifested by disregarding physical limits that have been set and focusing only on the present. As the adolescent becomes more aware of his sexuality, certain tensions may arise. These may be relieved by homosexual play, masturbation or sexual feelings toward the opposite sex.

Hospitalization for the adolescent can be a positive variable during his attempts to establish a sense of identity. The care given by the nursing staff should be comprehensive. If the nurse bases patient care upon an understanding of the adolescent and the developmental tasks involved, she will have served as a force during a crisis.
REF. Tiedt E.: The Adolescent in the Hospital: An Identity-Resolution Approach. Nursing Forum xi:120-140, 1974.

62. Q. How can nurses better understand and care for adolescents who are hospitalized?

A. Adolescence is a time of striving to achieve social, emotional and physical maturity; it is characterized by strife, confusion, conflict but also the capacity for change. A nurse who understands the characteristics of a normal adolescent can use this knowledge to make hospitalization a positive growing experience.

An adolescent is frequently self-centered and over-concerned with himself, interpreting lack of attention as rejection. It is also a time of developing values and standards of behavior. He wants honest, straightforward answers to his questions and is sensitive to lying or "stretching the truth". Rebellious behavior can often be the result of concern and frustration from inadequate information from those caring for him.

He is also searching for independence and control, while still needing guidelines for security and consistency. An adolescent responds well to being given responsibility, such as choosing his diet, cleaning his room, or scheduling a treatment.

Adolescence is a time of peer-group acceptance. Hospital rules frequently prohibit young teenagers or friends his age from visiting. Perhaps, a little "bending" of the rule for special visitors will increase the patient's self-confidence and independence.

Body image is a prime concern at this time. Any procedures that blemish the body are major concerns, such as full body casts or shaving of the head. With all the sexual changes and new feelings about his own body, the adolescent needs privacy. Nurses need to understand this, and to provide it. Masturbation, which is often a source of guilt and conflict, should not be punished but rather seen as a clue to reassure the adolescent that it is not harmful.

Nurses who understand, respect, and accept the adolescent can make hospitalization not only pleasant, but also a time of maturing, solving conflicts, and planning for the future.
REF. Lore A.: Adolescents: People, Not Problems. American Journal of Nursing 73:7, 1232-1234, July 1973.

63. Q. What might be some important characteristics about unwed pregnant adolescents?

A. According to a study done by a nurse who works in an adolescent guidance clinic for pregnant girls, there are differences between these adolescents and non-pregnant adolescent females from similar socioeconomic levels. Some of her findings include:

(1) The pregnant girls had fewer close relationships with anyone in their immediate family; father was mentioned only once and mother nine times (total sample was 30). However, 19 of the 20 non-pregnant girls named a family member as their "closest" person; father was listed twice and mother 12 times. The boyfriend was the closest person to 12 pregnant girls, and to only one from the other group.

(2) Non-pregnant girls seemed much more interested in games and sports, while the other girls had a tendency toward solitude and inactivity. All the non-pregnant girls had at least one hobby, while 21 of the pregnant adolescents had no hobbies. Much of their free time was spent sleeping and watching television. The non-pregnant girls seemed involved in community recreation centers, participating freely and believing these group activities were important.

(3) Reasons for pregnancy ranged from eleven girls who saw it as a way of escaping home to 12 girls who said it was accidental. Of these 12 girls, it is interesting to note that 9 of them had hobbies.

(4) The non-pregnant group seemed to be more realistic and goal directed, having already made plans for the future.
REF. Curtis F.: Observations of Unwed Pregnant Adolescents. American Journal of Nursing 74:1, 100-102, Jan. 1974.

64. Q. What crises arise for the pregnant adolescent?

A. A documentary study of 71 pregnant adolescents revealed the types of crises that are experienced. The crisis for the pregnant teen-age girl is three-fold: maturational or developmental, maternal, and pregnancy.

The first and most intense crisis was that of informing parents of the suspected or confirmed pregnancy. This was an upsetting period for the girl and her parents. Dread, fear of telling parents, embarrassment, grief, and remorse for having disappointed parents were all typical reactions. The critical nature of the parental encounter was due to fears of anger, reproach, punishment or rejection by parents.

Parents usually responded with feelings such as shock, grief, disbelief, self-reproach and questioning of the adolescent. With the passage of time, identification of mother and daughter of their shared femininity and paternal protective feelings relieved tension and restored disturbed relationships. As familial tension decreased, concrete plans concerning the pregnant adolescent were then made.

A major concern of the girls and their parents was the necessity of withdrawal from school. School is the occupation of the adolescent which is essential to and supportive of ego development in the adolescent. It is also a goal-oriented, steadying and sustaining influence that provides a focus and framework for effort. For many girls, school withdrawal represented rejection and punishment. For others, it meant interruption of hopes and plans and loss of self-esteem.
REF. LaBarre M.: Emotional Crises of School-Age Girls During Pregnancy and Early Motherhood. Journal of Child Psychiatry 11:537-555, 1972.

65. Q. What type of nursing intervention for the pregnant adolescent is appropriate?

A. Because of the developmental stage of the pregnant adolescent, the nursing process interventions must be different than those utilized in caring for and counseling a mature pregnant woman. For example, the physical setting should be decorated in a manner that is appealing to the adolescent, in order to put her at ease. Topics such as diet, smoking, and the present pregnancy must be approached in a genuine and non-judgmental manner that is not condescending. Genuine empathy will help in gaining the adolescent's trust.

The girl may be unusually suspicious, belligerent, hostile, apathetic or casual about her present pregnancy and the nurse's attempt to elicit information. Such responses should be met with understanding and support so that these feelings can be worked through.

Other personnel and significant persons such as the school nurse, teachers, school officials must be encouraged to support and understand the pregnant adolescent's plight and behavior. Her pregnancy must be perceived as a health problem, not a moral issue. She should receive the support given to any student with a health problem. The key factor in providing nursing care for the pregnant adolescent is gaining her trust. When this objective is met, the support and counseling necessary during pregnancy can be done.
REF. Curtis FL.: The Pregnant Adolescent. Nursing 74, 77-79, March 1974.

66. Q. How can nurses help counsel pregnant adolescents?

A. Pregnant adolescents are confronted with the conflict of growing up, finding identity and bearing the responsibility of an adult. It is no wonder that these young woman need help to cope with this additional crisis. One process used to help these adolescents is group therapy and crisis intervention. The major emphasis of teaching is using the group to share experiences and provide learning. Initially, the girls are preoccupied with the pregnancy. However, relating information is not enough. Their curiosity is so emotionally laden that time must allow for assimilation of the facts. An implication of this is that facts related to the pregnancy need to be repeated several times, and discussion encouraged through an unstructured approach.

Another major theme postnatally is birth control. Initially, the topic is greatly entwined with emotion. Besides providing information, the nurse needs to remember the girl's feelings, thoughts, and desires. It is too easy to simply prescribe a birth control method rather than to provide an atmosphere that allows the adolescent to make her own decision. Culture plays a big part here because incongruity between use of contraception and freedom of sexual activity can prevent a girl from using the device. For example, use of a contraceptive before the act denotes planning, which may seem promiscuous to some.
REF. Davis L, Nand GH.: Anticipatory Counseling of Unwed Pregnant Adolescents. Nursing Clinics of North America 6:4, 581-590, Dec. 1971.

67. Q. How does having an abortion influence the adolescent female?

A. Characteristic behavior patterns were observed in 24 adolescent girls who had voluntary abortions performed.

Girls who identified strongly with the infant allowed their mothers to make decisions and provide their care throughout the pregnancy and abortion. It was believed that this dependent, passive behavior helped the girl to vicariously recapture her own infancy. By contrast, girls who identified strongly with a maternal role were more independent. They made their own plans for the abortion and provided self-care. For this group, pregnancy and abortion seemed to be an organizing experience and a motivating force for further development.

Among adolescent girls, pregnancy that is followed by abortion heightens already-present developmental conflicts. The one most uniformly aroused conflict was found to be mothering vs. being mothered. Either regressive attachment to mother or new independent growth may be activated in the adolescent.
REF. Schaffer C, Pine F.: Pregnancy, Abortion and the Developmental Tasks of Adolescence. Journal of Child Psychiatry 11:511-536, 1972.

68. Q. How can formal education be provided to the adolescent during pregnancy?

A. Traditionally, the adolescent female has been excluded from public school during pregnancy. In selected situations, homes or school settings specifically designed for pregnant teenagers were the only alternatives available to limited numbers of teenagers. Recently, however, school boards and communities throughout the country have recognized the rights of pregnant students to continue their education in their regular schools. If a student wishes to transfer to another setting, plans can be made for her to transfer to home instruction in a maternity home, a community center or a special center.

The goals of education must be expanded beyond teaching basic learning. Specifically, they should include courses geared toward employment, family living, sex education, and family sex roles. In addition, if the teenage mother is to remain in school, facilities must be made available that provide infant care while she is being educated.
REF. McMurray G.: Continuing Education for Pregnant Teenagers. Nursing Outlook 17:66-69, Dec. 1969.

69. Q. Do the cities meet the needs of the pregnant adolescent?

A. A survey of 130 cities revealed many unmet needs in providing comprehensive services for pregnant adolescent girls. Since pregnant teen-agers represent a high-risk group, priority should be given to multi-service pre-natal care. The most frequent unmet need reported was for education services. General and administrative services were second, health services third, followed by social

services, financial assistance, vocational assistance and nutritional
services, respectively.

A relationship was found between city size and the degree of compre-
hensive services offered. That is, the larger the city the more like-
lihood that special services were available for pregnant adolescents.
REF. Wallace HM, et al.: A Study of Services and Needs of Teenage
Pregnant Girls in the Large Cities of the United States. American
Journal of Public Health 63:28, Nov. 1973.

70. Q. What might be some causes for the rising incidence of V.D.?

   A. Presently in the U.S. gonorrhea is the number one report-
able communicable disease and accounts for more than one-half of
all venereal diseases. Syphilis is also on the increase, with esti-
mates of 20,000 to 85,000 new cases reported each year. Several
factors have been proposed to explain this increase:

(1) Social factors have been afforded much importance because of
the generally more permissive attitude toward sex. The contraceptive pill has had its effect by adopting the ideology of sex separated
from reproduction. It has taken the worry of pregnancy out of sex,
and has influenced the liberation of women. Exactly what sexual influence the pill has had is debatable, but it is certain that it has allowed parents to choose their family.

Other social pressures of rapid change, inflation, overcrowding,
fewer jobs have affected young people. Many are searching for identity, acceptance, and belonging. Emphasis on brotherly love has increased communal living, where sexual freedom is seen as sharing
and gaining closeness.

(2) Inadequate educational programs certainly should accept some
blame. Dissenters of these programs use arguments such as children are too young to know those things, or talking about it implies
condoning and encouraging sexual acts, or teaching about the quick
easy treatment for V.D. deemphasises its seriousness, or those
who get V.D. deserve it. Because V.D. education has not been
openly presented, it enhances an attitude of secrecy about the detection of V.D., stifling the possible eradication of the disease.

(3) Physiologic factors are also affecting the rising incidence. For
example, the pill reduces the vaginal pH, making the woman almost
100% susceptible to contracting the disease. Also some strains of
V.D. are becoming resistant to treatment.
REF. Ahern C.: I Think I Have V.D. Nursing Clinics of North
America 8:1, 77-90, March 1973.

71. Q. What developmental characteristics are present in fatherless daughters that differ from daughters with a father?

A. One study of 72 adolescent girls divided into three groups showed several differences in the females' relationship with men. The groups consisted of girls, aged 13 to 17 years, who presently had fathers, whose fathers had died, or whose fathers were absent because of divorce. Some differences can be summarized as follows:

(1) There were no differences in sex-role typing among girls without fathers. The observed deviations were in the fatherless girls' interaction with males. Girls whose parents had been divorced sought more attention from male adults than the other two groups. Girls, whose fathers had died, seem to avoid males. When this group was subdivided into those-who had lost their fathers before the age of five years and those who had lost him at a later age, it was found that early separation seemed to have a greater effect on the avoidance behavior.

(2) Both groups who had no father, admitted anxiety around males, but exhibited the insecurity and apprehension differently. Girls whose parents were divorced reported more heterosexual activity. They dated earlier and more frequently than the girls whose fathers had died. There was some evidence that the girls whose parents were divorced harbored adverse feelings toward their fathers, while the other group often described their fathers as warm and competent.

(3) There seemed to be little difference in all three groups' relationship with their mothers. Mothers from broken homes tended to be overprotective and solicitous of their preadolescent daughters and reported more conflicts. The widowed mothers reported the least conflicts with their daughters.

In summary, it seems that effects of loss of a father are greatest when the daughter is young (under five years of age), and behavioral deviations appear in the adolescent years.
REF. Hetherington E.: Girls Without Fathers. Psychology Today 6:9, 47-52, Feb. 1973.

72. Q. What are some causes of juvenile delinquency?

A. Delinquents usually have low self-esteem, low status among peers and feel rejected by their families. The perceived disturbed family relationships force the adolescent to seek social groups outside of the family--his peers. The group sought is one that can meet the adolescent's need for decreased tension, enhanced self-concept and peer admiration.

Many sociogenic factors impinge upon adolescents. They easily yield to peer pressure, and sacrifice social for antisocial values. This appears to be an attempt to meet needs not fulfilled within the immediate family.
REF. Didato SD.: Some Recent Trends in Juvenile Delinquency. Mental Hygiene 53:545-549, Oct. 1969.

73. Q. What is the most recent type of care established for juvenile delinquents?

A. The institutions for rehabilitation of the juvenile delinquent are few, understaffed and provide inadequate treatment. As a result, many youngsters are sent to training schools which are true institutions. There, the psychopathological problems become worse. Most of these children show no improvement in behavior during their incarceration. In fact, many gain more knowledge about crime.

A sociologic approach, using a day type facility away from the homes of the delinquent boys is being used in one setting in Utah. The boys receive various types of rehabilitation as directed by the courts.
REF. Didato SD.: Some Recent Trends in Juvenile Delinquency. Mental Hygiene 53:545-549, Oct. 1969.

74. Q. What are the psychosocial problems of adolescents with epilepsy?

A. The psychosocial problems in 17 adolescents age 14 to 16 were investigated. A major goal of the study was to elicit the perceived problems of the teenagers and their parents. Interviews were used for problem exploration. Parents saw behavior problems (depression, moodiness, hostility and irritability) as the major form of difficulty and biggest problem with the teenager. Various school problems were next in importance. The teenagers' primary concerns were peer relationships and "being different" because of their epilepsy.

Most of the teenagers were restricted in social activities by their parents. Athletic restrictions such as prohibition of bicycle riding, gym and skating were demanded by parents.
REF. Richardson DW, Friedman SB.: Psychological Problems of the Adolescent Patient with Epilepsy. Clinical Pediatrics 13:121-126, Feb. 1974.

75. Q. What is the self-concept of the adolescent with epilepsy?

A. In a study of seventeen adolescent patients with epilepsy, aged 14 to 16 years, a variety of psychosocial problems were uncovered. A major objective of the study was to identify problems perceived by the family and the adolescent. The study found that most families had psychosocial problems including prolonged exclusion from school, serious social restrictions, depression and behavior problems. The adolescents saw their major problems as difficulty with peer relationships and "being different".
REF. Richardson DW, Friedman SB.: Psychosocial Problems of the Adolescent Patient with Epilepsy. Clinical Pediatrics 13:121-126, Feb. 1974.

76. Q. How can parents be prepared for the adolescence of a retarded child?

A. Parents should be educated regarding the developmental aspects of retardation with the goal of preparing the adolescent for the future. Such a goal can be met by utilization of the "normalization principle." That is, "making available to the mentally retarded patterns and conditions of everyday life which are as close as possible to the norms and patterns of the mainstream of society."

As the retarded child is reared, behaviors necessary for adult life should be fostered. Social skills, independence, emotional, maturation skills and interests as well as social adaptive behavior necessary for adult functioning should be encouraged. In the activities of daily living, parents can help the child as he begins to acquire acceptable and constructive behaviors. Parents and others need guidance in order to understand that, although the child or adolescent's intellectual functioning is abnormal, the experiences that will guide the child toward adulthood are those normally provided for the non-retarded.

REF. Hillsman G, O'Grady D.: Helping Adolescents with Mental Retardation. Children Today 1:2-6, May-June 1972.

77. Q. What is a cause of the "Generation Gap"?

A. Alienation of middle-class youth has become a growing phenomenon in the United States. Although it is not new, it is only recently that a substantial number of alienated young people have existed to form a subculture.

Alienation among the young may in part be caused by the American philosophy that espouses upward mobility as the only acceptable way of meeting one's aspirations. In most middle-class families, children are expected to equal or surpass parental social status. When the child fails to meet parental standards, parents may react with hostility. The child begins to experience a sense of failure and may drift toward an alienated group, which soothes his sense of failure; thoroughly a new philosophy.

The philosophy of alienation perceives society's flaws as wrong; e.g. racist, materialistic, war-mongering, insensitive, etc. Thus, the alienated adolescent feels justified in having rejected the "bad" standards of the parents. When there is family conflict about the failure of the adolescent to meet parental standards, the situation should be examined. Further, family counselling may be needed to resolve the conflict and perhaps prevent alienation.

REF. Ross C, Jr., Ross C, Sr.: Youthful Alienation and Social Mobility. Clinical Pediatrics 12:22-27, Jan. 1973.

78. Q. What factors minimize the hazards of hospitalization for the pre-school child?

A. In many cases the stress of hospitalization is an overwhelming experience for the pre-school child. The sudden separation from mother and introduction to a new environment and strange people has potential for causing psychological damage to the child.

Two approaches can be considered which can minimize or eliminate emotional trauma to the child due to hospitalization. Hospital confinement should be avoided whenever possible; hospital practice should be designed based upon the needs of the child. These goals can be met in several ways:

(1) The child can be treated on an outpatient basis.
(2) Sick children can be nursed at home by parents and a visiting nurse.
(3) Admit mother and child to the hospital.
(4) Permitting liberal or unrestricted visiting hours.
(5) Shortening the child's hospital stay.
(6) Giving consideration to the possible psychological consequences of hospitalization.

REF. Millar TP.: The Hospital and the Pre-school Child. Children 17:171-176, Sept.-Oct. 1970.

79. Q. What are reactions of parents when their child is hospitalized?

A. To answer this question, the author visited the home of 25 mothers to discuss the effects of hospitalization of the child, the mother, and the family. Some of her findings included the following:

(1) All the mothers reported that their child (ages ranged from 15 months to 9 years) showed various degrees of negative behavior such as crying, screaming, or anger toward hospital personnel.

(2) Two young children between the ages of one and five years were separated from their mothers. One child showed the typical protest and despair stages of separation anxiety, as described by John Bowlby. The other child had been in several foster homes and showed typical detachment behavior only.

(3) After hospitalization, many mothers reported that their child had difficulty recuperating from the hospital experience and illness, and developed negative behaviors, such as demanding more attention.

(4) All of the parents reported some degree of fear, uneasiness, and anxiety, and eighteen mothers mentioned specific incidents which were especially difficult for them. These included observing procedures such as lumbar puncture, electrocardiogram, starting intravenous feedings, and blood tests. Mothers also reported that not being with the child during a procedure but hearing him scream was frightening.

(5) Lack of information was a major concern of most of the mothers. Several also felt guilty about their child's illness and feared long-term aspects.

(6) All the mothers reported that family life was disturbed. Siblings missed the hospitalized child or their mother, and didn't want to stay with a relative or baby sitter.

(7) Many mothers shared some criticisms of the staff, such as nurses not spending enough time with patients; nurses sarcastic to mother or child; child taken to O.R. while awake; child given an injection while asleep; etc.
REF. Freiberg K.: How Parents React When Their Child is Hospitalized. American Journal of Nursing 72:7, 1270-1272, July 1972.

80. Q. Is pre-operative parental rooming-in beneficial?

A. Observations of 144 children between one and eight years of age were made. All of these children were scheduled for elective surgery. The emotional state of each child was evaluated by an investigator, prior to being moved into the operating room. Each child was classified as "awake", "asleep", "calm" or "crying".

Parents were interviewed within two days following the surgery. Parents were categorized as "rooming-in", "present before surgery", or "no contact" if parents left the evening prior to surgery and did not return until the post-operative period.

Approximately 62% of the children were awake but calm when they arrived in the operating suite, 14% were crying and 24% were asleep. No statistical difference between emotional state and parental contact was found. Age, however, played a significant role in the emotional state. 47% of the parents roomed-in with younger children while 22.8% of the parents roomed-in with older children. There was a greater incidence of crying in the children whose parents roomed in.

The authors conclude that parental-rooming-in is not emotionally beneficial to children prior to surgery. Rather, it appears to be of emotional benefit to doctors and nurses. Also, the authors suggest that elective surgery needs to be re-evaluated in light of the findings of this study.
REF. Lee JS, Greene NM.: Parental Presence and Emotional State of Children Prior to Surgery. Clinical Pediatrics 8:126-130, March 1969.

81. Q. How does a day-time hospital for children work?

A. A day-time hospital which eliminates overnite stays and separation from parents has been successful, according to this author. Children admitted to this six-bed unit are having elected procedures such as tonsillectomies, adenoidectomies, cystoscopies, various dilatations, etc. or are having chemotherapy or transfusions.

Before admission, the child and parents are invited to attent a "pre-op party", where equipment such as blood pressure cuffs, masks, gowns, stethoscopes, etc. are available to play with. A short slide show demonstrates the routine admission procedure, and refreshments are served. All the routine laboratory work, X-rays, and admission forms are completed on the day before admission. This procedure alone helps screen out patients who might have minor illness that prevent elective surgery. On the day of admission, parents and patient arrive on the unit at 7:00 AM, where last minute admission procedures such as vital signs are done. Surgeries are not scheduled before 9:00 AM to allow the patient time to get acquainted. Parents are encouraged to stay and help with as much care as possible. They accompany the child to the door of the O.R. When the child returns, post operative care is similar to inpatient procedures. Surgeons recheck the child and write discharge orders. Approximately three percent of the patients require extended stays.

The only change that has been made, according to the author, is that "patients or parents who would require continuous reassurance and support, or for whom continuous, rapid-pace environmental activity would not be beneficial are scheduled as in-patients". Otherwise, the program has met with much success from parents, children, nurses, and physicians.

REF. Condon S.: Day-Time Hospital for Children. American Journal of Nursing 72:8, 1431-1433, Aug. 1972.

82. Q. How does mental hospitalization affect the child?

A. While some children and youth need hospitalization in a mental institution, it is an experience that can be potentially harmful. The chief dangers of hospitalization of children and adolescents are cited as "development of a negative self-concept, reduced social competence and coping skills outside the institution, and, most importantly, falling victim to social stigma and its correlates of rejection and reduced opportunities for self-determination."

Mental hospitals should only be used to admit juveniles whose conditions justify admission and should only admit them when there are adequate treatment resources. By all means, they should not be used as a dumping ground for the young rejects of society.

REF. Weiss HH, Pizer EF.: Hospitalizing the Young: Is It for Their Own Good? Mental Hygiene 54:498-502, Oct. 1970.

83. Q. Is neonatal health insurance necessary?

A. At present, many insurance policies exclude newborn infants from birth up to 30 days. Because of this general policy, it is assumed that newborns are perceived by these companies as a high-risk group. Due to the general lack of neonatal health coverage, parents of a sick or premature baby must assume financial burden for the infant's health care.

Only two states, Florida and California, now require insurance companies who issue family policies to include coverage of the infant from the moment of birth. Such legislature can be enacted in other states through action of private citizens and health professionals.

REF. Schulkind ML, et al.: Neonatal Health Insurance. Clinical Pediatrics 13:209-210, March 1974.

84. Q. What are the myths in the pediatric implications of the battered baby syndrome?

A. (1) "Spare the rod and spoil the child". Parents feel that discipline and control are reasons enough for battering young children. Corporal punishment is an accepted way of raising a child in the western world. Aggressive delinquents have many more histories of batterings than non-aggressive delinquents. Most violent adult citizens have been severely battered as infants. These citizens view their childhood as being desirably strict, but the battered child grows up to be the battering parent. It is regrettable that strictness, discipline and battering get mixed up together when these matters are considered; (2) "Be it ever so humble, there is no place like home". A firmly identifiable mother figure is needed. It does not have to be the biological mother who mothers the baby though there has to be a mothering person for every child; (3) "A man's home is his castle". The rights of the child for reasonable care and protection must be balanced against the right of parents to be free to raise their children in their own image. But the child does no longer belong to his parents, he belongs to himself in the care of his parents unless he receives insufficient care or protection.
REF. Kempe C.: Pediatric Implications of the Battered Baby Syndrome. Archives of Disease in Childhood 46:245, 28-37, 1971.

85. Q. How is the diagnosis of the battered child syndrome made?

A. It is not necessary to be absolutely sure about abuse or neglect, since the law provides for cases of suspected abuse to be reported. The neglect and abuse of children denotes a situation ranging from deprivation of food, clothing, shelter and parental love, to instances in which children are physically abused, resulting in obvious physical trauma and often leading to death. A more descriptive term that could be applied to this entity is that of the "Maltreatment-Syndrome".

The diagnosis of the maltreatment syndrome in children must encompass the physical examination of the child, the questionable history as to the cause of the physical condition and diagnostic x-ray findings. The child's appearance may reflect neglect for his welfare if he is inadequately dressed for the weather, wearing torn or unwashed clothes, or if the child is unbathed and has body odor. The parents may be aggressive and abusive when approached, but may also be apathetic and unresponsive and may show little or no concern about the child. The index of suspicion would include:

History: multiple hospital visits, story at variance with clinical findings, family discord, parents' inappropriate reaction to severity of injury, child brought with complaint other than one associated with abuse e.g. cold, headache, etc.
Physical Examination: signs of general neglect, bruises, abrasions, burns, hematomas, old healed lesions, evidence of fracture and or dislocation of extremities, coma, convulsions, death, symptoms of drug withdrawal.

Differential Diagnosis: scurvy and rickets, infantile cortical hyperostosis, syphilis of infancy, accidental trauma.
Radiologic Manifestations: subperiosteal hemorrhages, epiphyseal separations, periosteal shearing, metaphyseal fragmentation, previously healed periosteal calcification.

Colored photographs particularly of the areas of injury, should be taken on admission. This will be of assistance if it becomes necessary that court action be taken to protect the child from further abuse.
REF. Fontana V, M.D.: The Diagnosis of the Maltreatment Syndrome in Children. Pediatrics 51:4 Part II, 780-782, 1973.

86. Q. What are some clues to determining suspected child abuse?

A. Some clues are: (1) conflicting stories about the "accident" from the parents on different occasions; (2) an injury inconsistent with the history; (3) signs of neglect or old scars; (4) inappropriate concern for degree of injury, either exaggerated concern or apathy toward child; (5) absence of parent for questioning or refusal of parent to sign consent for treatment or tests.
REF. Shydro J, et al.: Child Abuse. Nursing '72 2:12, 37-41, Dec. 1972.

87. Q. What are some characteristics of parents who abuse their children?

A. Often, these parents were products of abuse as a child, and know no other way of being a parent. For them, love means ridicule, neglect, abuse, which they pass on to their child. Often they learn mistrust of others, rarely building friendships. They may show a high vulnerability toward criticism, disinterest or abandonment from others. Such a crisis leads them to expect their own gratification from a child. Therefore, their views of children are distorted and unrealistic, and the child's failure to accomplish the parent's wishes leads to punishment.
REF. Shydro J, et al.: Child Abuse. Nursing '72 2:12, 37-41, Dec. 1972.

88. Q. Is group therapy and home visiting effective in working with abusive parents?

A. One such program of group therapy and home visiting is being conducted at UCLA Neuropsychiatric Institute. It is based on the "self-help approach" because these parents, who are often immature, impulsive people, need assistance in learning to set limits. They are depressed and self-deprecating and desperately need a "good" mother surrogate. In the group therapy session, the therapists are a child psychiatrist and a public health nurse. Evening meetings are held once a week, and both parents are required to come. Initially, the group shows strong feelings of outrage toward the injustice society has caused them. Eventually, they are able to discuss the problems which ultimately led to the abusive act or to discuss problems of being a parent. Those who benefit most from the session are the parents who become able to talk about the abusive acts themselves.

The public health nurse also visits the home at the parent's request. Here care can be individualized, and teaching can be begun. These parents are usually skeptical of any "help" and the nurse's first objective is forming a trusting relationship. Abusing parents are sensitive to domination and control, yet need "mothering". Therefore, as the nurse listens, she also gives only minimal attention to the child because the home will only be safe for the child if the parents can learn new ways of coping with crisis and dealing with children.

Because these parents know little about children, the nurse's role is teaching by example. She needs to stress normal growth and development and to show ways of dealing with behavior, such as jealousy or temper tantrums. In this program, the nurse uses the techniques of behavior modification to help parents handle undesirable behavior, because previously, punishment was the only known control.
REF. Savino A, Sanders R.: Working with Abusive Parents: Group Therapy and Home Visits. American Journal of Nursing 73:3, 482-484, March 1973.

89. Q. What is the nurse's role in working with parents of abused children?

A. The nurse needs to assume an active role in helping to identify battered children, and in establishing a relationship with the parents. It is essential that she understand the dynamics of this family, and not become punitive or hostile toward the parents. Because a crisis often provokes battering, it is helpful to express sympathetic understanding toward the parent. Since these parents frequently don't know what aspects of good mothering or care are, the nurse needs to take every opportunity to show by her example, not by lecturing or dictating, what children need both physically and emotionally. Because the parents may be hostile and defensive, it is especially important to realize one's own feelings and to understand the parents need help if the child is to return to a safe home.
REF. Shydro J, et al.: Child Abuse. Nursing '72 2:12, 37-41, Dec. 1972.

90. Q. Does child behavior invite adult abuse?

A. Forty-two families in which children were abused were studied. Its purpose was to characterize abused children and abusing parents.

The children tended to use violence in order to attain adult recognition. Their ability to channel aggression into more acceptable modes of behavior was limited. Many of the children manifested aimless, awkward behavior. Some of the behavior was so marked that it suggested brain damage. The presence of an adult who recognized the child acted as a catalyst in attaining vitality.

Most mothers perceived their abused child as the embodiment of
their own instinctual life. However, no comfort was derived from
the child. The perception and behavior of the child was distorted,
and the child was seen as devil or saint. The mothers abused their
children because they were reminders of the past and of personal
frustration. Unable to displace anger and violent behavior they
struck back at what was offensive--the child.
REF. Galdston R.: Violence Begins at Home. Journal of Child Psychiatry 10:336-350, 1971.

91. Q. What guidelines can we use when caring for a child who is
dying?

A. These authors extract from their background and experience
with terminally ill children some principles that seem to apply to all
children (and maybe to all patients) regardless of age:

(1) treat the child as normally as possible whenever feasible; build
on your own knowledge of growth and development and childhood tasks
so that the child is living life to his capacity; caution parents against
whispering in front of him which increases the feeling of secrecy and
fear;

(2) set reasonable limits on behavior, particularly demanding behavior because all children need the security derived from consistent,
yet flexible rules; parents need help to learn the importance of this
principle from the very beginning of the diagnosis so that anticipatory guidance prevents future problems;

(3) keep reassurances realistic, yet hopeful by relating treatment to
symptom relief and feeling better, rather than recovery;

(4) solicit the child's participation in treatment and care, especially
when his cooperation can decrease his feelings of helplessness;

(5) before responding to questions, make certain that you know the
precise nature of what he is asking; using open-ended statements
and reflection can allow the child to express his true concern in an
atmosphere that permits honesty and trust;

(6) always try to convey hopefulness and utility in relation to the
child, and in his concern for others on the unit who are critically
ill.
REF. Bright F, France Sister M.: The Nurse and the Terminally
Ill Child. Nursing Outlook 15:9, 39-42, Sept. 1967.

92. Q. How do children perceive death?

A. According to most studies, children's thoughts about death
fall into conceptual boundaries. The manner in which death is conceptualized and accepted varies with the child's age and developmental stage.

Before the age of three, children lack abstract thought and do not understand death as a concept. From 3-5, children have a limited concept of death and are learning the difference between animate and inanimate objects. As they observe living and dying, children between 5 and 9 years become aware of death and the sorrow that accompanies it. However, they do not believe it is universal. By 9, most children have witnessed death and wondered about it. They also realize that in the very distant future they too, will die. Around the age of 12, death is understood to be a universal and inevitable event. REF. Miller PG, Ozga J.: Mommy, What Happens When I Die? Mental Hygiene 57:21-22, Spring 1973.

93. Q. Are children aware of their fatal illness?

A. Several investigators have reported their findings about how children view death at various ages. One conclusion usually agreed upon is that up until the ages of 9 or 10 years, children do not have a realistic adult's view of death. Rather, they may fear the separation or mutilation associated with this concept. However, does that mean that they are unaware of what is happening to them, even if they have not been told their diagnosis or prognisis?

According to this author, who tested 64 children between the ages of 6 and 10 years, some who were terminally ill, chronically ill, briefly ill, or healthy, there is evidence that the children who were dying knew it and were scared and anxious. Some of her specific findings included:

(1) Scores of anxiety level were twice as high for the children with fatal illness, than for other hospitalized children, although only 2 of the 16 children knew their prognosis.

(2) Children with poor prognoses told more stories relating to threat to body integrity and pain than those in the comparison groups, suggesting that the "denial" was not effective in minimizing fear or anxiety.

(3) Children in the terminally ill group told of loneliness, separation, and death in their fantasy stories. A striking finding was that although only 2 of the 16 knew their diagnosis, more than half told stories of death, with facts that related the make-believe character to themselves. This supports the theory that allowing the child to discuss his condition openly need not enhance anxiety, but may help with his acceptance and adjustment.

(4) Although there was not a significant correlation between religious belief and previous experience with death versus present attitude, both of these variables affected how the children coped with their fears.

(5) Statements of anger and hostility from the children demonstrated their concern of being unsupported, yet incapable of escape. Feelings of punishment and guilt also colored their stories.

REF. Waechter E.: Children's Awareness of Fatal Illness. American Journal of Nursing 71:6, 1168-1172, June 1971.

94. Q. What implications for nursing care are present in the care of a dying child?

A. One of the most important considerations for a nurse to make is what does the child know and understand about death, for his age? The child under six years of age denies death, views it is impermanent and reversible, but fears the idea of separation. He reacts primarily to physical pain and to the clues that something is wrong with his body. His dependency needs and attachment to significant caregivers is heightened. The child between the ages of six and ten still does not see death as permanent or irreversible, but rather as a "person" with human often wicked, qualities. They usually fear and protest diagnostic and treatment procedures. Children, who are nine or ten years old, have an adult concept of death.

Although approaches toward caring for the dying child differ, some guidelines exist. For example, children seem to need some understanding of their illness, such as the need for hospitalization, blood transfusion, blood tests, and drugs with severe side effects. Adjustment to the illness and development of beneficial coping mechanisms seem more likely to occur when the child has some awareness of his illness. Parents need help, not only in their own grieving process, but also in learning to help the child accept his illness.

Another area of concern is that of providing information. The child and family go through periods of "doctor shopping" and questioning of personnel to find errors or inconsistencies. Often, a staff conference is necessary to provide correct information that conveys realistic hope. Still another area of concern is helping siblings understand the child's illness. Playmates or siblings of a similar age tend to develop anxiety and fear that they too will become ill and die.

Lastly, a most difficult decision faces health professionals - the moral and ethical question of when and how to prolong life.
REF. Chinn PL.: Child Health Maintenance. C. V. Mosby Company, St. Louis, 1974, pp. 435-439.

95. Q. How can parents be helped when this child is dying?

A. Parents of a dying child are overwhelmed with anger, grief, bewilderment and sorrow. Hospital personnel can help by recognizing, understanding and accepting parental behavior during this crisis period. Because parents feel guilty and bewildered, they should not only be provided knowledge about the illness but also an opportunity to express their feelings. Parents who are able, should be permitted to care for the child as much as possible; it provides a sense of contributing to the child's care, and helps relieve feelings of guilt, and gives support to the child. Withdrawal from the child by the family and friends should be carefully watched for and prevented or postponed by staff.

REF. Smith A, Schneider L.: The Dying Child. Clinical Pediatrics 8:131-135, March 1969.

96. Q. How can nurses help parents whose child has died from Sudden Infant Death Syndrome (SIDS)?

A. When parents lose a child to SIDS, they are stricken with acute grief, bewilderment, and painful guilt. Because of the nature of this mysterious disease, nurses can play a vital part in allaying the worst fears and anguish of these parents. The first contact the nurse usually has with the parents is in the emergency, where she should be alert to signs of SIDS that distinguish it from child neglect, abuse, or accident. SIDS infants are usually well-nourished, well-hydrated, and between the ages of two and four months. They may have blood-tinged, frothy fluids in the mouth, emesis on the face, and a diaper wet with urine and feces. The parents need immediate reassurance that there was nothing they could have done to prevent this. Assure them that although SIDS is not fully understood, it is a disease process just like pneumonia or cancer. Repeatedly reaffirm that nothing can prevent or predict this syndrome.

Parents need emotional support. In the emergency room, try to provide them with a private room, a priest or rabbi if they desire, and offer them a last opportunity to see their infant. Although each person grieves differently, they should be offered a chance for a last good-bye.

One very important aspect is the consent for autopsy. Because the cause of SIDS is still unknown, evidence from post mortem examination is essential to research. The autopsy report can also be a consolation to the parents concerning the diagnosis.

Follow-up care should be as soon as the autopsy report is ready, preferably a home visit about one week after the infant's death. This is a time for the nurse to help the parents express their feelings, ask questions and seek information. They may also be encouraged to join parents groups to gain comfort and solace from others who have experienced this tragedy.

REF. Patterson K, Pomeroy M.: Sudden Infant Death Syndrome. Nursing '74 4:5, 85-88, May 1974.

97. Q. How can we help a young child understand and accept the death of an expected baby?

A. Parents often find it difficult to explain death to children. When a newborn dies, they may be overcome by grief and unable to meet their child's needs. Often, too, they want to spare the child sad tidings, or believe he is too young to understand. However, children absorb the feelings and reactions of their parents. They are quick to realize a conspiracy of silence, that certain subjects are taboo. Their fantasies of the death are usually more terrifying than the real tragedy. Children under five years engage in animistic, magical thinking. They believe that wishing someone dead means he will die. These young children need to be reassured that their wishes cannot come true. Children's reactions to a death in the family can be classified according to age:

(1) 0-5 years: The child reacts to changes in his parents' behavior. He senses their withdrawal, and greatly fears separation and loss of their love.

(2) 5-10 years: The child worries about the implication of death for himself, and fear for his safety.

(3) 10-12 years: The child is generally supportive, but may have guilt that he is alive, while his sibling is dead.

To help a family, a nurse must know the children's ages, what they have been told, not only about the death, but about pregnancy and birth, and how the child responded to this information. Often, the nurse can assess the child's coping by identifying the parents' grieving. She can ask an older sibling what he thinks his little brother knows. Using a non-directive approach by asking open-ended questions helps the parents explore ways of helping the child understand death. Euphemisms only confuse the child. Honesty and openness can ease the pain of loss while strengthening bonds of communication. REF. Hardgrove C, Warrick L.: How Shall We Tell the Children. American Journal of Nursing 74:3, 448-450, March 1974.

98. Q. Has any progress been made in discovering the etiology of Sudden Infant Death Syndrome?

A. Recent research at Upstate Medical Center in Syracuse, New York, has provided data which support the hypotheses that prolonged apnea, a physiological component of sleep, is part of the final pathway resulting in sudden infant death. The observation that most cases of SIDS occur during sleep, led the researchers to study sleep patterns of five infants about one month of age. The infants had been referred because of cyanotic episodes of undetermined etiology. These patients were observed on an apnea monitor, as well as having respirations and eye movements recorded. The five patients demonstrated frequent apneic episodes during sleep, mostly brief and self-limited. However, a number of these episodes were severe enough to require prompt and vigorous resuscitation and two of the infants studied ultimately died during similar severe apneic episodes.

This study demonstrated that prolonged periods of apnea can occur in otherwise well infants, beyond one month of age. The occurrence of these apneic episodes appears to be influenced by some of the factors known to be related to SIDS, for example respiratory tract infections. Further research is needed, directed toward greater understanding of the variables influencing sleep apnea and its biochemical and neurological basis. This study suggests that perhaps in the future, there may be some way of identifying those infants who are at risk of becoming victims of SIDS.

REF. Steinschneider A, M.D., Ph.D.: Prolonged Apnea and The Sudden Infant Death Syndrome: Clinical and Laboratory Observations. Pediatrics 50:4, 646-653, 1972.

99. Q. What is the nurse's role in SIDS?

A. Sudden, unexpected death of an infant is a tragic event for any family. Guilt, anguish, and bewilderment always occur. The nurse who is able to care for such a family after the infant's death can be invaluable in helping parents in this time of grief. Encouraging parents to talk about their grief and the events preceding the infant death is of great therapeutic value. The nurse can help allay guilt feelings by reassuring the parents that they could not have prevented the child's death.

Through interviewing, the feelings of family members about the death of the infant can be established. At this point, the nurse could explain the disease process in an effort to provide accurate information and perhaps prevent one parent from blaming another for the infant's death.

Follow-up of the family for several weeks will give the family an opportunity to express their feelings. Siblings of the dead infant will be affected by the emotional responses of their parents. Toddlers may be frightened and act out. Older children may have guilt feelings and should be encouraged to verbalize.
REF. Patterson K, Pomeroy MR.: Sudden Infant Death Syndrome. Nursing '74 85-88, May 1974.

100. Q. What are some differences between chronic grief and acute grief?

A. Grief can be summarized as "the response to the loss of a loved object". When parents give birth to a defective child, they experience the loss of the fantasized and valued "perfect baby". Not only must they grieve for this acute loss, but they must also sustain the painful acceptance of a defective child. Unlike parents who experienced an acute loss, these parents in their chronic loss cannot complete the final phase of mourning.

The first stage of mourning is shock and disbelief. In chronic mourning, this stage is characterized by learning of the deformity, feelings of inadequacy and doubt, and hesitancy in one's ability to care for the child. In the second stage of grief, the feelings of guilt, anger, and failure are prevalent, with both parents trying to search for clues as to why this happened to them. They frequently need praise and repeated assurance that they are caring adequately for the child, especially if the child's physical health is deteriorating as well. In the third stage of grief-restitution, parents experiencing chronic grief do not have the rituals of a funeral and family to console them. Rather, they have the daily rituals of caring for their child to ever remind them of the imperfection.

When the child dies, the parents go through all three stages again, although the phase of shock and disbelief is shortened and the restitution phase, easier.
REF. Jackson PL.: Chronic Grief. American Journal of Nursing 74:7, 1289-1291, July 1974.

101. Q. Is neonatal mortality related to the sex of the infant?

A. Male infants born in the U.S. have an excessive risk of neonatal death when compared with females. In an analysis of 2,735 consecutive newborn autopsies, the ratio of males to females was 128:1. The ratio for all U.S. live births is 1.05:1, which is a significant difference. There was a nearly equal male to female ratio for most disorders in stillborn infants, but disorders arising after birth demonstrated a strong male disadvantage. The stillborn ratios presumably reflect the maternal influence, but after birth and removal from the maternal environment, the inherent biological disadvantage of being male is uncovered. This disadvantage is not related to specific disease processes, a fact which is born out by the finding of several disorders in which sex ratios for stillborns are different from ratios for liveborn infants.
REF. Naeye R, et al.: Neonatal Mortality, The Male Disadvantage. Pediatrics 48:6, 902-906, 1971.

102. Q. Is there a relationship between chromosome abnormality and perinatal death?

A. In the early phases of pregnancy wastage (preimplantation loss and spontaneous abortion), at least 35% of fetuses are chromosomally abnormal. By contrast, the frequency of chromosomal abnormalities in liveborn infants is only 0.5%.

A survey of unselected necropsied infants dying in hospitals was done. Chromosome results were obtained from 500 of the 726 infants examined. There were 28 infants with chromosome abnormalities which is 9% of macerated stillbirths, 4% of fresh stillbirths, 6% early neonatal deaths for which results were obtained; 13% of infants had lethal malformations and 2.5% died from other causes. The incidence of E18-trisomy in this survey indicates that this abnormality is more common at birth than is generally accepted. Chromosome abnormalities are most commonly found in infants where the maternal age exceeds forty years.

It is suggested that a chromosome analysis on all infants dying in the perinatal period would contribute toward the understanding of etiology, and provide a useful indication for preventive action in future pregnancies.
REF. Machin GA.: Chromosome Abnormality and Perinatal Death. The Lancet 1:7857, 549-551, 1974.

## II. MEDICAL AND SURGICAL PROBLEMS OF CHILDREN

103. Q. What is functional intestinal obstruction in the infant?

A. Intestinal obstruction is one of the most common conditions responsible for the admission of an infant to a surgical pediatric unit in the first 4 weeks of life, only spina bifida and congenital heart disease being more common.

An anatomical abnormality which causes an organic obstruction sooner or later gives rise to the 3 classical signs of repeated vomiting, abdominal distention, and failure to pass normal meconium or stool. This combination of signs may also occur in the absence of an organic lesion because of a disturbance of intestinal peristalsis or when meconium is abnormally viscid. Such a disturbance has been called "functional intestinal obstruction". Hirschsprung's disease and meconium ileus have been excluded because they have an organic basis. REF. Howat JM, Wilkinson AW.: Functional Intestinal Obstruction in the Neonate. Archives of Disease in Childhood 45:244, 800-804, 1970.

104. Q. What are some causes of functional intestinal obstruction?

A. The history of the pregnancy: were ganglion blocking agents given? was there heroin addiction, ruling out maternal hydramnios? The infants suffered from respiratory distress, born after less than 37 weeks' gestation and delivered by cesarian section. Sepsis-either alimentary or generalized.

The exclusion of Hirschsprung's disease should raise the suspicion of hypothyroidism as a possible cause before 3 months. REF. Howat JM, Wilkinson AW.: Functional Intestinal Obstruction in the Neonate. Archives of Disease in Childhood 45:244, 800-804, 1970.

105. Q. What is the treatment for functional intestinal obstruction?

A. Meconium obstruction can be overcome by (1) rectal examination or enema; (2) oral feeding within 24 hours of admission; (3) intravenous fluids; (4) blood transfusions in the case of bronchopneumonia and septicemia; (5) x-ray examination of the abdomen in the supine and erect position showed typical gaseous distention of the whole intestine with no fluid levels in the dilated loops of intestine of different sizes. Features of obstruction can resolve spontaneously. REF. Howat JM, Wilkinson AW.: Functional Intestinal Obstruction in the Neonate. Archives of Disease in Childhood 45:244, 800-804, 1970.

106. Q. What is a rare complication of phototherapy?

A. Phototherapy is a common treatment for neonatal hyperbilirubinemia and is used extensively in hospital nurseries. Several cases of complications in the newborn due to phototherapy have been reported. After 24 hours of phototherapy, these infants had developed dark oily-brown color skin, urine and serum. The serum bilirubin remained elevated at 20 to 30 percent direct bilirubin level for three weeks. Serum SGOT, alkaline phosphatase and LDH were moderately elevated and returned to normal within a month.

The authors suggest that "a rare complication of phototherapy for neonatal hyperbilirubinemia might be hepatocellular damage associated with cholestases." If light therapy is immediately discontinued upon discovery of this complication, the infant is not permanently damaged.

REF. Sharma RK, et al.: A Complication of Phototherapy in the Newborn: The Bronze Baby. Clinical Pediatrics 12:231-233, April 1973.

107. Q. What is the significance of an elevated hematocrit in the newborn?

A. Thirty infants with Down's Syndrome had hemoglobin, hematocrit and prothrombin levels measured. Twenty-nine of the infants had elevated hematocrits. The investigators concluded that "a high hematocrit seems to be a characteristic of newborn with Down's syndrome." The high blood viscosity may be part of the cause for the peripheral cyanosis often found in infants with Down's syndrome. Fluid shift from vascular to intervascular space, caused by slow capillary circulation, helps raise the hematocrit higher.

Although the prothrombin was relatively low, the author recommends abstaining from giving vitamin K during the newborn period. It is felt that extra vitamin K might increase the danger of thrombosis when the hematocrit is 70 or more.

REF. Lappalainen J, Kouvalainen K.: High Hematocrits in Newborns with Down's Syndrome. Clinical Pediatrics 11:472-474, Aug. 1972.

108. Q. What are common causes of dehydration in children?

A. Two common causes are diarrhea and vomiting, although another very important consideration is the effect of surgery on water loss. Diarrhea and vomiting, as well as other conditions, can cause three different types of dehydration:

(1) Isotonic dehydration occurs when water and salt are lost, producing simple dehydration that is easily corrected by replacing water. In diarrhea, the lost intestinal secretions are alkaline, and lack of food will intensify the production of acid metabolites, from cell breakdown causing metabolic acidosis. In vomiting, hydrogen ions are decreased from loss of hydrochloric acid, causing metabolic alkalosis.

(2) Hypertonic dehydration results when water loss exceeds sodium loss, causing hypernatremia. This type of dehydration results from severe diarrhea, low water intake, high solute intake, insensible water loss from sweating or rapid respirations, or poor renal function. Distinguishing signs for this type include avid thirst, parched mucous membranes, normal to decreased urine output, but normal skin turgor, due to the shift of fluid from intracellular to extracellular compartments. Metabolic acidosis may occur from the kidney's failure to excrete nonvolatile acid metabolites quickly enough.

(3) Hypotonic dehydration results from water loss that is proportionately less than the salt loss. Hyponatremia can result from large ingestion of fluids, intravenous fluids without electrolytes, and profuse sweating. Clinical signs range from lethargy to coma; skin turgor is very poor and mucous membranes are clammy; blood pressure is generally lowered. Low sodium levels can impair cardiac and renal functioning, and can cause cerebral edema, resulting in seizures.
REF. Lee J, Gregory A.: The ABC's and mEq's of Fluid Balance in Children. Nursing '74 4:6, 28-36, June 1974.

109. Q. What is the immediate treatment of severe dehydration due to diarrhea?

A. A critical stage in diarrhea occurs when a volume of fluid equal to about 10% of body weight is lost over a period of a day or two. At this stage anorexia or vomiting usually occurs, precluding oral feedings. Parenteral therapy should be instituted. Even if severe undernutrition exists, the first 6-8 hours should be a period of brief starvation with parenteral glucose providing emergency calories. In considering the first 24 hours of treatment, the first hour involves immediate infusion of a volume of fluid over 10-15 minutes, to expand the intravascular compartment. Whole blood, plasma, 5% albumin or 10% glucose with 75 mEg/L of sodium and 20 mEg/L of bicarbonate and 55 mEg/L of chloride have been used successfully. After initial infusion, the remaining fluid and electrolytes can be combined as a single solution administered over the following 24 hours. A glucose concentration of 5% with appropriately calculated electrolytes can be given. After 8 hours, some patients may take glucose and electrolyte solutions by mouth. The more severely dehydrated patients will remain on infusion. Ideally, after proper hydrations, the patient should show a 7-10% gain in body weight after 24 hours. Whether, on the second day, oral feedings containing calories and carbohydrates can be given, depends on the state of nutrition and the etiology and duration of the diarrhea.
REF. Fineberg L.: The Management of the Critically Ill Child with Dehydration Secondary to Diarrhea. Pediatrics 45:6, 1029-1036, 1970.

110. Q. How does hypernatremic dehydration occur?

A. Any child with diarrhea will lose proportionately more water than sodium. Diarrheal stool produces water loss with 50-60 mEq/liter of sodium. Skin losses are approximately 40 mEq/liter and water lost through respiration is virtually sodium free. Therefore, in diarrheal dehydration water is always lost in excess of sodium. If a child's diet is inappropriately high in sodium or solute, hypernatremic dehydration could result. This is especially true when children have gastroenteritis and solutions of water, salt and sugar are mixed incorrectly, reversing the amounts of salt and sugar. Also, powdered formulas mixed in too high a concentration, or boiled skim milk which is boiled to the point where significant concentration occurs, can be causes of diet-induced hypernatremia.

REF. Haddow J, M.D., Cohen D, M.D.: Understanding and Managing Hypernatremic Dehydration. Pediatric Clinics of North America 21:2, 435-441, 1974.

111. Q. How can a nurse recognize fluid imbalances in a child?

A. Fluid requirements for children are more specific and exactly calculated than for adults. Although an infant has more fluid per body mass (70-80%) than the adult (50-60%), he also has less reserve for conservation of fluid loss. His increased metabolic rate and his immature kidneys are just two reasons for this deficiency. Another is that his fluid requirement is greater: a month-old infant requires 100 ml./kg. of water while the adult needs only 30-40 ml./kg.

Several conditions cause fluid and electrolyte imbalances, but the signs are similar for dehydration and change according to the ion lost. These include:

(1) behavioral changes such as irritability, lethargy, or refusal to eat;
(2) loss of tissue turgor, particularly on the abdomen;
(3) dry mucous membranes, particularly the tongue and lips;
(4) weight loss, especially a comparison of admission or preadmission weight with present weight which can be a guide to degree of dehydration:
    mild:      2-4% loss of body weight
    moderate: 5-9% loss
    severe:    over 10% loss
(5) sunken eyeballs and depressed fontanel which usually occur with 10% weight loss;
(6) temperature which may be elevated from the cause of dehydration or decreased especially in hypovolemia;
(7) urine output decreased; the normal range is:
    6 months:  12ml/hr.
    1 year:    22ml/hr.
    5 years:   28ml/hr.
    12 years:  33-35ml/hr.
(8) thirst, which may be present, but difficult to evaluate, absence of tearing and salivation is a better indicator;

( 9) respirations which vary according to cause of fluid imbalance, hyperpnea or kussmaul breathing results from metabolic acidosis as a result of diabetic coma, salicylate poisoning, or diarrhea;
(10) decreased blood pressure from hypovolemia which can cause shock, (B.P. usually not an early sign in children);
(11) neurological signs, particularly from electrolyte imbalance: for example, decreased potassium causes muscle irritability and cardiac arrhythmias, and calcium deficiency can cause muscle twitching and convulsions;
(12) laboratory values vary: dehydration causes an increased hematocrit, urine specific gravity will increase, blood gases and serum electrolytes can be abnormal.
REF. Lee J, Gregory A.: The ABC's and mEq's of Fluid Balance in Children. Nursing '74 4:6, 28-36, June 1974.

112.  Q. What signs can alert a nurse to anaphylactic shock?

A. Anaphylactic shock, or complete circulatory collapse, is an acute antibody-antigen reaction to a foreign substance such as penicillin, horse serum, or insect bites. One of the first clues to this life-threatening reaction is a hive somewhere on the body other than the site of injection. Severe pruritis of the hands and feet occur, as well as a severe burning sensation of the rectum and vagina. Blood pressure falls rapidly, until pulse and respirations are absent. Immediate treatment is epinephrine, 1:1000 dilution at the dosage of 0.01 cc./kg. until 0.3 cc. for children or 0.5 cc. for adults, administered subcutaneously. At the same time cardiopulmonary resuscitation procedures should be begun if vital signs are absent.

Besides these medical treatments, nursing measures should be employed which help decrease the patient's fear and anxiety. For example, the patient may fall into an unconscious state, but evidence seems to prove that patients hear very well. In fact, severe shock may cause hearing to be exaggerated, so that loud voices cause irritability, when soft voices can calm the patient. A patient's sensitivity to tactile stimuli may also be heightened. Therefore, softened voices and warm tactile stimulation can help reduce fear and loneliness of the patient. The nurse needs to remind others in the room of these comfort measures, and she needs to be aware of any unnecessary rough movement of the patient, as well as good positioning to decrease pressure areas.
REF. Craven RF.: Anaphylactic Shock. American Journal of Nursing 72:4, 718-721, April 1972.

113.  Q. What parental teaching should the nurse do when the diagnosis of the infant is Pierre-Robin Syndrome?

A. Pierre-Robin syndrome is a triad of congenital anomalies: micrognathia (underdeveloped mandible), glossoptosis (backward dropping of the tongue), and cleft palate. Infants born with these defects have difficulty breathing and swallowing because of the obstruction of the pharynx and airway from glossoptosis. A variety of procedures have been advocated for maintaining the tongue in the forward position. One procedure is to tie the tongue surgically to the lower lip, and remove a section of mucosa from under the tongue, gum and lower lip so that adhesions will form, artificially creating a tongue tie until the mandible increases with size, and the tongue tie can be released. Another procedure is to create a type of traction at the tip of the tongue, which forces the tongue forward.

Parents need to be taught two main procedures; proper feeding, which is complicated by a cleft palate and maintenance of a clear airway. The infant needs to be fed in an almost vertical position, so that the tongue and jaw are forced forward. Asepto syringe or nasogastric tube feedings may be needed; a suction machine should be available because of the danger of aspiration. Proper positioning is essential for a patent airway. If traction is used, the infant is placed on his back; if a tongue tie is created, a prone position will keep the jaw and tongue forward. If cyanosis can be prevented and adequate nutrition maintained, these infants will do well because growth of the mandible will adequately house the tongue. The cleft lip can be repaired at about 18 months of age, so that proper speech should not become a problem.

REF. Agrafiotis P.: Teaching Parents About Pierre-Robin Syndrome. American Journal of Nursing 72:11, 2040-2041, Nov. 1972.

114. Q. What nursing care is required in Landry-Guillain-Barré Syndrome?

A. Landry-Guillain-Barré syndrome is actually two clinical entities: Landry's ascending paralysis and the Guillain-Barré syndrome. Both are classified as forms of acute idiopathic polyneuritis. The cause is unknown, but the symptoms begin with tingling paresthesia and slight weakness of legs, progressing to complete paralysis of legs. This immobility ascends to the arms and trunk causing respiratory failure. The oral, pharyngeal, and laryngeal muscles are paralyzed, making talking and swallowing difficult. All of this occurs in the space of 12-24 hours.

Physical care is aimed at maintaining respiratory function. A tracheostomy is done, and the patient is placed on a volume respirator. He needs frequent suctioning, chest percussion, and change of position. Feeding is done by gavage, and frequent oral suctioning is needed to remove saliva because of swallowing difficulty. Skin integrity must be maintained through physical therapy and hygiene. Gastrointestinal problems, particularly constipation, are common and laxatives or enemas are needed. Atony of the smooth muscle of the urinary tract causes stasis and pyelonephritis.

One major problem is communication - often the only voluntary movement intact is the blinking reflex. Questions can be asked with one blink for "NO" and two for "YES", or one can ask the patient to "spell" by narrowing down letters until a word is formed. Recovery

is usually complete with good supportive medical and nursing care.
Rate of recovery can be from a few weeks to a year.
REF. Glenn J, et al.: Pediatric Paralysis in Bogota. American
Journal of Nursing 73:2, 299-301, Feb. 1973; House M, et al.:
Coma, Hope Makes a Difference in Nursing Care. Nursing '74 4:5,
24-29, May 1974.

115. Q. What physical characteristics help one in identifying Down's
Syndrome in an infant?

A. Down's syndrome is an inherited disorder, characterized
by several physical findings: the head is small, the face flat, and
the eyes are slanted upward (hence, the other term, Mongolism).
Strabismus and Brushfield spots on the iris are common. Cataracts
are also seen after age ten. The nose is small and flat, the lips are
broad, dry and fissured, and the tongue is large and protruding. The
neck is broad and short, and the chest is usually deformed with flat
nipples. The abdomen protrudes; diastasis recti and umbilical hernia are not uncommon. The extremities are usually short, and der-
matoglyphics include a transverse palmar line on the hand (simian
crease). Hypotonicity and hyperextensibility of the joints are common.

However, some investigators have identified another clinical sign
that may be helpful in diagnosing this syndrome. These children
seem to have smaller ears than the general population. Values for
ear length (the vertical axis of the pinna, including the lobe) are
commonly below two standard deviations for normal length. In this
study the range of ear length for normal newborns was 3.2 cm. to
4.6 cm. All of the newborns with Down's syndrome had ear lengths
between 2.6 cm. and 3.4 cm., with a mean of 3.0 cm.

Although no one clinical finding is diagnostic of Down's syndrome,
ear length is another clue toward early detection of this chromosomal abnormality.
REF. Aase J, et al.: Small Ears in Down's Syndrome: A Helpful
Diagnostic Aid. Journal of Pediatrics 82:5, 845-847, May 1973.

116. Q. Is there a relationship between long-term antiepileptic drug
therapy and the development of rickets?

A. According to several investigators, long term treatment
with anticonvulsive medication can lead to the development of vitamin D deficiency. What the exact mechanism is that leads to this
depletion is not clearly understood. It is known that dilantin and
phenobarbital enhance hepatic enzyme activity, which may act to
accelerate the degradation of vitamin D. Another nutritional defect
associated with anticonvulsant drug therapy is folate deficiency.

Nurses can be alert to signs of vitamin D deficiency by looking for
symptoms of rickets or osteomalacia. The skeletal system is most
severely affected with the formation of the "rachitic rosary" of the
ribcage, pigeon breast deformity of the chest, and bowlegs or knock

knees (genu varum or valgum). The deformity of the tibia causes the femora to externally rotate, causes instability of the hip joints with a resulting waddling gait. Other manifestations of severe rickets are poor muscle tone, abdominal distention, and lordosis.

Treatment of rickets is replacement of vitamin D. The dosage has varied according to different clinical reports. The present authors prescribed from 2,000 to 50,000 units for one patient, and approximately 10,000 units for the other. Vitamin D supplements of 200-800 units daily did not prevent the development of rickets in either patient. (Normal daily requirement of vitamin D is 400 units).
REF. Borgstedt A, et al.: Long-Term Administration of Antiepileptic Drugs and the Development of Rickets. Journal of Pediatrics 81:1, 9-15, July 1972; Barnett H.: Pediatrics. Appleton-Century-Crofts, New York, 1968, pp. 374-376.

117. Q. What are some basic positions for effectively doing postural drainage?

A. Postural drainage, percussion, and vibration can effectively remove secretions that block the airpassages and provide a medium for bacteria to multiply. The positions conducive to drainage are based on the anatomy of the bronchial tree, but because the bronchi are so segmented, a few basic positions accomplish the drainage with a minimum of exhaustion.

(1) Anterior apical segments: Place the patient in a semi-Fowler's position, using a pillow for support under his back. Percuss the upper left and right lobes.
(2) Posterior segments: Place the patient in a sitting position, but leaning forward on a bedtable, placing a pillow under his chest. Percuss the upper left and right lobes.
(3) Anterior basal segments: With the patient supine, elevate the hips with three to four pillows. The patient's knees are flexed, but his feet and shoulders are flat on the mattress. Percuss the basal lower lobes of right and left lungs.
(4) Posterior basal segments: Same position as above but with the patient prone.
(5) Right lateral basal segment: Position the patient on his left side, elevating his hips on three to four pillows so that the hips are higher than the shoulders. Percuss over the lower lateral rib cage for the right basal lobe.
(6) Left lateral basal segment: Place the patient on his right side with his hips elevated and proceed as above.

Percussion should be done for one to minutes followed by vibration during expiration for three to five deep breaths.
REF. Foss G.: Postural Drainage. American Journal of Nursing 73:4, 666-669, April 1973.

118. Q. What kind of preparation is necessary for patients who are undergoing lymphography?

A. Lymphography is the delineation of lymph vessels (lymphangiography) and nodes (lymphadenography) by injection of a radiopaque dye, such as alphazurine, into the lymph vessels and tracing their path via x-ray. Such conditions as lymphosarcoma, a type of cancer which can attack children, can be diagnosed through this test.

The procedure often takes from three to ten hours to complete. While the physician tries to locate the tiny lymphatic vessels between the toes, the patient must lie very still. In trying to evaluate the preparation patients received for this procedure, the authors explored patients' feelings about what they had been told. The patients recommended including information about the reason for the test, the use of local anesthesia, the part of the body involved, the possibility of pain, and especially the length of time involved. Patients felt that the presence of someone to talk to during the procedures helped the time pass. This is particularly true of children who may need their mother to read or play with them during the test. Patients also felt that they should know about the blue discoloration of the skin from the dye, the possible side effects of the dye, and what the post procedural care involved.

Since this test is often done to diagnose cancer, patients and family need support in accepting the final diagnosis.
REF. Nebe D, Gavaghan M.: Lymphography and Patients' Reactions. American Journal of Nursing 73:8, 1366-1368, Aug. 1973.

119. Q. What nursing interventions are involved in the care of a child with esophageal varices?

A. Portal hypertension with esophageal varices occurs when there is any major block along the portal system. Normally, blood from the digestive tract empties into the portal or liver circulation for purification and detoxification of various substances before returning to the heart via the inferior vena cava. When a major blockage occurs, backup of blood and increased pressure result, forcing the body to form alternative or collateral circulation. The most common type of portal obstruction in children is subhepatic or blockage of blood flowing to the liver. Although the cause is unknown, omphalitis, an inflammation of the umbilicus, has been identified as a contributing factor.

Besides the presence of esophageal varices from the increased pressure, other problems associated with liver disease can also be present, such as jaundice, ascites, peripheral edema, spider nevi, splenomegaly and hepatomegaly. Hepatic coma is also a threat from increasing ammonia levels in the blood. Medical and nursing care is aimed at control of the bleeding episodes from the esophageal varices. The medical procedures employed have several nursing implications:

(1) Pitressin, a posterior pituitary hormone, is given which causes smooth muscle constriction (vasoconstriction) and seems to allow a clot to form at the site of bleeding. Side effects such as colicky abdominal cramps, evacuation of bowels, increased blood pressure, and facial pallor indicate that the drug is working. Therefore, the nurse needs to observe for these signs because absence signifies ineffective results. Also, the increased pressure can mask signs of impending shock from hypovolemia.

(2) The Seng Staken-Blakemore Tube, a nasogastric tube with separate esophageal and gastric balloons, may be inserted to exert pressure against the walls of the esophagus. Once passed through the nose or mouth, each balloon is inflated (gastric balloon to a pressure of 75 mm. and esophageal balloon to about 30 mm.), and traction is applied to the tube so that the gastric balloon fits tightly against the cardioesophageal junction. Maintaining traction of the tube either by attaching the end to a pulley or by having the child wear a football helmet and attaching it to the nose guard is essential to prevent the balloon from dislodging and covering airway. Also, with the tube in place, the child cannot swallow saliva and will need oral suctioning or will need to be taught how to spit out the saliva. The balloons are usually kept inflated for 24 to 48 hours; any longer treatment necessitates periodic deflation to prevent mucosal necrosis.

(3) Because of free blood in the gastrointestinal tract, several enemas may be given to clear the blood and the bacteria, which normally breaks down the protein into ammonia. Tap water enemas are never given because of water intoxication. Because high blood ammonia levels are a potential danger, antibiotics are given to inhibit the normal flora from breaking down protein. When the normal flora is absent, vitamin K must be administered intramuscularly.

(4) Teaching is also essential in helping prevent future attacks of this life-threatening disorder. Aspirin is to be avoided; foods which are rough and can irritate the esophageal walls are excluded so a soft, bland diet is recommended; any physical straining or hard play is also discouraged. Parents and child need a great deal of support not only during the acute attack, but also in maintaining daily living. Since surgery is indicated in severe, uncontrollable cases, anticipatory preparation may also be needed.

REF. Altshuler A.: Esophageal Varices in Children. American Journal of Nursing 72:4, 687-693, April 1972.

120. Q. What is the current thinking regarding febrile convulsions?

A. Febrile convulsions, known since the time of Hippocrates, remain one of the most common pediatric problems and one of the most controversial topics in pediatrics with disagreement about definition, prognosis and therapy. Two distinct definitions are currently advocated regarding seizures with fever in children between the ages of 6 months and 6 years. The first definition is that febrile convulsion is an epileptic event occurring in the context of febrile illness regardless of type of seizure, duration or previous CNS abnormalities.

The second definition is that such seizures are not alike, but fall into two categories: simple febrile convulsion, occurring in previously normal children and seizures with fever occurring in previously abnormal children. These are considered to be epileptic seizures precipitated by fever.

Most febrile convulsions are generalized, occur in children between 6 months and 6 years and are rare after the age of 3 years. They occur more frequently in males. Most febrile convulsions are brief, lasting from less than 5 minutes to 20 minutes and all are associated with fever over 102° F. Most febrile convulsions occur with viral infections such as tonsillitis, otitis and roseola infantum. Febrile convulsions appear to be inherited as an autosomal dominant with incomplete penetrance. Treatment focuses on the cause of the fever and prompt reduction of the fever by tepid sponging and antipyretics. If seizure occurs, adequate oxygenation and treatment is with diazepam (Valium) or Phenobarbital I. V.

Children who have prolonged and recurrent seizures with fever or febrile status epilepticus should be treated with anticonvulsants on a long-term basis. It does not appear warranted by present evidence, to place previously normal children with a single simple febrile convulsion on long-term anticonvulsant therapy. It is hoped that further studies on febrile convulsions will distinguish patient populations, type and duration of seizures and report data in such a way that the question of prognosis and need for prolonged treatment can be established without a doubt.

REF. Ouellitte E, M. D.: The Child Who Convulses With Fever. The Pediatric Clinics of North America May 1974.

121. Q. Does fever in the child always require treatment with antipyretics?

A. Fever frequently is the only or perhaps the best prognostic or diagnostic sign to follow. For this reason, antipyretics should sometimes be withheld. Granted that febrile convulsions in children are a concern, there is evidence that it is the rapidity of temperature change rather than the level which determines whether febrile convulsions are likely to occur. Febrile seizures should be avoided where possible and those who have had febrile seizures should be treated immediately for febrile illness. The questionable case is the run of the mill, mildly febrile illness in an otherwise healthy child.

Fever per se is not usually of any significant danger to the child, provided that the increased insensible water loss is replaced, but all antipyretics possess some toxicity and side effects. Frequently, the need for antipyretic therapy can be minimized by simply assisting the body itself to maintain its own temperature. Rather than "bundling up", the child should be uncovered as much as possible to promote heat loss. Sponging, when cautiously performed with tepid water is probably the safest way of reducing fever. It must be cautioned that excessively rapid reduction of fever can be dangerous and can lead to vascular collapse. Procedures such as sponging with ice water or alcohol or the use of ice water enemas are contraindicated in the highly febrile, seriously ill or very young child. Tepid sponging used in conjunction with aspirin or acetominophen is the treatment of choice when antipyresis is deemed indicated. REF. Done AK, M.D.: Antipyrectics. Pediatric Clinics of North America 19:1, 167-177, Feb. 1972.

122. Q. What are some important facts about hypothermia?

A. Hypothermia or reduction of body temperature is usually accomplished by three methods: drug combinations, surface cooling, and extracorporeal cooling. Each of them uses the principles of radiation, conduction, convection, and evaporation for heat loss. Radiation is the loss of infrared heat rays from the body to the environment. Conduction is loss of heat from within the body to the air: convection is the same principle but aided by air currents. Evaporation is heat lost by converting water on the skin to vapor.

Surface cooling is the oldest and simplest method of hypothermia, which involves bathing in cold water, sponging with ice or alcohol, and placing ice bags or hypothermia blankets on the body. Several complications can result from surface cooling. Temperature drift refers to the continued decrease of body temperature even after the surface coolants have been removed. This can continue from a couple of degrees to as much as 10 degrees in deep hypothermia. Such temperature changes place stress on the heart muscle and may lead to cardiac arrhythmias, fibrillation, and eventually arrest. Shivering is another problem because it increases metabolic activity at a time when conservation of energy may be the aim of therapy. It may also lead to exhaustion of liver and glycogen stores causing hyperventilation.

Burns and frostbite can occur from excessive cooling in one area and can be prevented by lubricating the skin and rotating placement of coolants. Fat necrosis develops from solidification of subcutaneous fat at sites of hypothermia application. This is especially prevalent in young children who have a thin layer of fat and skin.

Precautions during hypothermia include frequent monitoring of temperature, pulse, blood pressure, respirations, shivering, and skin color.
REF. Devney A, Kingsbury B.: Hypothermia: In Fact and Fantasy. American Journal of Nursing 72:6, 1424-1425, Aug. 1972.

123. Q. What nursing intervention is required when a patient with systemic lupus erythematosus is receiving cyclophosphamide?

A. Systemic lupus erythematosus (SLE) is a diffuse inflammatory disease of connective tissue which can affect many organ systems. It occurs predominantly in woman of young adulthood, and can occur in children, particularly in adolescence. Symptoms vary greatly, but intermittent fever, arthritis, skin lesions such as the characteristic "butterfly rash" on the face, endocarditis, and central nervous system lesions are common. The ominous complication and cause of death from SLE is progressive renal damage. The etiology of this disease is unknown, but evidence strongly supports an antigen-antibody reaction.

Because of the suspected involvement of the immune system, prednisone, a steroid, is the first drug of choice. This seems to be effective in treating most manifestations of the disease, except the nephritis. Recently, cyclosphosphamide (Cytoxan), an alkylating agent of the nitrogen mustard group, has been successfully used in treating the progressive renal involvement. Patients treated with this drug, as with prednisone, suffer several side effects. Cytoxan can cause leukopenia, severe nausea, anorexia, vomiting, hemorrhagic cystitis, and alopecia. Several nursing interventions arise because of these side effects, in addition to the patient's adjustment to a potentially fatal disease. One primary objective is prevention of infection since both prednisone and cytoxan cause myelosuppression. The severe nausea and vomiting often make eating impossible, and patients need meals that are attractive and appealing. Most important is the administration of an antiemetic prior to giving cytoxan. Body image is a crucial concern, first because of prednisone's effects of cushing-like symptoms and second the hair loss from cytoxan. Usually, the hair will grow back, but in the meantime wigs are good substitutes.

REF. Sato F.: Trials with Cyclophosphamide in SLE. American Journal of Nursing 72:6, 1077-1079, June 1972.

124. Q. What factors influence wound healing?

A. Essentials in the care of wounds necessitate promoting those factors that favor wound healing and preventing those factors that hinder wound healing. General factors influencing the healing process include: (1) age, youth favors healing, (2) deficiency diseases such as anemia, malnutrition, avitaminosis (especially vitamin C) inhibit cellular restructure, (3) circulatory impairment, (4) excessive mobility, which can lead to delayed union of edges and hemorrhage, and (5) certain drugs such as steroids, which mask infection. Local ischemia, hematoma, or foreign body can hinder healing. Probably the greatest threat to wound healing, however, is infection. Several factors concerning care of wounds can help prevent infection, such as:

(1) The environment should be as clean as possible. Dusting, floor mopping, and bedmaking should be done before dressing changes.
(2) To eliminate droplet infection, face masks should be worn, and conversation kept to a minimum during the procedure.
(3) Unnecessary exposure both of the wound and clean dressing should be avoided, so that good organization of time and equipment is essential.

(4) Avoiding contamination of the wound is paramount by protecting the surroundings, patient's skin, and clean dressing. Sterile technique should always be used, and sterile gloves and/or forceps employed to apply dressings.
(5) Rough handling and unwise use of antiseptics can damage new tissue.
REF. Powell M.: An Environment for Wound Healing. American Journal of Nursing 72:10, 1862-1865, Oct. 1972.

125. Q. What immunosuppressant drugs can be used to reverse the rejection process?

A. One immunosuppressant is Azathioprine (Imuran), a 6-mercaptopurine derivative, which is thought to block DNA and RNA synthesis and the production of the sensitized lymphocyte clone. Another drug, prednisolone, an adrenocortical, steroid has three effects: (1) it interferes with the lymphocyte's ability to recognize a transplant antigen, and to form a clone, (2) it has a lymphocytolytic effect, and (3) it interferes with the inflammatory process in the graft.
REF. Tunner W, et al.: Compulsive Post-op Care. Nursing '72 2:12, 30-35, Dec. 1972.

126. Q. Physiologically, what occurs during the rejection of a transplanted organ?

A. The rejection of a transplanted organ, such as a kidney, is an immunological response in which a delayed hypersensitivity reaction is evoked. Transplantation antigens from the donor kidney circulate to the host's lymph nodes, where they trigger the production of a lymphocyte clone, which contains specific antibodies to the foreign antigen or kidney. These antibodies attack the graft, producing an inflammatory process in the endothelial spaces of the graft. The inflammatory process brings platelets and fibrin to the area, infiltrating vascular walls. Lymphocytes migrate through the walls into the renal parenchyma, further reducing blood flow. If the process continues, fibrinoid degeneration takes place, markedly reducing the functioning parenchyma.
REF. Tunner W, et al.: Compulsive Post-op Care. Nursing '72 2:12, 30-35, Dec. 1972.

127. Q. In caring for a child who has received a kidney transplant, what are some signs to alert you to organ rejection?

A. Hyperacute rejections of kidney transplant can occur within minutes of completed vascular anastomosis in surgery, or within the first few postoperative hours. Some common warning signs are:

(1) an abrupt fall in urine output
(2) a concomitant febrile episode
(3) cloudy or smoky urine from lymphocytes and red blood cells, if the urine had previously been clear

(4) graft tenderness as internal edema increases
(5) laboratory values of proteinuria, increased BUN and serum creatinine, with a concomitant fall in creatinine clearance
(6) malaise, irritability, or lethargy.
REF. Tunner W, et al.: Compulsive Post-op Care. Nursing '72
2:12, 30-35, Dec. 1972.

128. Q. Is rheumatic fever still considered to be a major childhood
health problem in the U.S.?

A. The decline in the incidence of first attacks of rheumatic
fever over the past 30 years has not been significant, according to
a study done in Baltimore. The incidence of rheumatic fever is much
higher among low income groups and may be seen very infrequently
by the private physician. In contrast to the small decline in incidence, the decline in mortality has been marked, as has been the
incidence of recurrent attacks. Even though rheumatic fever is preventable, the complacency in treating streptococcal infections on the
part of some physicians and the low priority given to care of respiratory infections by the population at risk, have caused it to remain
prevalent in this country.
REF. Gordis L, M.D., Markowitz M, M.D.: Prevention of Rheumatic Fever Revisited. Pediatric Clinics of North America 18:4, 1243-
1253, 1971.

129. Q. What are some of the problems in the primary and secondary prevention of rheumatic fever?

A. Primary prevention involves diagnosing a streptococcal infection of the throat. A reliable diagnosis can be achieved only with
the aid of throat culture. This simple diagnostic test is sometimes
overlooked or unavailable. A simple screening test using sheep blood
agar can detect the presence of Beta-hemolytic streptococci without
the need to identify nonpathogenic bacteria. In clinics where patient
recall is difficult, it is often justified to start treatment without culture on the basis of clinical judgement. When treated, inappropriate
drugs, insufficient dosage or inadequate length of treatment, are
common causes for failure to prevent rheumatic fever. Penicillin is
the drug of choice and must be given for 10 days to insure maximum
effectiveness in doses totalling 0.6 to 1.2 million units. Recurrent
attacks of rheumatic fever make up 15% of all cases. Secondary
prevention may fail because children and adolescents are lost to
follow-up, patients take prophylactic medication irregularly and prophylaxis is thought not important for adults. If children do not take
oral medication regularly closer follow-up is necessary and perhaps,
monthly intramuscular injections should be substituted. For patients lost to follow-up, greater use should be made of public health
nurses and the school health system to provide medical supervision.
Patients who have had rheumatic fever should be maintained on prophylactic medication well into adult life even if they have no rheuma-

tic heart disease and had no carditis during the acute phase of rheumatic fever. The ultimate eradication of rheumatic fever is probably dependent upon the development of a method which is more biological and less cumbersome to prevent streptococcal infections.
REF. Gordis L, M.D., Markowitz M, M.D.: Prevention of Rheumatic Fever Revisited. Pediatric Clinics of North America 18:4, 1243-1253, 1971.

130. Q. Is there a relationship between social class and the prevalence of rheumatic fever?

A. An investigation of the relationship between special tendencies to familial rheumatic fever and social class was done. A total of 378 patients and 1,486 of their relatives were studied. Rheumatic fever was found in 15.6% of these. Among the siblings the rate was 19.6%. Among the controls, only 3.4%. Of the siblings 3.1% were affected.

From these data the investigator concludes that genetic predisposition to rheumatic fever and rheumatic heart disease is an important factor. Social class did not influence the prevalence of rheumatic fever. However, those in the lower social class were more liable to develop severe heart disease with rheumatic fever.
REF. Winter ST.: Familial Rheumatic Fever. Clinical Pediatrics 11:252-253, May 1972.

131. Q. How can the location of an endotracheal tube be determined?

A. During the immediate phase of endotracheal intubation, auscultation of the chest and stomach and observation of the movements of the chest wall and abdomen provide some clues to the proper placement of the tube. However, often these procedures do not provide quick assurance of accurate placement because of the widespread, uneven transmission of sounds particularly in young infants and asymmetric movements of the chest wall, which may be hardly discernible. Repeated laryngoscopy is traumatic, wastes valuable time, and often causes more airway obstruction during the procedure. Radiographic study is valuable, but frequently unavailable and impractical during an emergency situation.

The author proposes two easy, rapid tests to determine proper endotracheal intubation.

(1) Introduce a small French feeding tube nasally or orally, depending on the position of the ET tube, into the esophagus. While 100% oxygen is administered through the ET tube, draw a gas sample from the feeding tube and analyze it immediately. (Author used the Beckman Model 0-2 Oxygen Analyzer). If the $O_2$ concentration from the feeding tube is greater than 50%, the endotracheal tube is probably in the esophagus. (Immediate resuscitation by bagging and mask using 100% oxygen can alter these results, by forcing a high $O_2$ concentration into the stomach and esophagus).

(2) Instill 0.5 cc. of a dilute solution of methylene blue (1.10 methylene blue to sterile isotonic saline) into the feeding tube. At the same time, aspirate the ET tube. The presence of any methylene blue in the endotracheal tube confirms its placement in the esophagus or stomach.

REF. Scanlon J.: Rapid Maneuvers to Determine Location of Endotracheal Tube in Newborn Infants. Journal of Pediatrics 82:6, 1091-1092, June 1973.

132. Q. What are the signs of lomotil toxicity?

A. Lomotil (diphenoxylate hydrochloride and atropine sulfate) is a commercial preparation widely used for the treatment of diarrhea. Its dangers to children have not been well recognized.

Overdosage or sensitivity to the drug will produce symptoms like those of atropine toxicity; e.g. hyperreflexia, flushed skin and tachycardia. The child may have pinpoint pupils, early convulsions, hypotonia and loss of deep tendon reflexes. These signs will last for two to three hours.

Following this phase, a second phase, lasting for approximately 30 minutes begins. There is an abrupt drop in temperature, disappearance of flush and progressive central nervous system depression. Respiration is slow and may cease. There may be convulsions.

When there is lomotil intoxication, emesis or gastric lavage should be performed. Activated charcoal, via nasogastric tube should be given in order to prevent further lomotil absorption. Other appropriate treatment includes maintenance of adequate ventilation, a narcotic antidote at the bedside for 48 hours following ingestion, close supervision and observation for the first 24 hours. The bladder should be kept empty in order to prevent reabsorption of the medication.

REF. Snyder R, et al.: Toxicity from Lomotil. Clinical Pediatrics 12:47-48, Jan. 1973.

133. Q. How significant is a single umbilical artery?

A. Reports and analysis of children born with a single umbilical artery (SUA) have been done. All agree that SUA is usually accompanied by other congenital anomalies that are often life-threatening. The child with SUA has a one in two chance of surviving and being normal.

The newborn with SUA is considered high-risk and should be treated as such. Follow-up through school age is essential in order to detect undetected anomalies and functional problems.

The most common anomalies found among 203 infants with SUA were polydactyly, inguinal hernia, and cardiovascular malformations. In most infants several organ systems were involved.

REF. Johnson CF.: The Single Umbilical Artery and What It Means. Clinical Pediatrics 12:367-371, June 1973.

134. Q. How should the drug imferon be administered?

A. Imferon, a parenteral form of iron replacement therapy, is a dark viscous medication, which if not injected deeply into the muscle causes pain and staining of the skin. Because of these properties, intramuscular injection using a Z-track technique is recommended. To insure deposition of the medication deep in the muscle, a long needle should be used. (For children about one and one-half inches according to the child's size. For adults, about two or three inches). The gauge should be about size twenty. One needle should be used to withdraw imferon, and another needle used for the injection, which prevents any deposition of the drug along the line of insertion. Before injecting the medication, 0.25 or 0.5 cc. of air (depending on needle length) should be drawn into the syringe. This air, which rises toward the plunger, acts as an irrigant to clean the needle of medication, thus preventing leakage along the needle track when the needle is withdrawn. The procedure for Z-track is to pull the skin and subcutaneous fat to one side before the injection, inject the needle and medication slowly wait ten seconds, withdraw the needle, and immediately release the skin tension. Apply light, steady pressure over the site but do not massage, as this can force medication into surrounding subcutaneous tissue. In children, the vastus lateralus muscle should be used.

REF. Hays D.: Do It Yourself the Z-Track Way. American Journal of Nursing 74:6, 1070-1071, June 1974.

135. Q. What is another use for Menghini's Biopsy Needle?

A. Lymph nodes, which are involved in various diseases, offer an excellent and easily accessible tissue for diagnostic purposes. There have been reports of aspiration biopsy of lymph nodes by hypodermic injection needle and by the Vim-Silverman biopsy needle. But aspirated material which is smeared and examined, loses its original architecture and histological interpretation is difficult. Failure rate amounted to about 40%.

The Menghini biopsy needle was successful in 84% of cases in this study. The procedure appears to be simple, safe, and does not require strong sedation or general anesthesia. It can be performed at the bedside and in the out-patient department quickly and with a minimum of trauma to the lymph node, the child, and the parents. Failure may be due to small size of the node. Partial failures were mainly due to aspiration of caseated and necrosed material.

REF. Bhandari B, Jain AM.: Lymph Node Biopsy in Infants and Children. Archives of Disease in Childhood 45:242, 510-512, 1970.

136. Q. What are some signs of hypovolemic shock in children?

A. In older children and adults, hypovolemic shock is often the result of hemorrhage. In younger children particularly between the ages of 6 months and 3 years, diarrhea or vomiting is the usual cause of hypovolemic shock. Children of this age group can develop electrolyte imbalance very rapidly, necessitating immediate treatment.

Nurses can recognize hypovolemic shock by cold, clammy skin, rapid weak thready pulse, rapid swallow respirations, but hypotension may be a later sign, and can be missed because of the difficulty in reading accurate blood pressures on small children. More significant are signs of dehydration such as sunken eyes, dry mucous membranes, poor skin turgor particularly of the testes or vulva, depressed fontanel, and decreased urinary output.

A notable exception to the above signs is when an infant loses fluid but retains electrolytes in hypertonic diarrhea. The resulting edema rather than dehydration makes it essential that the nurse look for signs such as doughy skin, elevated body temperature, central nervous system irritability, lethargy, and seizures.
REF. Hunt J.: Thermal Burns. Nursing '74 4:5, 46-52, May 1974.

137. Q. What are some common errors in the treatment of neonatal shock?

A. There are three main types of shock in newborns: cardiogenic shock, hypovolemic shock, and septic shock. In treating all three, doctors and nurses need to be careful of the following errors:

(1) Failure to keep the baby warm. Bathing and shampooing may cause undue exposure and cold. Keep him in dry linen in a warmed isolette.
(2) Failure to start a peripheral I.V. at the first sign of shock. Nurses should have equipment ready if they themselves do not start the infusion.
(3) Lack of precision, especially intake and output.
(4) Lack of equipment, which enhances lack of precision. These newborns need an ultrasonic blood pressure monitor, pediatric drip chambers for I.V., and a constant infusion pump.
(5) Giving too much oxygen. Give oxygen only when needed; as skin turns pink, administer a lower concentration.
(6) Too vigorous suctioning. Suction briefly only when withdrawing the catheter. Vigorous suctioning can trigger a vagal response causing apnea and bradycardia.
REF. Hunt J.: Thermal Burns. Nursing '74 4:5, 46-52, May 1974.

138. Q. Is central venous pressure monitoring used in children?

A. The determination of Central Venous Pressure (CVP), has become an established technique for monitoring massive fluid and blood replacement in infants. A properly determined CVP is an accurate measure of effective filling pressure of the right heart and thus of circulating blood volume. Arterial blood pressure is a less

accurate measure of peripheral circulation because both cardiac output and peripheral resistance are variable. The superior vena cava is the preferred site for CVP monitoring, although the external jugular veins may also be used.
REF. Haller AJ, M.D.: Monitoring of Arterial and Central Venous Pressure in Infants. Pediatric Clinics of North America 16:3, 637-642, 1969.

139. Q. What is the current thinking regarding T&A surgery?

A. Tonsillectomy is the most frequently performed operation in the U.S. There exists a general feeling among critical observers that the majority of these operations are unnecessary and may even be harmful. There exists appreciable difference in attitude among physicians regarding tonsil and adenoid surgery. Some, aware of the potential anesthetic, immunologic and psychological risks, may refuse to consider tonsillectomy for their patients. Others, having cared for children who were helped, perhaps dramatically by tonsillectomy, adenoidectomy or both, continue to recommend surgery for selected patients. Less disagreement exists concerning adenoidectomy. Most authorities advocate such surgery for children with recurrent otitis media or with hypertrophied adenoids which interfere with nasal breathing. Large scale comprehensive studies are necessary in order to resolve the conflict regarding T&A surgery.
REF. Paradise J, M.D.: Why T&A Remains Moot. Pediatrics 49:5, 648-650, 1972.

140. Q. What is the frequency and cause of duodenal ulcer in children?

A. The incidence of duodenal ulcers is rare in children, many hospital centers reporting 1-2 cases yearly. The cause of peptic ulcer in children is unknown, however various problems have been implicated in the etiology. Among the possible causes are CNS damage, sepsis, trauma, circulatory changes in the G.I. tract, burns, congenital heart disease, steroids, salicylates and emotional factors. Many times the evidence as to etiology is circumstantial and most peptic ulcers occur without any obvious reason.
REF. Rosenbind ML, M.D., Koop E, M.D.: Duodenal Ulcer in Childhood. Pediatrics 45:2, 283-286, 1970.

141. Q. Can intussusception be treated other than surgically in children?

A. The management of intussusception is controversial. Some authorities advocate surgery as the primary treatment, while others consider barium enema reduction the treatment of choice. A series of 288 patients with intussusception was studied. Most had a short duration of illness and presented with intermittent abdominal pain and/or vomiting. Bloody stools and palpable abdominal masses can also be symptomatic of intussusception.

It is felt by the authors that the diagnosis of intussusception, especially in its early stages, can not be made by reliance on clinical findings alone. Barium enema is necessary for early and accurate diagnosis. It is also felt that barium enema treatment is simple and safe with low morbidity. Upon confirmatory evidence of intussusception, reduction is attempted immediately under fluoroscopic control. Barium in physiological saline is administered as an enema from a height of 90 cm. If reduction is unattainable, the height is increased to 150 cm. Several attempts are made if the intussusception remains, allowing the bowel to evacuate spontaneously following each attempt. The outcome of this treatment was successful in 81-87% of the cases.

The only contraindication to barium reduction is marked intestinal obstruction or peritonitis. The main indication for surgical correction in the patients studied, was failed barium enema reduction. REF. Gierup J, M.D., et al.: Management of Intussusception in Infants and Children: A Survey Based on 288 Consecutive Cases. Pediatrics 50:4, 535-545, 1972.

142. Q. What advice do parents have about the home care of a child with a tracheostomy?

A. John and Hilary Kaler, parents of a four year old boy with a tracheostomy since infancy suggest several excellent clues:

(1) a list of necessary equipment (mist tent, nebulizer, suctioning equipment, catheters, track tube, etc.) should be given to the parents much earlier than at discharge, and the list should be very detailed, right down to a description of scissors and tracheostomy tape sizes.
(2) parents may need help in obtaining equipment, and in planning for a large backup supply of disposable items, such as catheters and tracheostomy tubes.
(3) supplies can sometimes be purchased through a local visiting nurse association, and later repaid by Medicaid.
(4) when a child begins to feed himself, a contoured, tight-fitting bib helps prevent crumbs and spills from entering the tube.
(5) never assume that a new tracheostomy tube will fit, because of possible mislabeling of a new tube; remove the old tube by its wings to keep it sterile in case it needs to be replaced immediately. Never discard the entire supply of old tubes when you buy new ones.
(6) providing humidity in a mist tent can be difficult when the child crawls and walks; closing the tent flaps to the mattress with wooden clothespins from the outside helps solve this problem.
(7) to protect the child from cold winter wind and particles flying into the tracheostomy opening, tie a "cowboy handkerchief" at the back of his neck as a protective flap.

(8) one danger that can only be overcome by careful supervision, is the danger of falling into any depth of water. Swimming pools and bath tubs were always off limits.

(9) the parents need the availability of a nurse for guidance not only in tracheostomy care, but also in normal growth and development, and perhaps most important, the contact with other parents who have been through the same experience.

REF. Kaler J, Kaler H.: Michael Had a Tracheostomy. American Journal of Nursing 74:5, 852-855, May 1974.

143. Q. Is surgical management of children with hiatus hernia indicated?

A. The less delay in surgical intervention when a child is not responding to medical management might reduce the number of children who develop strictures as a result of gastro-esophageal reflux and might improve the development of the child. A gastric fixation with gastrostomy not only improves the nutrition of the child before a major corrective procedure, but in a few cases may avoid more drastic operation. Though maximal acid secretion tests do not help to identify those cases likely to develop a stricture, it is, however, a useful procedure in indicating whether or not vagotomy should be added to fundal plication.

REF. Lari J, Lister J.: Some Problems in Surgical Management of Children with Hiatus Hernia. Archives of Disease in Children 47:252, 201-206, 1972.

144. Q. Are there factors other than environmental hazard involved in poisoning in children?

A. Early studies of poisoning in children emphasized the importance of factors such as hazards in the environment and insufficient parental supervision as causal factors. More current research indicates that these factors are not significant and that psychosocial factors such as behavior problems, "risk-taking" patterns, abnormalities in the parent child relationship and family stresses are causal factors in childhood poisoning. Also there has been found a relationship among childhood poisoning, accident proneness and pica. In a 5 year follow-up study of 52 families with incidents of childhood poisoning, the poisoned children, especially repeaters, were found to have more behavior problems than control children. These children were characterized as hyperactive, "aggressive-impulsive" and "passive-anxious". The study indicates that a parent-child relationship with elements of a power struggle, misdirected anger, and developmental characteristics such as oral exploratory behavior, mimicry and negativism predisposes toddlers to ingest poisons. Implications for prevention of poisoning point to concentration on the parent-child relationships rather than environmental hazards.

REF. Margolis J, M.D.: Psychosocial Study of Childhood Poisoning: A 5-year Follow Up. Pediatrics 47:2, 439-444, 1971.

145.  Q. Can "accidental" self-poisoning in children be considered suicidal behavior?

A. Suicide attempts in school age children are considered to be almost non-existent, although the National Clearinghouse for Poison Control Centers classifies all ingestions by children over age 5 as non-accidental unless specifically reported to the contrary.  In a study of 1,103 cases of poisoning in the 6-18 year age groups, 13% were considered unintentional, 13% "trips", 26% suicide attempts and 48% suicide gestures or affect reactions.  The estimate by the National Clearinghouse for Poison Control Centers of 115,000 self-poisonings annually in the U.S., ages 6-18, defines this as a mental health problem of significant magnitude.
REF. McIntire M, Angle C.: Suicide as Seen in Poison Control Centers.  Pediatrics 48:6, 914-921, 1971.

146.  Q. Should ipecac syrup or apomorphine be given to induce vomiting after ingestion of poisons?

A. The first principle of treatment for most poisons other than caustic agents or petroleum distillates is ridding the body of the substance either by vomiting or gastric lavage.

Ipecac syrup is usually given as the preferred emetic, but it has the disadvantages of oral administration which requires the child's co-operation, slow onset of action, and failure to induce vomiting at all. Some investigators have suggested the use of apomorphine as a substitute.

This study looked at the advantages and disadvantages of each medication by administering either drug to a group of 86 children who had ingested poison and were brought to the emergency room.  Forty-four patients received ipecac, 15-30 ml. per os, which was repeated in 20-30 minutes if vomiting had not been induced.  Forty-two children received apomorphine, 0.07 mg. per kilogram subcutaneously. Each child's pulse, respiratory rate, blood pressure, pupil size, level of consciousness, and degree of central nervous system depression were rated, as well as time elapsing between administration of the drug and onset of emesis, number of times of emesis, and failure of vomiting to occur at all.

Results indicated that forty of the forty-four children vomited after receiving ipecac; the onset of vomiting was 14 minutes (mean). The other four children received second doses of the drug, and three vomited after a total elapsed time of 30 minutes, the fourth after 50 minutes.  Thirty-six of the children in the other group vomited within a mean time of 4 minutes after receiving apomorphine.  The duration of vomiting was highly variable (a mean of 3 emesis from ipecac and 6 from apomorphine).  However, the side effect of central nervous system depression occurred in more than half the children given apomorphine.

Although the results of the study show that apomorphine induces vomiting faster than ipecac, the authors feel that the disadvantages of central nervous system depression and that it cannot be given at home outweigh its advantages. They also state that although the central system depression was not life-threatening, it could mask signs of toxicity from the ingested poison.

REF. MacLean W.: A Comparison of Ipecac Syrup and Apomorphine in the Immediate Treatment of Ingestion of Poisons. Journal of Pediatrics 82:1, 121-124, Jan. 1973.

147.  Q. What is the treatment of acute poisoning in a child?

A. The elimination of the ingested poison from the child's stomach is the immediate treatment. There is a lack of agreement as to whether this should be achieved by gastric lavage, by emesis with ipecacuanha (ipecac), or by administration of adsorptive charcoal.

A study was done to compare ipecac-induced emesis with gastric lavage. The most important complication of gastric lavage is impairment of pulmonary function. Additional problems created are: gastric hemorrhage, esophagus perforation, cardiac arrest; psychologically an adverse effect of the crying child on relatives and also nursing and medical personnel; and treatment is laborious and time consuming.

When 30 ml. or less of ipecac syrup is given the child, vomiting occurs in 98% of the patients. The efficiency of syrup of ipecac and gastric lavage can be estimated by the percentage recovery of ingested poison. Gastric lavage was inefficient and often valueless. The drug removed varied from 3-12%. When ipecac was given, 39% of the ingested poison was recovered. Adsorbitive charcoal may be administered to patients who do not respond to ipecac.

In unconscious patients syrup of ipecac is contraindicated. Gastric lavage may also be contraindicated in comatose patients.

Syrup of ipecac has measurable advantage over gastric lavage in evacuating children's stomachs, in terms of safety, effectiveness, and rapidity of action. The average period for action with ipecac is likely to be 17 minutes, or 82 minutes depending on whether the child is treated at home or in the hospital. In contrast, the mean delay to completion of gastric lavage is estimated at 126 minutes, and this procedure has little place in the treatment of the child with poisoning.

REF. Reid DHS.: Treatment of the Poisoned Child. Archives of Disease in Childhood 45:241, 428-433, 1970.

148.  Q. How is accidental poisoning with delayed-release tablets different from those of most childhood poisoning?

A. Delayed-released (timed release) tablets have a special coating which delays the release of the active ingredients. A major problem is that after ingesting, symptoms may not arise until 6-16 hours have elapsed. By this time the tablets have passed beyond the stomach and cannot be retrieved by either forced emesis or gastric lavage.

The surgical procedure laparotomy is ruled out and would only be successful if the tablets were extremely hard; a soft mass of semi-digested tablets would be difficult to find and remove. A combination of oral purges with magnesium sulphate, soap and water enemas and saline colonic wash outs is used, and these retrieved a considerable proportion of the tablets before they were completely absorbed. Peritoneal dialysis may be indicated only if dialysis will accelerate the body's elimination of the poison, and that the poison is dialysable. Severe seizures would be treated cautiously with paroldehyde.
REF. Meadow SR, Leeson GA.: Poisoning with Delayed-release Tablets. Archives of Disease in Childhood 49:4, 310-312, 1974.

149. Q. What is the American Association of Poison Control Centers?

A. The APPCC is a national voluntary association organized in 1958. Its' goals are threefold; to prevent poisonings, to assemble information on potential hazards of household products and medicines in the home and to advise on the prevention, diagnosis and treatment of acute poisonings. The functions are carried out by education of health professionals and the public.

All members centers sponsor Poison Prevention week. The association has helped get safety legislation regarding poisoning passed. An annual meeting is held to disseminate information about poison prevention. Visual aides for lay education about poisoning are available through the Association.
REF. Mofenson HC.: The American Association of Poison Control Centers. Clinical Pediatrics 13:305-306, April 1974.

150. Q. How serious is the problem of lead poisoning in this country?

A. In addition to children with clinically apparent lead poisoning, between five and ten percent of children ages 1 to 5 have lead poisoning as defined by blood levels over 50 mcg. per deciliter. Most cases of lead poisoning are caused by ingestion of paint containing lead, the peak incidence being 2 years of age. Most houses built before 1950 contain some lead paint, the danger being greatest where buildings are old and deteriorated with peeling paint. Intake of more than 150 mcg. of lead a day exceeds the daily permissible intake and begins to be accumulated in the bones. As the disease progresses, 10% of children develop vomiting. Later in the disease, anemia and incipient encephalopathy appear. Encephalopathy is characterized by increasing lassitude, semi-coma, convulsions and possible death. Children with lead poisoning who are not

treated until encephalopathy develops have a 30-40% chance of gross
brain damage if they survive treatment. This may manifest itself
as spasticity, quadraplegia, blindness, deafness, convulsions, etc.
Probably all have some form of brain damage, though this may be
subtle as in behavior problems or learning disability.

Treatment is with chelating agents: EDTA for children without signs
of encephalopathy and BAL plus EDTA for children with signs of encephalopathy. Penicillamine is used when acute treatment does not
return blood levels to normal. Since treatment of children only after
signs of lead poisoning have developed can result in 30% suffering
brain damage, it is obvious that these children must be discovered
before symptoms appear. Screening for lead poisoning can be done
by using micro samples of capillary blood. Children should be screened at least annually from ages 1-5.

REF. Klein R, M.D.: The Prevention of Lead Poisoning in Children.
Pediatric Clinics of North America 21:2, May 1974.

151. Q. What are some facts nurses should know about lead poisoning?

A. Lead poisoning or plumbism is an insidious disease, sometimes fatal, that occurs because of the acute or chronic ingestion of
lead, found in paint chips, plaster, putty, dirt and colored pages of
magazines. It is a disease of young children, particularly between
the ages of one and three because of the practice of "pica", a habit-
ual, selective, purposeful ingestion of nonfood stuffs. The habit of
oral exploration is normal between these ages, but in lead poisoning,
unsupervised pica leads to chronic, insidious poisoning.

Lead is a cellular toxin that inhibits certain enzymatic reactions,
particularly in the renal, nervous, and hematological systems. In
the kidneys, lead damages the cells of the proximal tubules, resulting in abnormal excretion of amino acids, protein, glucose, and
phosphate. In the hematological system, leads interferes in the biosynthesis of heme, causing an increase of its precursors, delta-
aminolevulinic acid, coproporphyrin, and protoporphyrin. Reduction
of the heme molecule leads to anemia, one of the signs of this disease.

However, the most serious and irreversible side effects of lead
poisoning are on the nervous system. Death from encephalopathy
occurs in about 5% of children with severe lead levels. Mental retardation, neurological deficits, seizure disorders, and behavioral
and learning disturbances may occur even with mild lead intoxication.

History taking is the clue to detecting this potential problem and
laboratory test of blood lead level is the diagnostic tool.

REF. Reed A.: Lead Poisoning: Silent Epidemic and Social Crime.
American Journal of Nursing 72:12, 2181-2184, Dec. 1972.

152. Q. How can lead poisoning among children be eradicated?

A. Lead poisoning or plumbism has been identified as a disease that mainly occurs in children between 1 and 6 years. Generally, they live in urban housing where there is accessible lead-based paint which the child ingests.

Lack of awareness of the prevalence of lead poisoning, poor housing, absence or poor enforcement of health and housing codes have been major deterrents in eliminating lead poisoning. The most effective means of eradicating plumbism is to provide adequate housing for the poor, free of paint and plaster containing lead. Equally as important, education of the public concerning the signs, symptoms and treatment of the disease is vital. Health professionals should also be well-informed about the problem, its early detection, treatment and follow-up. Most important, the child involved should be placed in a lead-free environment following detection of high lead blood levels.
REF. Si Lin-Fu J.: Childhood Lead Poisoning-An Eradicable Disease. Children 17:2-7, Jan.-Feb. 1970.

153. Q. What is an unsuspected source of lead poisoning in children?

A. The author's help was enlisted to find the source of lead ingested by a nine year old suburban child with pica. The child did not have access to leaded paint. However, soil, grass, newspaper and magazines were eaten by the child.

The lead content of the colored pages of the magazine contained "substantially more lead than those printed in black and white." The ink used on the color pages were the source of lead. The authors conclude that "ingestion of one twentieth of a colored magazine page containing .28% lead would raise a child's lead intake to a potentially hazardous level.
REF. Hankin L, et al.: Lead Poisoning from Colored Printing Inks. Clinical Pediatrics 12:654-655, Nov. 1973.

154. Q. What effect could asymptomatic lead poisoning have on children?

A. It is a well-known fact that severe lead poisoning can cause brain damage manifest by mental retardation, convulsions, hemiparesis, blindness and deviant behavior. Children with lead poisoning may also show subtle signs of brain injury such as deficits in visual-motor perception or behavior, while general intelligence remains normal.

But what happens to children with lead levels that are clinically borderline, and who exhibit no acute signs of lead poisoning? According to this study's findings, subtle abnormalities may also be present. The authors found that overall intelligence scores were normal and comparable with the control group's scores, but that deviations in behavior ratings occurred three times as often in children with lead exposure. The most frequent deviations were extreme negativism, distractibility, and constant need for attention. Although both groups most frequently failed five motor tests, the lead exposed group failed the tests, twice as often.

These findings have implications for health workers who care for such children, and implications for screening programs, which might miss these potential problem children.
REF. de la Burde B, Choate M.: Does Asymptomatic Lead Exposure in Children have Latent Sequelae? Journal of Pediatrics 81:6, 1088-1091, Dec. 1972.

155. Q. Is there any relationship between blood-lead levels and behavior in children?

A. The determination of the concentration of lead in blood has limitations but is generally considered the most reliable biochemical index of lead exposure and absorption. A lead concentration of 40mg. or more per 100ml. whole blood is suggestive of excessive exposure.

In this study, distance of the place of residence to lead polluting factory showed greater blood absorption. Because of inappropriate feeding habits in disturbed children, hyperkinetic children, these had higher lead levels than non-hyperkinetic controls.

A group of children with pica will have poorer fine motor control and greater degrees of psychological disturbance than matched controls without pica. This is readily explained on basis of the fact that if a child has one sign of emotional disturbance (pica) he is much more likely to have other signs of disturbance.

Findings of the study seem to indicate that moderately raised blood-lead level implies that the child has come in contact with a contaminated environment and this should be investigated.

Secondly, if the child has inappropriate feeding habits as part of a pattern of general behavior disturbance or delayed mental development, it is most unlikely that increased lead absorption was an etiological factor unless there had been a definite episode in the past of encephalopathy or other signs of intoxication.

Study suggests that psychological deficiencies following lead poisoning relate more to the mother-child relationship than to the presence of encephalopathy or height of the blood-lead level.
REF. Lansdown RG, et al.: Blood-Lead Levels, Behavior, and Intelligence: A Population Study. The Lancet 1:7857, 538-541, 1974.

156. Q. What role do nurses play in the diagnosis and treatment of lead poisoning?

A. Before treatment for lead poisoning can be begun, detection of its presence is essential. Because lead interferes with the proper functioning of several systems, its signs and symptoms may mimic other conditions. Also, many of its signs, such as behavioral changes can go unnoticed unless the nurse specifically asks the mother about them. For example, as lead levels rise, the child becomes lethargic, clumsy, apathetic, and irritable. He may lose skills previously learned. He may complain of stomach aches, and lose a previously good appetite. Mothers need to be asked about the practice of pica, which they may think is normal. Questions need to be asked in an unjudgmental manner because parents are perceptive and sensitive of criticism. The socioeconomic status needs exploration, such as housing conditions, supervision of the children, and financial resources for food.

Confirmation of the diagnosis is made by blood lead levels. Generally, blood lead levels of 60 micrograms per 100 ml. of blood are treated with chelating agents. These agents bind lead to reduce its concentration in soft tissue and to promote its rapid excretion. Two chelating agents commonly used are calcium disodium edathamil (ca-edta) and dimercaprol-1-propanol (bal). Treatment usually consists of five days of therapy, and necessitates several painful injections. Nurses need to plan carefully for the rotation of sites and the preparation of the child. A complication of these drugs is convulsions, because of the depletion of calcium, and seizure precautions should be available.

Comprehensive care is not only drug therapy but also environmental change, so that the source of lead is removed. Nurses need to help parents understand the dangers of chipped paint and ways to improve housing.
REF. Reed A.: Lead Poisoning: Silent Epidemic and Social Crime. American Journal of Nursing 72:12, 2181-2184, Dec. 1972.

157. Q. How serious is the problem of accidental falls in children?

A. Children account for 4% of fatal falls and 42% of non fatal falls requiring hospitalization nationally. However, in large cities such as New York, children may account for up to 20% of the accidental deaths from falling. The preponderance of high rise buildings account for the greater incidence of accidental falls. This study indicated that falls from heights are a hazard primarily to preschool boys, in the warmer months and in the afternoon hours. The incidence of fatal falls is also greatest among preschoolers. There are 2 definite groups of children who have falling accidents. The first are preschool children who fall exclusively from windows and fire escapes with little regard for height and the second are older children who fall shorter distances from a variety of hazardous play areas. These findings are consistent with the development of judgement in children. The preschooler does not sense the dan-

ger at higher elevations, whereas the older child becomes less care-
less in his play. It is obvious that safe and effective window guards
would greatly lessen the hazard of falls to children in urban areas,
especially slums.
REF. Sieben RL, et al.: Falls as Childhood Accidents: An Increasing Urban Risk. Pediatrics 47:5, 886-892, 1971.

158. Q. What are the best automotive restraint devices for children?

A. A properly designed restraining system can greatly reduce
morbidity and mortality in vehicular accidents. It is recommended
that children from birth to 12 lbs. be transported in a rear seat bassinette, held in place by seat safety belts in the front and rear. The
bassinette should be parallel with the long axis of the car and the infant should be in a feet forward position. Children from 12 to 24
lbs. should be placed in a rear seat safety harness or toddler seat.
Children from 24 to 48 lbs. should be placed in a rear seat shield-
type system. Children weighing more than 50 lbs. should use the
adult type lap belt and when they are taller than 55 inches the shoulder harness should be used as well. Infants of less than 12 lbs. may
also be transported in an infant carrier on the front seat, secured
with a safety belt and facing the back of the car.
REF. Burg L, et al.: Automotive Restraint Devices for the Pediatric Patient. Pediatrics 45:1, 49-53, 1970.

159. Q. Are there any guidelines for school bus safety?

A. No one state is following all the recommended safety precautions for school buses. The physicians for automotive safety
recommend: (1) a physical exam for school bus drivers prior to employment, (2) bus drivers aged 25-60 years, (3) job training for drivers before they are allowed to drive passengers, (4) school bus de-
signs should include all available safety features, (5) seat belts to
be worn by drivers, (6) uniform bus signal lights and bright yellow
color, (7) crash padding on all guard rails and exposed steel and
seat belts for passengers, (8) better protection for front seat passengers, (9) standing in buses should be prohibited, (10) adult mon-
itors on all bus rides. Also highway safety and road crossing drills
should be taught to children from kindergarten to 12th grade.
REF. Charles S, M.D., Shelness A.: How Safe is Pupil Transportation. Pediatrics 45:1 Part II, 166-185, 1970.

160. Q. Does atmospheric pollution with tobacco smoke endanger
the health of non-smokers?

A. Admissions to hospital during the first year of life were
recorded in a prospective study of 10,672 infants whose mothers'
smoking habits were known. The infants of mothers who smoked
had significantly more admissions for bronchitis or pneumonia, especially in the winter, and more injuries. More admissions were
for upper-respiratory-tract infections, gastroenteritis, childhood
infectious diseases, and other diagnoses.

The excess of bronchitis and pneumonia in the group exposed to smoke increased with increasing number of cigarettes smoked by the mother. It occurred within subgroups of birth-weight, social class, and birth order. It was seen mainly in infants aged 6-9 months, while at older and younger ages there was no significant effect of maternal smoking.

The findings support the hypothesis that atmospheric pollution with tobacco smoke endangers the health of non-smokers.
REF. Harlap S, Davies MA.: Infant Admissions to Hospital and Maternal Smoking. The Lancet 1:7857, 529-532, 1974.

161. Q. What tools are available for early diagnosis of sickle cell disease?

A. Sickle cell trait and sickle cell anemia can be diagnosed by several screening methods. In the past, the sickle cell preparation was used extensively. It is an inexpensive test but it has many false positive results. A more contemporary test is the Sickledex Test. The test is simple but expensive and can be performed by persons who do not have technical training.

A major disadvantage of these tests is that they do not distinguish between people with sickle cell trait and sickle cell anemia or other abnormal hemoglobins. They only indicate whether or not sickle cell disease (trait or anemia) is present.

In order to specifically diagnose the type of sickle cell disease present hemoglobin electrophoresis can be employed. The technique is reliable, accurate and inexpensive.
REF. Pearson HA, M.D.: Progress in Early Diagnosis of Sickle Cell Disease. Children 18:222-226, Nov.-Dec. 1971.

162. Q. What are the clinical manifestations of sickle cell anemia?

A. Children with sickle cell disease, always have anemia, but its severity may vary. Sickle cell disease is associated with an accelerated hemolytic process which produce the symptoms of pallor, weakness, and fatigability. In addition to these features of chronic anemia, unique clinical aspects of sickle cell disease result from occlusion of blood vessels and subsequent tissue infarction, by distorted sickled red blood cells which are found in large numbers in the blood of these patients. The clinical and hematological manifestations of sickle cell disease thus reflect two processes: (1) severe hemolysis and the compensatory mechanisms which this hemolytic anemia evoke and, (2) widespread vaso-occlusive phenomena involving many tissues and organs.
REF. Pearson H, Diamond L.: The Critically Ill Child: Sickle Cell Disease Crises and Their Management. Pediatrics 48:4, 629-635, 1971.

163. Q. What is a sickle cell crisis?

A. There are 4 types of episodic events which are called crises. They are:

(1) Aplastic crisis - diminished red cell production, triggered by viral or other infection, superimposed on the usual rapid destruction of RBC's, is the basis of aplastic crisis.
(2) Hyperhemolytic crisis - In association with certain drugs or acute infections, the rate of hemolysis may increase, causing pallor, weakness and possible abdominal pain.
(3) Splenic sequestration crisis - This may be acute or chronic. Acute sequestration crisis in young children between 8 months and 5 years of age is most dangerous and may result in death within hours. These children whose spleens are not infarcted and fibrotic may suddenly pool (sequester) vast quantities of blood in the spleen, causing a drop in hemoglobin and hypovolemic shock. The chronic manifestation of this crisis is termed functional asplenia. Because of damage to the spleen it ceases to function despite splenomegaly.
(4) Vaso-occlusive crisis - these are the most common crises and the only painful ones. Obstruction of blood vessels by tangled masses of sickled cells causes vasospasm and occlusion. This may occur as swelling and pain of the hands and feet in infants (hand-foot syndrome), in the joints and extremities and the abdomen. In some cases occlusion of the vessels in the CNS may cause hemiplegia or monoplegia.
REF. Pearson H, Diamond L.: The Critically Ill Child: Sickle Cell Disease Crises and Their Management. Pediatrics 48:4, 629-635, 1971.

164. Q. What is the treatment of sickle cell crisis?

A. The treatment for aplastic crisis is transfusion of fresh packed cells, given slowly in a dose of 2-3 ml/kg every 8 hours until the hemoglobin is increased by 5 Gm/100 ml. In hyperhemolytic crises, the treatment consists of finding the site of infection and treating with antibiotics. Also dehydration and acidosis must be corrected and adequate blood transfusions given. Treatment of sequestration crises is directed toward prompt correction of hypervolemia with plasma expanders and blood transfusions. Splenectomy may be indicated after one or two sequestration crises. In chronic asplenia, penicillin therapy is indicated for any significant unexplained fever, due to the susceptibility to pneumococcal infections.
There is no specific drug therapy for vaso-occlusive crises. Dehydration should be combatted, usually with parenteral fluids. Acidosis must also be treated and a well oxygenated atmosphere provided. Transfusion with blood is not routinely used in vaso-occlusive crises.
REF. Pearson H, Diamond L.: The Critically Ill Child: Sickle Cell Disease Crises and Their Management. Pediatrics 48:4, 629-635, 1971.

165.  Q. What is the role of the nurse in providing care for the child
with sickle cell anemia?

A. In general, the nurse's role consists of providing anticipatory guidance, coordination and continuity of care of the child and
family and health education and casefinding.

Specifically, the nurse should assess the family in order to evaluate
their knowledge and attitudes about the child's illness.  In this way,
the child's feelings and behavior can be better understood and his
needs more accurately assessed and cared for.  This can be done
through discussion, open-ended interviews, listening and role-play-
ing by the child, family and nurse.

In addition, parental counseling regarding the child's growth and development can help them recognize, anticipate and meet the child's
needs.  With increased understanding, the parents will be better
able to understand the child and provide support, especially during
traumatic experiences and hospitalization.  Continuity of care and
coordination of health services is crucial.  The nurse should be able
to make parents aware of their importance for the health of the child.

As a community member, the nurse's role as a casefinder and health
educator can help give parents and young adults valid facts regarding
sickle cell anemia.
REF. Suckett C.:  Caring for Children with Sickle Cell Anemia.
Children 6:227-231, Nov.-Dec. 1971.

166.  Q. What preoperative precautions are essential when the patient has sickle cell anemia?

A. Sickle cell disease is an autosomal recessive disorder
characterized by the body's inability to carry oxygen to the tissues
because of abnormal hemoglobin.  When an individual has the trait,
he ordinarily exhibits no evidence of the disease, unless subjected
to extreme stress or limited oxygen.  The disease, however, has
several manifest characteristics because of defective Hemoglobin
S.  In an environment of decreased oxygen supply, Hb-S will not
readily dissolve in fluids and forms a sickled-shape red blood cell.
This crescent shape with jagged ends causes RBC to stick together
forming a thrombosis.  This thrombosis in the capillaries causes
decreased blood flow to surrounding tissues, which in turn causes
swelling and severe pain.  When this pathophysiological change occurs, a sickle cell crisis is present.

Such crises can be precipitated by infection, stress, dehydration,
hypoxia and other conditions causing extra strain on the body.  Surgery is often one such precipitating factor, and special precautions
are essential to prevent a crisis.

Since sickling occurs when oxygen tension is low, every effort must
be made to prevent hypoxia.  This includes administering oxygen (a
croupette may be used for young children), checking for signs of

upper respiratory infection that could cause severe complications post surgery, avoiding sedatives that depress the respiratory center such as barbiturates and narcotics, keeping the patient well hydrated before and after surgery, and avoiding stress and fatigue as much as possible.

It is not unusual for these patients to need transfusions to maintain an adequate hemoglobin level. Before surgery, packed red cells are given because the plasma from whole blood could cause hypervolemia, and lead to congestive heart failure. During surgery, whole blood may be replaced if blood has been lost. Nurses need to be especially alert to signs of transfusion reactions because of multiple previous replacements.
REF. Doswell W.: Sickle Cell Disease: How It Influences Preoperative and Postoperative Care. Nursing '74 4:6, 19-22, June 1974.

167. Q. What postoperative nursing care is required for the patient with sickle cell anemia?

A. The same main objective is present postoperatively as preoperatively-prevention of hypoxia. Hypoxia presents the greatest threat to the patient with the disease, but certain operative procedures such as cardio-pulmonary bypass and hypothermia can present risks to the carrier as well. Postoperatively, the patient needs frequent respiratory therapy, such as coughing, deep breathing, postural drainage, repositioning, administration of oxygen and humidity. Blood gases need to be monitored and the nurse should be aware of values indicating decreased $pCO_2$ or $pO_2$, as well as oxygen saturation. Incisional pain may cause hypoventilation which will cause the $pCO_2$ to rise. An early indication of this disturbance is restlessness. Deep breathing and oxygen should be primary interventions.

Vital signs can also be clues to impending danger. Abnormal pulse rate can indicate hypoxia; decreased breath sounds can lead one to suspect respiratory depression or atelectasis. Cyanosis should not be relied upon because often these patients are black, and chronic anemia can lead to tissue compensation. Immobility carries special risks, too, because stasis of blood enhances thrombosis formation. Passive exercises may need to be done for the patient in order to conserve his energy, thereby lowering his metabolic rate. Hydration is essential because decreased circulatory fluids also predispose to thrombosis. Intravenous lines need careful monitoring, and oral fluids should be encouraged as early as possible.
REF. Doswell W.: Sickle Cell Disease: How It Influences Preoperative and Postoperative Care. Nursing '74 4:6, 19-22, June 1974.

168. Q. What is hemophilia?

A. Hemophilia is a bleeding disorder usually inherited as a sex-linked recessive trait. However, about 25% of patients have no known family history of the disease, so that the defect is usually attributed to mutation. There are several types of hemophilia, classified according to factor deficiencies: Classic hemophilia or hemophilia A is a deficiency of factor VIII; hemophilia B or Christmas disease is a deficiency of factor IX. The blood coagulation mechanism is abnormal, but the exact defect is unknown. There are no defects in vasculature of blood vessels or platelet function so that the following tests are usually normal: bleeding time, platelet count and prothrombin time.

Diagnosis is usually made on a history of bleeding episodes, sex-linked inheritance, and laboratory findings. Hemophiliacs can be classified into three general groups according to the severity of the factor deficiency: (1) severe defects, less than 1% of the normal amount of factor VIII or IX, (2) moderate defects, levels of about 5% or more, and (3) mild defects, level of about 25-50% (normal values for factor VIII is 60-120%, and for factor IX 60-130%.) Hemophiliacs with severe deficiencies bleed spontaneously or from minor trauma. Those who are moderately affected have trouble only with injury and mildly affected individuals usually require therapy only after severe injury or surgery.

Bleeding is the most common manifestation of this disorder. Hemarthrosis, bleeding into the joints, presents the most complications, including crippling, muscular atrophy, synovitis, osteoarthritis, and retarded growth. Life-threatening complications include intracranial bleeding, hemorrhage into the neck or pharynx causing airway obstruction, intestinal obstruction, and paralysis due to hemorrhage and compression of deep nerve roots.

Therapy is aimed at controlling the bleeding by replacing the deficient factor. Some replacement products available for factor VIII include: cryoprecipitate, lyo concentrate, hemophil, and humafac. Factor IX replacements are fresh frozen plasma, konyne concentrate. The concentrates are made from normal human plasma, which ordinarily contains small amounts of the factor, as well as isohemagglutinins. Multiple replacement therapy carries the risk of transfusion reactions from the isohemagglutinins.

Replacement therapy alone is not enough to help these patients and family cope with all the problems created by this disease. A joint approach which aims at prevention as well as management of orthopedic, medical, neurological, and psychological problems is essential for optimal adjustment of the individual.

REF. Sergis E, Hilgartner M.: Hemophilia. American Journal of Nursing 72:11, 2011-2017, Nov. 1972.

169. Q. Can hemophilia occur in a female?

A. Antihemophilic factor deficiency (Factor VIII deficiency, hemophilia A) in the female is rare since this disease is transmitted by sex-linked inheritance. However, hemophilia A can occur in females and may be the expression of one of several phenomenon:

(1) offspring between a hemophiliac male and a carrier female,
(2) a "symptomatic carrier" of hemophilia A with a moderate decrease in AHF activity,
(3) a phenotypic female who has inherited one gene for hemophilia and lacks a second normal X chromosome as in Turner's syndrome (XO) or XX/XO mosaicism,
(4) a female with an autosomally dominant transmitted form of AHF deficiency such as von Willebrand's disease or combined Factor V and VIII deficiency,
(5) a genotypic female with severe AHF deficiency whose parents do not carry a gene for hemophilia.

The first four possibilities are usually discernible through family history (1 and 2), chromosome analysis (3), or factor analysis (4). Type 5, however, has no simple explanation for its occurrence. At least eight well documented cases have been reported. Theoretical possibilities for this occurrence might be:

(1) a spontaneous mutation of a normal X-chromosome,
(2) nondysjunction of the maternal X-chromosome with loss of the paternal sex chromosome,
(3) inactivation of all normal X-chromosomes early in embryonic development.

REF. Czapek E, et al.: Hemophilia A in a Female: Use of Factor VIII Antigen Levels as a Diagnostic Aid. Journal of Pediatrics 84:4, 485-489, April 1974.

170. Q. What role do nurses play in the home care of hemophiliac patients?

A. Because of the long term problems of this bleeding disorder and the advantage of immediate replacement of the deficient factor during a bleeding episode, home care programs have been started which allow the patient the freedom to initiate his own therapy without hospitalization. In the home care program, hemophiliac patients and family (parents or spouse) are taught how to administer the replacement factor and how to control or prevent bleeding episodes. Generally, the physician assumes responsibility for referring and screening the patient, but the nurse does the actual teaching with the patient. Some criteria used for selecting patients include: (1) expression of a willingness to learn venipuncture technique, (2) an ability to follow instruction, (3) an ability to manage and monitor transfusions, (4) a willingness to accept the necessity for home care, and (5) sufficient emotional stability to accept the responsibility.

Although the preparation and instruction of each patient is individualized, some general guidelines are established to help the nurse systematize her instruction:

(1) In the first session, the nurse reviews the philosophy of the home care program, and tries to elicit from the patient what he expects to accomplish, what he already knows about the disorder and the

medications, and what experience he has had in preparing or administering the concentrates. This initial interview gives the nurse a data base from which to plan for the patient at his level of readiness and knowledge.

(2) In the first teaching session, aseptic technique of drawing up medication is reviewed, with emphasis on handwashing and sterile precautions.

(3) Second procedure is demonstration and practice of venipuncture, emphasizing sterile technique, use of tourniquet, selection of a vein, and preparation of the skin. Patients must be able to do this procedure with either hand and arm.

(4) Finally, the preparation and administration of cryoprecipitate and plasma concentrates are demonstrated. Patients are taught how to recognize transfusion reactions, and are cautioned against too rapid infusion rate.

(5) After a patient has mastered all these steps, he performs the entire transfusion under the supervision of the teaching nurse.

So far, these programs have been successful, allowing the patient freedom and independence. Some studies show that school attendance among these children is higher. One precaution is the continued need for medical supervision at regular intervals.
REF. Sergis E, Hilgarten M.: Hemophilia. American Journal of Nursing 72:11, 2011-2017, Nov. 1972.

171. Q. What is the pathophysiology of Disseminated Intravascular Coagulation (DIC)?

A. DIC is a disease process characterized by intravascular consumption of clotting factor and platelets, widespread deposition of fibrin thrombi within the vascular periphery and generalized hemorrhagic diatheses. Several events can trigger the DIC process and cause activation of the coagulation mechanism by tissue thromboplastin which leads to the formation of fibrin. Certain factors are lowered or depleted during active DIC; they are antihemophilic factor, proaccelerin, platelets, prothrombin, and fibrinogen as fibrin is deposited in small vessels, the fibrinolysin system is activated. The fibrinolysin splits the fibrin into fragments. These fibrin split products or FSP, circulate and cause thrombi and emboli, depletion of clotting factors, hemolytic anemia and finally shock and death.
REF. Hathaway W, M.D.: Care of the Critically Ill Child: The Problem of Disseminated Intravascular Coagulation. Pediatrics 46:5, 767-773, 1970.

172. Q. In what conditions can DIC occur in children?

A. Any severely ill child may develop the complication of disseminated intravascular coagulation. A critically ill child should be suspected of having DIC if evidence of the following signs are present: (1) the potential for the presence of a triggering substance such as endotoxin, damaged tissue (tissue thromboplastin), endothelial damage or proteolysis, (2) multiple system involvement producing coma, renal shutdown, respiratory disease and shock, (3) a bleeding diathesis, (4) hemolytic anemia associated with fragmented or burred RBC's. Laboratory confirmation includes evidence of depletion of coagulating factors. Treatment consists of heparinization, replacement of depleted factors and supportive care.

REF. Hathaway W, M.D.: Care of the Critically Ill Child: The Problem of Disseminated Intravascular Coagulation. Pediatrics 46:5, 767-773, 1970.

173. Q. What is hemorrhagic disease of the newborn?

A. Classical hemorrhagic disease of the newborn is due to vitamin K deficiency. The vitamin K dependent clotting factors (II, VII, IX, X) are physiologically depressed in the premature and normal infant, which results in prolongation of the prothrombin time. The incidence of this condition has been greatly reduced by the practice of prophylactic administration of 1 mg. of vitamin K to all newborn infants. This can be given to the mother during labor or to the infant immediately after delivery. Hemorrhagic disease of the newborn, should it occur, can be treated with 1-2 mg. of vitamin K which results in rapid correction of the clotting defect and cessation of hemorrhage within 4-8 hours.

REF. Hathaway WE, M.D.: Coagulation Problems in the Newborn Infant. Pediatric Clinics of North America 17:4, 929-941, 1970.

174. Q. Do children with Cooley's anemia have retarded mental development?

A. A study was done of 138 consecutive cases of Cooley's anemia (homozygous beta-thalessemia) for evaluation of mental status. Although there is a large amount of information regarding severe retardation of physical growth in this disease, little had been said regarding mental development. The present study indicated that although these children commonly had abnormalities in affective state, behavior and character, the intellectual function remained within normal range. In 125 of the patients over the age of 5 years, intelligence tests revealed no significant deviation from the expected norms. Ninety-six patients demonstrated abnormal behavior and 67 presented abnormal emotional responses, mainly depression and anxiety.

REF. Logothetis J, et al.: Intelligence and Behavior Patterns in Patients with Cooley's Anemia (Homozygous beta-thalassemia): A Study Based on 138 Consecutive Cases. Pediatrics 48:5, 740-743, 1971.

175. Q. What are some complications of blood transfusion?

A. In supervising the administration of blood transfusions, nurses have the responsibility of knowing how to observe for complications. Some adverse reactions include:

(1) Hemolytic reactions is the lysis of cells by an antigen-antibody combination resulting from A-B-O, Rh, or other group incompatibilities. With the hemolysis, free hemoglobin is released into the serum, and enters the kidney, causing severe renal damage. The onset may be acute, or may be insidious, diagnosed by the presence of jaundice. Physiological signs include fever, chills, dyspnea, decreased urine output followed by possible acute renal failure, hypotension which can be evidence of shock, and flank and leg pain.

(2) Febrile reactions result when donor leukocytes are transfused into a recipient who has antileukocyte antibodies. This antigen-antibody reaction releases pyrogens, producing fever. Multifused and multiparous patients are especially at risk. Symptoms, which may occur within the first 15 minutes of administration, include fever, chills, and occasional lumbar pain.

(3) Overload of electrolytes is another potential danger. The breakdown of red blood cells releases potassium into the blood. This increased potassium can be particularly critical if the patient has renal or cardiac disease. Signs alerting the nurse to hyperkalemia include vague muscle weakness especially in the extremities, slow possibly irregular pulse, paresthesia of hands, feet, and tongue, and gastrointestinal hyperactivity characterized by nausea and diarrhea. If these symptoms go unnoticed, paralysis of the respiratory and cardiac muscles can lead to arrest and death.

(4) Another electrolyte complication is hypocalcemia, caused by the preservative and anticoagulant, acid citrate dextrose (ACD). The sodium citrate anticoagulant binds with the calcium ions to remove them from circulation. Hypocalcemia causes neuromuscular irritability, muscular cramps, hyperactive muscle reflexes, and carpopedal spasm of the hands. Convulsions and cardiac arrest can eventually occur.

(5) Circulatory overload can occur if transfusions are given too rapidly. Children and infants are particularly at risk, especially if other factors such as renal or cardiorespiratory problems exist. Signs include left heart failure and pulmonary edema. Hemorrhage into the lungs and gastrointestinal tract are also possible.

(6) Hypothermia can result from the transfusion of cold blood (usually stored at $1^0$ to $6^0$ Centigrade). Besides complaining of chills, the patient is in danger of cardiac arrest. This can easily be prevented by allowing blood to remain unrefrigerated for a short time (less than one hour) or using a warming coil.

(7) Anaphylaxis, can also occur, which is an antigen-antibody reaction of a patient to allergens in the donor's blood. This is recognized by chills, urticaria, vertigo, bronchospasm, edema, headache, decreased blood pressure, weak thready pulse. Severe reactions may require the use of a bronchodilator and a vasoconstrictor.

(8) Infectious contamination is always a danger, and infections such as hepatitis, malaria, and syphilis can be carried in the donor's blood.
REF. Child J, et al.: Blood Transfusions. American Journal of Nursing 72:9, 1602-1605, Sept. 1972.

176. Q. How can nurses help prevent and manage iron deficiency anemia?

A. Many authors have studied the possible effects of malnutrition on a developing young child, and some evidence has been accumulating that poor nutritional intake during infancy results in decreased brain growth. Among children, iron-deficiency anemia is the most common type of nutritional anemia, and usually results from inadequate daily ingestion of iron. Iron is an essential component of the hemoglobin molecule. Heme, the iron-containing portion, is responsible for the oxygen-carrying capacity of blood, allowing for the oxidative processes in cell metabolism to occur. About two thirds of the body's iron is found in hemoglobin, and about one third is stored in the liver, spleen, and bone marrow.

Levels of iron in the body are measured by many laboratory tests, but two common ones include hemoglobin level and hematocrit. Exactly what values of iron can be considered inadequate varies, but a guideline is from 10.0-11.5 gm. hemoglobin per 100 ml. of blood or less.

Nurses have a particular role in preventing this disorder because of their close contact with families. Some of the interventions available to them include:

(1) identification of the anemia through dietary history taking, and physical assessment of family members, confirmed by laboratory values,
(2) preventive teaching of pregnant mothers about the importance of their nutrition during pregnancy, which can provide the newborn with about a six month store of iron; also teaching the mother about proper infant feeding, such as the use of iron-supplemented formulas, early introduction of fortified cereals, and a proper limited amount of whole milk, which contains minute amounts of iron,
(3) counseling of families whose children are anemic by planning meals based on the financial budget, cultural pattern, and food preferences; this is often a most difficult job and requires a nurse who has formed a trusting relationship with the mother, and who is willing to shop with the mother if necessary, praise her efforts, offer recipes, and encourage her in her efforts.
REF. Wilson P.: Iron-Deficiency Anemia. American Journal of Nursing 72:3, 502-504, March 1972.

177. Q. Is there a relationship between anemia and scholastic achievement?

A. According to a study done by these authors, there is a correlation between low hemoglobin levels and intellectual performance. Subjects were students, aged 12 to 14 years from a junior high school. Ninety-two students comprised the "anemic" group because of hemoglobin levels between 10.1 to 11.4 gm. per 100 ml. For comparative study, the 101 students in the control group had hemoglobin levels between 14.0 to 14.9 gm. per 100 ml. Intellectual performance was evaluated by the Iowa Tests of Basic Skills. Results showed that scholastic performance of all subjects in the anemic group were below those of their peers, but that the greatest deterioration of performance was among anemic males. (The authors point out that this difference may be a consequence of normally rising hemoglobin levels in males of this age group, but not among females).

The poor performance of these students is a complex problem, because who is to say what factor leading to decreased iron-levels could have caused the deterioration. However, iron deficiency is generally considered to be a reflection of poor general nutritional intake. Also, the anemic children could have come from poorer families, which resulted in poor nutrition, as well as less guidance and educational stimulation.

REF. Webb T, Oski F.: Iron Deficiency Anemia and Scholastics Achievement in Young Adolescents. Journal of Pediatrics 82:5, 827-830, May 1973.

178. Q. What are the major causes of burns in children?

A. Burns are the third leading cause of accidental death in childhood. Two million patients a year are hospitalized with burns and yet the great majority of burns are preventable. In the toddler stage the most common accident occurs when the child reaches up and pulls a pot handle on the stove. Usually scalding of the arms, chest and shoulder result. In summer many burns occur from outdoor barbecues. These are flash flame burns of the hands, face, arms, and chest, usually in boys, resulting from flammable substances poured on the fire. In the autumn when leaves are being burned, pant-leg burns are common. At all seasons burns caused by nightclothing catching fire on stoves, gas ranges or candles are encountered.

REF. Herrin J, Crawford JL.: Care of the Critically Ill Child: Major Burns. Pediatrics 45:3, 449-458, 1970.

179. Q. How do you evaluate the extent of burns in children?

A. The following chart provides a guide for evaluating the total percentage of the surface area burned.

| | Newborn | 3 Years | 6 Years | 12 Plus Years |
|---|---|---|---|---|
| Head | 18% | 15% | 12% | 6% |
| Trunk | 40% | 40% | 40% | 38% |
| Arms | 16% | 16% | 16% | 18% |
| Legs | 26% | 29% | 32% | 38% |

These percentage figures refer to front and back. For example, if an infant suffered burns of the anterior trunk, this would comprise 20% of his body surface.
REF. Herrin J, Crawford J.: Care of the Critically Ill Child: Major Burns. Pediatrics 45:3, 449-458, 1970.

180. Q. What is the protocol for the initial treatment of severe burns?

A. The following outline of initial evaluation and treatment is carried out at the Shriners Burn Institute in Boston. The order is approximate and several procedures may be carried out simultaneously.

( 1) Check adequacy of airway providing whatever assistance is necessary
( 2) Sedate only if necessary, using I.V. route
( 3) Remove clothing and weigh patient
( 4) Establish an I.V. line, preferably a central venous pressure line
( 5) Evaluate extent and depth of burn
( 6) Cover burns with wet dressings of 0.5% silver nitrate solution; Use sulfamylon on face
( 7) Splint areas of potential contractures
( 8) Obtain blood for baseline lab studies
( 9) Calculate fluid requirements and establish fluid regimen
(10) Insert foley catheter and obtain urine sample
(11) Commence charting of intake and output, vital signs and blood and urine values
(12) Initiate low dosage penicillin prophylaxis
(13) Give protection against tetanus
(14) Obtain a detailed diagnosis, also diagnosis regarding the injury
(15) Consider means of achieving temporary or permanent skin cover
(16) Plan nutritional support, treatment of anemia and hypoproteinemia, rehabilitation including physiotherapy and emotional support.

REF. Herrin J, Crawford J.: Care of the Critically Ill Child: Major Burns. Pediatrics 45:3, 449-458, 1970.

181. Q. What is the recommended method for the topical treatment of burns?

A. Continuous topical application of 0.5% silver nitrate or sulfamylon cream has been shown to give a high level and a broad spectrum of surface bacterial control. These agents are effective only when in close contact with residual viable tissue. They cannot penetrate thick eschar, and thus wet dressings or cream must be totally removed daily. The burn surface should be carefully debrided of necrotic tissue that separate easily from the granulating bed. Cultures should be taken from representative areas so that

the nature of the bacterial flora is constantly known. Silver nitrate 0.5% should be applied with gauze dressings, warm and wrapped loosely to a thickness of 1/2 inch. Cream can be applied without dressings.
REF. Herrin J, Crawford J.: Care of the Critically Ill Child: Major Burns. Pediatrics 45:3, 449-458, 1970.

182. Q. How do electrical burns of the mouth occur and what is the treatment?

A. Toddlers between the ages of 6 and 36 months are the most frequent victims of electrical mouth burns. The injury is usually sustained when the toddler puts the plug from an electrical appliance such as an iron, percolator or frying pan which is plugged into the wall, but disconnected from the appliance, into his mouth. The contacts are not exposed, but the electrolytes in the child's saliva complete the electric circuit and transmit current through the local tissues causing considerable destruction. The injury initially appears as a painless white parchment-like patch of skin. Within a few hours, considerable edema occurs and is followed within time by the formation of black eschar. Tissue necrosis follows and there is danger of hemorrhage. In a study of 54 cases, bleeding occurred between the first and twenty-first day in 25% of the cases. Observation in the hospital is recommended during this time. Treatment involves cleaning the wound and application of A&D ointment. Feedings are with a rubber tipped bulb syringe. Eighty-three percent of the cases required later plastic surgery performed at least one year after healing of the burn to allow for maturation and softening of the extensive scar tissue present.
REF. Gifford G, et al.: The Management of Electrical Mouth Burns in Children. Pediatrics 47:1, 113-119, 1971.

183. Q. What are common family reactions to a severe burn?

A. A patient, who has been burned, has psychological and physical problems that extend toward the family. Just as the patient deals with his crisis based on past learning, so do family members. It is essential in caring for patients and their families that nurses recognized these coping mechanisms. According to the authors, there are three common reactions of family members:

(1) Indecision - The feelings of hopelessness and helplessness often immobilize the family from making decisions or formulating actions toward a goal. The staff can neither make the decision for the family, which fosters their immobilization, nor demand a decision from them. Rather, their needs must be met and trust established, so that slowly their resources can be mobilized.

(2) Intensification of preexisting problems - Unresolved preexisting problems often become evident through quarreling and bickering in the unit. Attempts at control can take the form of undermining

the patient's control of his hospitalization and rehabilitation. Sometimes these long-existing problems cannot be solved by the staff; their effects, however, can be minimized for the patient's recovery and well-being.

(3) Guilt feelings - Feelings of responsibility and guilt can impede the rehabilitation of the patient. With a child, the parents try to make up for any real or imagined shortcomings by allowing the child excessive freedom. The child then becomes uncooperative, unmanageable, and demanding, which makes treatment more difficult.

Nurses need to recognize and understand the reasons behind these reactions before they can help families adopt new ways of coping. REF. Bowden M, Feller I.: Family Reactions to a Severe Burn. American Journal of Nursing 73:2, 317-319, Feb. 1973.

184. Q. What kind of discharge planning is needed for the patient with burns?

A. Patients with burns experience the problems, depressions, and anxieties of most hospitalized patients but also the crisis of disfigurement, long-term recovery, and extensive rehabilitation. Their recovery extends into the home, and discharge planning is essential. One burn care unit has developed a home care program, staffed by a nurse, who works with the entire health team and the community visiting nurse service.

When a patient is to be discharged she plans the care needed at home with the physician and other nurses. She gives direct care to begin to know the patient, his physical and emotional needs, and to gather data for her home care plan. If a child is going to a foster home, she will visit the foster parents to evaluate the care given to the child and his adjustment to the environment.

Not every patient receives a home visit. Often, all the teaching of wound care, physical therapy, proper positioning, and nutrition is done before discharge. If home visiting is required, the nurse evaluates the home environment for safety, cleanliness, adequate heat, etc. She may give direct care until the patient or other family member is able to assume responsibility. Frequently, she is asked several questions about scarring, need for grafting, or other disfigurements. These patients, who have already heard the answers, need reassurance and support.

When a school-age child is discharged, she visits him in school, and uses this opportunity to discuss any problems with the school nurse or teacher.

The home care nurse also attends burn clinic where patients who still need medical care come for treatment. One purpose of this visit is evaluation of the progress at home, and offering of any help or advice that is needed. So far, this program has been successful, although the author feels that almost every patient needs home visiting.

REF. Calleia P, Boswick J.: A Home Care Nursing Program for Patients with Burns. American Journal of Nursing 72:8, 1442-1444, Aug. 1972.

185. Q. How common is cancer in children?

A. The number one cause of death in children between 1 and 15 years of age is cancer. The incidence is approximately 10 per 100,000 children annually. Acute leukemia occurs in nearly 4 per 100,000 children. Mortality tables do not accurately reflect the total number of children who develop cancer, since the data are collected from death certificates and do not include patients who survive.

REF. Fernbach D, M.D., Starling K, M.D.: Acute Leukemia in Children. Pediatric Annals 3:5, 13-26, 1974.

186. Q. Have any advances been made in treating childhood cancer?

A. There has been a great deal of progress in the treatment of childhood cancer over the past 30 years. This progress can be attributed to:

(1) Better knowledge of the history and course of various diseases, which allows earlier and more thorough surgical treatment.
(2) The development of high energy radiation, which combined with increased knowledge of the spread of the disease has contributed significantly to the treatment of such diseases as Hodgkins and lymphomas.
(3) The use of intensive, intermittent short-course chemotherapy, usually with a combination of drugs. Chemotherapy as an adjuvant to surgery or radiation or alone has greatly increased survival and in some cases produced cures in many forms of cancer.

REF. Burchenal J, M.D.: Advances in the treatment of Childhood Cancer 1944 to 1974. Pediatric Annals 3:4, 9-12, 1974.

187. Q. How is leukemia diagnosed?

A. The symptoms which present in leukemia depend on the degree of bone marrow involvement and the extent and location of extramedullary infiltration. The child may have symptoms of pallor, infection, bleeding, organomegaly and bone pain as isolated complaints or in any combination or sequence. Leukemia is a great imitator of other conditions and symptoms may simulate fever of unknown origin, arthralgia appearing similar to rheumatoid arthritis or osteomyelitis, or anemia or purpura. The diagnosis is suspected on the basis of altered peripheral blood counts, but definitive diagnosis is made by examination of the bone marrow. Because the bone marrow specimen is so critical in making a correct diagnosis, it should be obtained and examined by those with expertise in this area. Aspiration of sternal bone marrow is not recommended in children, because the sternum is a thin structure in the small child and is near vital organs. Bone marrow specimens can be easily and safely obtained from the posterior iliac spine with only local anesthesia required.

REF. Fernbach D, M.D., Starling K, M.D.: Acute Leukemia in Children. Pediatric Annals 3:5, 13-26, 1974.

188. Q. What is the present treatment regime of childhood leukemia?

A. Today, more than half of the children with acute lymphoblastic leukemia who receive intensive therapy are alive three years after diagnosis. This prolonged survival rate is due to newer treatment regimes. Although much controversy exists about induction and maintenance therapy, some common features exist:

(1) Induce rapid induction of remission with prednisone and vincristine immediately after the diagnosis is confirmed. This combination drug therapy induces a complete remission in 90-95% of patients.
(2) Induce prophylactic treatment of the central nervous system with radiation and/or intrathecal methotrexate. This prophylactic treatment reduces the incidence of CNS involvement from 50% to less than 10% and appears to induce prolonged hematologic remissions.
(3) Continue maintenance therapy with a combination of two or more antileukemic drugs, such as methotrexate, cyclophosphamide (cytoxan), or 6-mercaptopurine.
(4) Discontinue chemotherapy after an extended period of 2 to 7 years of complete remission.

This protocol undoubtedly has risks. Transient alopecia and skin irritation are caused by radiation. Methotrexate may cause chemical meningitis, mucous membrane ulceration, and gastrointestinal symptoms. The other antileukemic drugs cause immunosuppression, exposing the patient to the risk of opportunistic infections which can lead to death. Other long-term complications include, sterility from cyclophosphamide, suppression of growth, drug-induced or radiation-induced malignancies, or pulmonary fibrosis and osteoporosis from methotrexate.

REF. McIntosh S, Pearson H.: Treatment of Childhood Leukemia. Journal of Pediatrics 83:5, 899-902, Nov. 1973.

189. Q. What are the chemotherapeutic agents used in leukemia and how are they used?

A. Many drugs are presently being used in the treatment of leukemia to induce remission or maintain remission. Various combinations of these drugs are being studied to discover the optimum method of inducing and maintaining remission. One recommended

therapy regimen used for induction of remission: vincristine, prednisone, daunomycin L-aspariginase adriamycin, for maintenance:
6-mercaptopurine, methotrexate, cyclophosphamide, cytosine ara-
binoside. These drugs are used in the following sequence:

1. Remission induction: Prednisone 60 mg per $m^2$ per day with a
   minimum dose of 20 mg and maximum of 60 mg, for 7 days de-
   crementally. Vincristine 2 mg/$m^2$ per week I.V. for 4 to 6 doses.
   Induction therapy is continued for 4-6 weeks until remission is
   achieved.
2. CNS therapy or prophylaxis: Methotrexate 15 mg/$m^2$ per week
   intrathecally X4 then every 8 weeks X5.
3. Maintenance therapy: 6-mercaptopurine 75 mg/$m^2$ per day orally.
   Prednisone for 28 days every 3 months.
4. Relapse: Induction with vincristine as in item 1. Maintenance
   with methotrexate 25 mg/$m^2$ daily. Reinforce with prednisone
   for 28 days every 3 months.

Further relapse or failure to respond to therapy may require the use
of cyclophosphamide or such investigational drugs as adriamycin.
REF. Fernbach D, M.D., Starling K, M.D.: Acute Leukemia in
Children. Pediatric Annals 3:5, 13-26, 1974.

190. Q. Has the life expectancy in acute leukemia of childhood been
increased?

A. Acute leukemia, the most common childhood neoplasm, had
a median survival of 4-5 months between first symptom and death,
before the use of folic acid antagonists. The advent of many new
chemotherapeutic agents and the use of intensive intermittent chemotherapy and intrathecal methotrexate, has altered the outlook for
survival, and possibly cure, drastically. Some studies are now projecting 5 year survival rates as high as 50%. These patients were
induced into remission with vincristine and prednisone in conjunction
with craniospinal irradiation and intrathecal methotrexate. Studies
have demonstrated that in cases of acute leukemia with a survival of
5 years, the patient has a 50% chance of remaining free of the disease for an indefinite period of time.
REF. Burchenal J, M.D.: Advances in the Treatment of Childhood
Cancer 1944-1974. Pediatric Annals 3:4, 9-12, 1974.

191. Q. What is Wilm's tumor?

A. Wilm's tumor or congenital nephroblastoma is one of the
distinctive forms of childhood cancer. It has been regarded as a
tumor with the best long-term survival rate, however, reclassifica-
tion of many reported cases of Wilm's tumor to nonmalignant meso-
blastic nephroma (mesenchymal hamartoma), has cast doubt on the
validity of survival figures. The presenting complaint is usually
that of abdominal swelling or a lump of mass observed by the parent.
The tumor occurs with equal incidence in either the right or left kidney. The tumor destroys or displaces kidney tissue. Therapy includes

surgical removal of the tumor and nephrectomy, radiation therapy and chemotherapy. Many patients have marked improvement for months or years and many can be cured, so that all cases even with metastases, should be treated.
REF. Porvars D, M.D.: Wilm's Tumor: Recent Advances and Unsolved Problems. Pediatric Annals 3:5, 55-70, 1974.

192. Q. What is the current treatment for the child with Wilm's tumor?

A. Wilm's tumor is a malignant tumor of the kidney. Its incidence in children under five is second to leukemia.

Once the diagnosis of Wilm's tumor is made the child's management must be perceived and treated as an emergency situation. That is, all diagnostic tests must be done within 24-48 hours following hospital admission. All palpation of the abdomen must be discouraged in order to prevent milking of cancer cells into the circulation. On admission to the hospital the following diagnostic tests should be done:

1. Blood studies
    (1) SGOT - serum glutamic oxalacetic
    (2) BUN - blood transaminase urea nitrogen
    (3) LDH - lactic dehydrogenase
    (4) Uric acid
    (5) Alkaline phosphatase
    (6) Bone marrow smears
2. X-rays
    (1) Abdominal
    (2) Intravenous pyelogram
    (3) Chest
    (4) Long bones
3. Isotope scans
    (1) Kidneys
    (2) Liver

Once these tests are completed, treatment will consist of surgery, radiation and chemotherapy. The involved kidney will be removed transabdominally. X-ray therapy will be instituted post-operatively in order to render nonviable any cells that may have escaped locally during surgery. In conjunction with radiation therapy, chemotherapy using actinomycin D (Cosmegen) is given. The aim is to destroy metastases. The drug is toxic. Therefore, careful and frequent observation of the child must be made.

Following surgery, X-ray therapy and chemotherapy, weekly blood counts, monthly chest X-rays, urinalysis and physical examinations should be done.
REF. Pochedly C.: Current Management of the Child with Wilm's Tumor. Modern Medicine 116-123, Jan. 26, 1970.

193. Q. What are the signs and symptoms of neuroblastoma?

A. Neuroblastoma is a neoplasm whose primary tumor arises in the sympathetic ganglia or adrenal gland and is metastatic in 70% of the cases at the time of diagnosis. There are 4 main areas of signs and symptoms:

1. Mass - a mass representing the primary tumor or metastatic distribution is either abdominal or in lymph nodes.
2. Neurologic signs - these are weaknesses in an extremity, a limp or paralysis.
3. Pain - usually pain occurs in the bone or joints and is most uncommon under the age of two.
4. Orbital signs - ecchymosis and proptosis may appear.

Other signs and symptoms include respiratory tract symptoms, diarrhea, epistaxis and hematuria. With the exception of orbital signs associated with abdominal mass, no other grouping of signs and symptoms is sufficient to constitute a pathognomonic syndrome. REF. Helson L, M.D.: Neuroblastoma: Early Diagnosis a Key to Successful Treatment. Pediatric Annals 3:5, 46-54, 1974.

194. Q. Can nephritis develop in children after irradiation and chemotherapy for nephroblastoma?

A. Nephrectomy is an essential part of the treatment of unilateral nephroblastoma. The tumor occurs in 10% of children. Radiotherapy, chemotherapy are available for treatment in addition to surgery. For children less than 1 year of age with unilateral disease, treatment complementary to surgery is probably unnecessary. Postoperative radiotherapy to the abdomen became conventional therapy because it seemed to reduce significantly the number of metastases in the abdominal wall and renal bed. Whether it remains necessary with today's surgical approach of wide exposure, early ligation of the renal vein, removal of the kidney and encapsulated tumor intact, has not yet been proven.

Chemotherapy has been added to routine management and actinomycin D is the chemotherapeutic agent most widely used. Cyclical chemotherapy has been added for many patients, and vincristine or actinomycin C has been the drug of choice.

In two children subsequent to nephrectomy for nephroblastoma, the single remaining kidney was given irradiation of 1500 and 2000 RAD, preceded by chemotherapy with actinomycin D and associated with vincristine therapy. Both children developed a radiation type of nephritis but have survived so far. The use of these two chemotherapeutic agents may increase the risk of radiation damage to the kidney of the child.

It seems that the above two drugs make the child's kidneys more vulnerable to nephrotoxicity from radiotherapy. The safe level for renal irradiation associated with chemotherapy is not known.

After nephrectomy for nephroblastoma a contralateral kidney shown to be "normal" on intravenous urography and on ultrasonography if available should be well screened if any irradiation is being given elsewhere. Irradiation and cytotoxic treatment together may be much more hazardous than either separately.
REF. Arneil GC, et al.: Nephritis in Two Children After Irradiation and Chemotherapy for Nephroblastoma. The Lancet 1:7864, 960-963, 1974.

195. Q. What are the clinical manifestations of heart disease in children?

A. It is often assumed that serious cardiac dysfunction will be very obvious clinically, however, this is not necessarily true, especially in the infant. When manifestations such as respiratory distress or liver enlargement appear in less than severe form, they may be disregarded or attributed to other causes. Significant clinical manifestations of serious heart disease will produce one or more, but not always each of the following abnormalities:

1. Symptoms - cyanosis, edema, growth failure, feeding difficulty, irritability
2. Physical Signs - severe cyanosis, liver enlargement, pronounced tachycardia gallup rhythm, profuse sweating, rapid breathing, skin pallor
3. Electrocardiogram - the EKG may be normal in patients with important heart disease, however, a properly recorded and interpreted EKG usually helps in separating benign from significant congenital heart disease
4. Chest X-Ray - roentgenography can help determine the shape of the heart and great vessels, the presence of cardiac dilatation, esophageal or tracheal compression, parenchymal abnormalities of the lung.
REF. McNamara D, M.D.: Management of Congenital Heart Disease. Pediatric Clinics of North America 18:4, 1191-1205, 1971.

196. Q. What impact does heart disease have upon the child and his family?

A. The child with a chronic heart disease lives within a family who is affected in many ways because of the anxiety of dealing with the problems of a cardiac defect. The impact on life style is multifaceted:

(1) The child and his family live with the constant uncertainty of the prognosis. Frequently, parents admit that this uncertainty of the future is the hardest aspect to bear. Children, too, are aware of their condition, and can fear death, separation, or pain because of their illness.

(2) Another constant source of anxiety is because of the chronicity of the illness. The whole family is usually caught up in living with this chronic condition, including siblings who may live in the shadow of the sick child. Normal development can be affected because the normal progression of dependency to independency is blocked by the parents' over-protectiveness and the child's security in continued dependency.

(3) Often some aspect of the heart disease necessitates partial isolation of the child from his peers, further affecting his social development. Cyanotic spells may severely limit activity levels and the risk of infection can present dangers to the already weak child.

(4) Financial burdens are also problems, even with help from federally funded programs such as Crippled Children's Services, because there are other expenses such as in time, travel, and energy. REF. Roberts FB.: The Child with Heart Disease. American Journal of Nursing 72:6, 1080-1084, June 1972.

197. Q. How can nurses effectively work with a child and his family when the diagnosis is heart disease?

A. Three aspects seem essential in the comprehensive care needed by these children. The first is a team approach of doctor, staff nurse, visiting nurse, school teacher, social worker and other personnel who are integrally involved. This team needs to communicate among themselves so that parents and child receive one message. Medical jargon is so diverse that one simple word can have several large technical synonyms. Care in the hospital and at home needs to be planned with the team, the child if old enough, and the parents so that each is working toward a mutual goal.

Secondly, the child can never be viewed alone, but must be seen as part of a family system. Often, the most important aspect of caring for the chronically ill child is working with his parents. Frequently, it is not possible to immediately advise, counsel, or teach parents because of their own anxiety and fears which block communication. Therefore, to be effective a nurse must first meet their needs before attempting to help the child. This is an aspect of care that can be taken too narrowly. For example, parents have their own social needs, their need to be loved by each other, and their need for time and intimacy alone. They may feel guilty about spending time and money for their own needs, but also need to understand that only when their emotional reserves are refilled can they give again.

The third major aspect of care is the child himself. The nurse needs to listen to him and to encourage him to express his feelings either verbally or nonverbally through play or drawings. It is clearly evident that all children at some age fear separation, mutilation, pain, anesthesia. How much more frightening for the sick, weak child who may also fear punishment as the reason for his illness.

REF. Roberts F.: The Child with Heart Disease. American Journal of Nursing 72:6, 1080-1084, June 1972.

198. Q. What are some of the special areas nurses should consider when caring for a child with heart disease?

A. Several factors need to be considered when caring for a child with heart disease: the child's age, his specific diagnosis, changes in life style because of the diagnosis, and parents' understanding of the illness. Depending on this assessment, several problem areas can be identified:

(1) Restriction of physical activity can often be necessary when the defect is cyanotic type. This immobility causes special problems for the toddler who is exploring and conquering his universe by mastering motor skills. For the older child, restricted activity may mean loss of peer group contact, and a feeling of "losing out on living". Besides immobility, cyanotic heart disease and other disorders such as rheumatic heart disease can cause physical abnormalities that affect a child's body image. For example, the latter disorder can cause obesity and moon face from taking steroids. For an adolescent female, this might be much more of a crisis than the actual disease itself.

(2) Besides hospitalizations, a child must also face each day at home. Here, the emphasis should be on normalcy, not sickness. One of the greatest problems parents face is discipline. They are often ambivalent about limit setting because of their own guilt feelings toward the child, yet become so angry and frustrated by the child's insatiable demands, that they realize discipline is essential. Prevention is the key to this vicious cycle that can plague a family. When the diagnosis is made, parents need anticipatory guidance about growth, development, and discipline. One good approach is the use of behavior-modification theory.

(3) Diet can become a grave concern to mothers, especially when the child is an infant. Feeding-gratification-mothering are so closely entwined that mothers often need help to maintain a positive image of themselves. Infants with cardiac problems frequently suck and feed poorly, because of easy tiring. They may wake up dissatisfied, yet still be too weak to feed enough to gain weight. Periodic evaluations of the mother's progress is essential since trying to please her infant may be fruitless yet exhausting.

(4) Many children with heart defects severe enough to warrant the above problems also need medication at home. One of the drugs frequently prescribed is digoxin, which can be potentially toxic. Parents need excellent teaching and supervision while the child is in the hospital. In rheumatic heart disease, penicillin is taken long after the child appears well. Parents need to understand the reason

for prolonged therapy. Whenever possible, the child should be encouraged to take his own drugs, not only to increase his feeling of responsibility, but also his feeling of control, when so frequently limitations are placed upon him.

REF. Roberts F.: The Child with Heart Disease. American Journal of Nursing 72:6, 1080-1084, June 1972.

199. Q. How does a child describe his heart?

A. Children have different conceptions of what the heart is and does according to their ages and various past experiences. For example, very young children about four and five years of age have usually heard the word "heart", know that it is located in the chest or back, and think it looks like a valentine shape. Until about the age of seven, they characterize it by its sound-tick tock, a drum or a pump.

Children between the ages of seven and ten had a better concept of the heart, knowing that it wasn't valentine-shaped and that it had veins and was associated with pumping and blood. However, they often erroneously associated other functions to the heart, such as breathing. They usually described the heart as "it makes you live" or you need it "to stay alive", associating life and death with the heart.

At about the age of 10 or 11, the children seemed to have a much more logical and scientific concept of its function. They described its pumping action in terms of veins, valves, and circulation, and were aware that death occurred if the heart stopped. Although why death occurred was still not well understood, the framework was complete for further comprehension.

REF. Reif K.: A Heart Makes You Live. American Journal of Nursing 72:6, 1085, June 1972.

200. Q. What is the incidence of ventricular septal defects in children?

A. Ventricular septal defects are the most common congenital heart lesions. They are responsible for 30-40% of all congenital heart disease at birth. Congenital heart disease occurs in about 1% of all live births in the U.S. Each year there are about 40,000 children born with congenital heart defects and about 12-16,000 of these children have ventricular septal defects. Ventricular septal defects may appear with other cardiac lesions or form an integral part of some complex lesion such as tetralogy of Fallot. Other lesions associated with ventricular septal defect include patent ductus arteriosus, atrial septal defect, coarctation of the aorta and transposition of the great vessels. If all of these are considered, then as many as 50% of all liveborn children with congenital heart disease have ventricular septal defect.

REF. Hoffman JIE.: Ventricular Septal Defect: Indications for therapy in infants. Pediatric Clinics of North America 18:4, 1091-1107, 1971.

201. Q. What are the symptoms of ventricular septal defect?

A. Initial symptoms are likely to be rapid breathing, easy and excessive sweating both of which may increase after feeding. Weight gain is low and is usually below the third percentile, while height may be in the tenth to twenty-fifth percentile. If the VSD is small the only abnormality may be a systolic murmur, grade 3-4. The heart is not enlarged and no other heart sounds are abnormal. In a big defect pulmonary hypertension is present causing an exaggerated pulsation along the left sternal border and an unusually loud pulmonic component to the second heart sound. If there is a large left to right shunt, the heart will be enlarged, both ventricles hyperactive, pulmonary hypertension will be present as well as a mid-diastolic murmur. Since these children with congestive heart failure are tachypneic, have rales and show intercostal and subcostal retractions, the diagnosis may be hard to separate from lung infection. If in doubt, the child should be treated for both diseases, since the most common reason for a child with heart disease developing CHF is pulmonary infection. EKG does not help to diagnose the nature of a congenital heart lesion, but once ventricular septal defect is diagnosed, it may help to indicate severity.
REF. Hoffman JIE.: Ventricular Septal Defect: Indications for therapy in infants. Pediatric Clinics of North America 18:4, 1091-1107, 1971.

202. Q. How soon are symptoms of ventricular septal defect apparent?

A. Infants with small ventricular septal defects have no symptoms. However, the infant who is asymptomatic should be seen frequently for at least the first 6 months since large defects may produce no symptoms for several months. If the ventricular septal defect is large, the child may be well for the first few months and then develop symptoms, or he may have symptoms which gradually increase from the first few weeks after birth. The difference in the appearance of symptoms may be due to the rate at which pulmonary resistance falls and the large left to right shunt forms. Congestive heart failure is rare under the age of 2 months in an infant with simple ventricular septal defect. The presence of congestive heart failure at this early age should be viewed as an alert to the likelihood of other associated heart lesions, anemia or severe infection.
REF. Hoffman JIE.: Ventricular Septal Defect: Indications for therapy in infants. Pediatric Clinics of North America 18:4, 1091-1107, 1971.

203. Q. What is the prognosis in ventricular septal defect?

A. Death in infancy from VSD is uncommon, especially under 2 months of age, although neonatal deaths may occur at a higher rate among premature infants. Infants with big ventricular septal defects have 2 major possible prognoses (1) spontaneous closure of the

defect, and (2) the development of pulmonary vascular disease. The total incidence of spontaneous closure is estimated between 25-50% of all ventricular septal defects in childhood. Complete closure occurs most commonly in small defects in 50-80% of the cases, and less commonly in 5-10% of severe defects. Sixty percent of those defects which are going to close in childhood, close by age 3 years and 90% by age 8 years. Even though complete closure is uncommon in larger ventricular septal defects, partial closure is quite common and may occur in about 50% of them. If both complete and partial closure are taken into consideration, 75-80% of children with VSD have a good prognosis. The greatest danger from septal defect lies in the development of pulmonary vascular disease and a premium is put on the early detection and treatment of children who are at risk of developing this complication. Surgical treatment involves either banding of the pulmonary artery or direct closure of the ventricular septal defect. The type of procedure depends on the age and size of the child. Open heart surgery in sick infants under 6 months has a mortality rate of 20%, whereas, banding has a rate of 6%.
REF. Hoffman JIE.: Ventricular Septal Defect: Indications for therapy in infants. Pediatric Clinics of North America 18:4, 1091-1107, 1971.

204. Q. What is transposition of the great arteries?

A. Transposition of the great arteries is a congenital heart defect in which unsaturated systemic venous blood is delivered via what is usually called the right ventricle into the aorta, and saturated pulmonary venous blood is delivered via what is usually called the left ventricle to the pulmonary artery. This defect may occur alone or in conjunction with other defects such as, ventricular septal defect, patent ductus arteriosus, and subvalvular pulmonic stenosis.
REF. Rashkind, WJ, M.D.: Transposition of the Great Arteries. Pediatric Clinics of North America 18:4, 1075-1090, 1971.

205. Q. Can children with transposition of the great arteries survive?

A. Until recently transposition of the great arteries was always a fatal lesion. It is now considered curable with proper medical and surgical management. Early detection is paramount, followed by careful regulation of body temperature, maintaining acid-base balance and the use of oxygen and anticongestive measures. Emergency cardiac catheterization with the use of balloon atrioseptostomy to open the atrial septum may be performed. The child is followed until the ideal time for corrective surgery, usually about 2 years of age. Current advances indicate that this surgery may be performed in the latter half of the first year of life, permitting these children to lead a normal life, free of cyanotic heart disease.
REF. Rashkind WJ, M.D.: Transposition of the Great Arteries. Pediatric Clinics of North America 18:4, 1075-1090, 1971.

206. Q. What is the postcardiotomy syndrome?

A. Postcardiotomy syndrome was first seen in patients following mitral valvotomy and it is now known that it may occur after any surgical procedure in which the pericardium is opened. The syndrome is characterized by fever, chest pain, pericarditis, pleural effusion and arthralgia. It usually occurs 1-8 weeks after cardiac surgery or pericardial injury and may occur as late as 4-6 months past surgery. Treatment with therapeutic doses of aspirin alleviates symptoms in 24-72 hours with continuation of therapy for 7-10 days. More severely ill patients may require corticosteroid therapy.
REF. Benzing G III, M.D., Kaplan S, M.D.: Late Complications of Cardiac Surgery. Pediatric Clinics of North America 18:4, 1225-1242, 1971.

207. Q. How can a nurse help prepare a child for cardiac catheterization?

A. Although cardiac catheterization is not a very painful procedure, it is long and tiresome, and the equipment used can be frightening to a child. Preparation for this procedure can be a two stage affair: precatheterization teaching and postcatheterization follow-up and evaluation. It is usually done with the child and his parent. In the precatheterization visit, the nurse should concentrate on describing the known facts that will happen to the child, leaving out details that can vary, such as the effect of the dye on the system. Puppets, dolls, or equipment such as masks can be used depending on the child's age and developmental level. In postcatheterization, the child is asked to describe how the test felt. Some of the important events and facts to tell the children include:

(1) The preparation for the test: "NPO" and what that means, the "I don't care shot" before he leaves the room, the bath with special soap, and the ride to the heart room on a stretcher with a man or woman dressed in a green gown. The child needs to know that his parents are usually not allowed past the elevator, but that they will wait for him.

(2) The test itself: how long it will take, what the room looks like, the big machines (X-ray) that take pictures, the special sounds, the people who wear masks and hats, the table with restraints, the EKG leads, the preparation of the site (usually the groin in a child) with a cold, brown soap, and a last shot in the leg so that there won't be any pain. Because children fear pain, mutilation, or intrusive procedures, the nurse should demonstrate the pushing on the leg that the doctor will do.

(3) Post-procedural care: bandage on his leg, bedrest for the rest of the day, and meals as usual.
REF. Tesler M, Hardgrove C.: Cardiac Catheterization: Preparing the child. American Journal of Nursing 13:1, 80-81, Jan. 1973.

208. Q. What are some behavioral characteristics of newborns with cardiac stress?

A. The investigator of this study found that abnormal behavior wasn't always related directly to cardiac malfunction but to illness as a general phenomenon. The behavior patterns fell into seven general categories:

(1) Respiratory status - Almost 90% of the infants demonstrated abnormal breathing such as tachypnea (sleeping respiratory rate over 60), mild to moderate intercostal and subcostal retractions, and hyperventilation (irregular rate of 100-120, which was a poor sign).
(2) Feeding behavior - The most common difficulty was incoordinated sucking, swallowing and breathing. Severe dyspnea while feeding sometimes necessitated gavage feeding in order to conserve energy and prevent aspiration.
(3) Activity level - Some of the babies were continuously restless even during sleep, while others were lethargic. While awake, neither group of infants seemed to show normal interest in their environment.
(4) The majority of the babies had generalized cyanosis, which fluctuated with positioning, usually worsening when supine. Although oxygen helped respiratory distress, it did little in improving color of skin.
(5) Muscle tone - Hypotonia seemed to increase with hypoxia. One of the first signs of lost muscle tone was loss of arm movement during feeding.
(6) Heart rate - Most babies had a cardiac rate between 140 and 160 while sleeping. As distress became most severe, the heart rate dropped.
(7) Cry - In general, the cry was frail and breathless, rather than lusty as in healthy babies. Lack of movement of the extremities during crying usually meant severe distress.
REF. Gillon J.: Behavior of Newborns with Cardiac Distress. American Journal of Nursing 73:2, 254-257, Feb. 1973.

209. Q. What is the etiology of cardiac failure in infants?

A. Infants under 1 year of age account for 90% of the pediatric patients who develop heart failure. The majority of these children have congenital heart defects. The congenital heart defects most commonly associated with heart failure are transportation of the great vessels, coarctation of the aorta, ventricular septal defect, aortic atresia, endocardial fibroelastosis, atrioventricularis cummunis, total anomalous venous return from the pulmonary vessels, single ventricle and patent ductus arteriosus. Atrial septal defects and tetralogy of Fallot, although relatively common defects, are seldom associated with congestive heart failure.
REF. Goldring D, et al.: The Critically Ill Child: Care of the infant in cardiac failure. Pediatrics 47:6, 1056-1063, 1971.

210. Q. What is the pathophysiology of cardiac failure in infants?

A. Most cardiologists would agree that heart failure may be simply defined as the inability of the heart to pump blood in accordance with body needs. Cardiac failure may result from a primary abnormality in the heart muscle or may be secondary to a structural defect such as stenotic valves. When the right ventricle fails it cannot eject as much blood as normally and the output is diminished while the residual volume is increased. The end diastolic pressure rises and there is a corresponding rise in the right atrial and venous pressure. Likewise when the left ventricular chamber fails there is an increase in the end diastolic pressure of that chamber as well as of the left atrium and the pulmonary veins. In most instances, right sided failure results from and is associated with left sided failure. In an effort to preserve cardiac output and to accomodate the large volume of residual blood in the chambers, there is cardiac dilatation. The more the heart is filled with residual blood in diastole, the greater the force of the following contraction. This principle operates until the myocardial fiber has reached its maximum length and no further cardiac dilatation is possible. The elevation of pressures, the disturbances in blood flow and the abnormal distribution of water and electrolytes which accompany and characterize heart failure, may be regarded as homeostatic mechanisms in which the body attempts to preserve cardiac output.
REF. Goldring D, et al.: The Critically Ill Child: Care of the Infant in Cardiac Failure. Pediatrics 47:6, 1056-1063, 1971.

211. Q. What are the signs and symptoms of congestive heart failure in the infant?

A. In the infant with congestive heart failure (combined right and left ventricular failure), the most common signs and symptoms are tachypnea, tachycardia, cardiomegaly, hepatomegaly, pulmonary rales and rhonchi, feeding difficulties, growth failure and cyanosis. Some less common symptoms are peripheral edema, ascites and gallop rhythm.
REF. Goldring D, et al.: The Critically Ill Child: Care of the Infant in Cardiac Failure. Pediatrics 47:6, 1056-1063, 1971.

212. Q. What is the prognosis for infants with congestive heart failure?

A. Mortality rates in children with cardiac failure range from 50-85%, partly because a significant number of these children have inoperable cardiac lesions. The range of palliative and corrective surgery is however, ever increasing. If a baby is to be saved by cardiac surgery, every effort must be made to diagnose and treat medically the heart failure. Medical treatment includes the use of monitoring, digoxin, oxygen and parenteral fluids. It is recommended that treatment and cardiac studies be done at medical centers with well equipped and well staffed intensive care units.

REF. Goldring D, et al.: The Critically Ill Child: Care of the Infant in Cardiac Failure. Pediatrics 47:6, 1056-1063, 1971.

213. Q. What is cor pulmonale and does it affect children?

A. Cor pulmonale, also known as pulmonary heart disease, is defined as right ventricular hypertrophy secondary to disease of the lung parenchyma or pulmonary vasculature, or resulting from abnormalities in pulmonary function. Pulmonary hypertension is basic to cor pulmonale and is responsible for the development of right ventricular hypertrophy. Although fibrocystic disease is the most common cause of cor pulmonale in children, a number of other conditions such as upper airway obstruction, neuromuscular diseases, deformities of the thoracic cage, respiratory center dysfunction, high altitude, pulmonary hypertension and thromboembolism may be causative factors.
REF. Noonan J, M.D.: Pulmonary Heart Disease. Pediatric Clinics of North America 18:4, 1255-1272, 1971.

214. Q. What nursing implications arise when a patient is on digitalis?

A. Digitalis is a widely used medication in treatment of heart disease in children and adults. A therapeutic and potentially toxic drug, digitalis has two main effects: it increases the force of contractions (positive inotropic) and it decreases the rate of contractions (negative chronotropic). Its therapeutic benefits include increased cardiac output, decreased venous pressure, decreased heart size, relief of edema, reversal of arrhythmias to normal sinus rhythm. It also has a diuretic effect by enhancing renal perfusion and by inhibiting sodium reabsorption.

Digoxin and digitoxin are the most commonly used digitalis preparations. Although their cardiac effects are the same, their speed, duration, and side effects differ. Digoxin (Lanoxin) is fast-acting (5 to 30 minutes), has a short half-life of one and a half days, and is excreted mainly by the kidneys. Digitoxin is slower acting (26 to 120 minutes), has a long half-life of 5 to 7 days, and is excreted by the liver.

There are many toxic effects of digitalis which should be well known by nurses who may be the first to detect them. Early symptoms include anorexia, nausea, and vomiting. Visual disturbances such as difficulty reading, seeing hazy or shimmering visions or halos around dark objects, blind spots or color distortions usually come later. Neurological symptoms such as headache, drowsiness, insomnia, vertigo, confusion or delirium can be present, along with fatigue and muscle weakness. Toxic cardiac effects include arrhythmias such as premature ventricular contractions and altered heart rate, especially a slowed rate.

When nurses administer this drug, they should always be mindful of its therapeutic effects so that they can evaluate the patient's response to its toxic effects. They must help patients and parents understand these side effects, and alert them to signs which call for reevaluation of the treatment regime. They need to be taught how to take their pulse, and at what range the drug should be withheld. They should take no other medication with digitalis except with the physician's knowledge. Correct dosage and correct time is essential, so that written schedules and instructions should be included.
REF. Winslow E.: Digitalis. American Journal of Nursing 74:6, 1062-1065, June 1974.

215. Q. Lo parents understand the risk factors involved in recurrence of congenital heart disease?

A. The authors attempted to ascertain the knowledge parents had about the specific heart defect and the recurrence risk involved. They interviewed 39 families whose child had one of three common congenital heart lesions (ventricular septal defect, atrial septal defect, or tetralogy of Fallot) and asked the following questions:

1. What is your understanding of your child's heart condition?
2. Do you know the name of your child's heart condition?
3. Have you thought, "Why this child?"
4. What do you know about the chances of this same condition occurring in a subsequent child of yours?
5. Do you plan to have more children?; or if more appropriate, why have you had no more children?

Results indicated that none of the parents were aware of the recurrence risk of their child's defect. (Nora and associates cite 4-5% recurrence risk for ventricular septal defect, and 3% for atrial septal defect or tetralogy of Fallot.) Less than half (15 of 39) knew the name of the defect. Only 13 knew enough about the disorder to describe it. Three families indicated their decision to have no additional children. Four months later, after the initial interview when correct information had been supplied, 9 of the 35 families (4 families were not reinterviewed) knew the potential mathematical risk and half of them could name their child's condition. This low percentage of recall appears to indicate that parents need more extensive counseling, which is repeated several times to insure that the parents understand the correct facts.
REF. Reiss J, Menashe V.: Genetic Counseling and Congenital Heart Disease. Journal of Pediatrics 80:4, 655-656, April 1972.

216. Q. How can a nurse best assess the relationship between neonatal cyanosis and arterial oxygen saturation (AOS)?

A. The authors of this study attempted to determine the relationship of clinical assessment of cyanosis (color of skin and mucous membranes of neonates) and arterial oxygen saturation. For each clinical assessment, observations were made of the infant's lips, ears, trunk, nailbed, hands, and region around the mouth for signs of cyanosis. Immediately following the clinical observations, arterial blood gas samples were taken.

The results showed that the trunk and ears had few false positive observations but many false negatives. The hands, nailbeds and circumoral area had many false positive observations (that is, cyanosis with an AOS greater than 90%) but few false negatives (cyanosis with AOS less than 80%). Over-all the lips or tongue were the most reliable sites studied.

According to the results, the only certain correlation that can be made is that acyanosis of the hands and circumoral region indicates an AOS above 80%, necessitating no additional oxygen. From this, it seems that nurses and physicians need to use both clinical assessment and arterial blood gas determination to effectively evaluate the blood oxygenation.

REF. Goldman H, et al.: Neonatal Cyanosis and Arterial Oxygen Saturation. Journal of Pediatrics 82:2, 319-324, Feb. 1973.

217. Q. Can primary endocardial fibroelastosis be inherited?

A. The condition is defined as a congenital condition of unknown etiology and can best be diagnosed at autopsy. These findings show the endocardium as smooth, porcelain-like, and greatly thickened with proliferation of elastic and fibrous tissue and these changes frequently extend to involve the valves - particularly the mitral and aortic. The papillary muscles and chordae tendineae are enlarged. The left atrium and left ventricle are most frequently affected. Myocardial hypertrophy or dilatation are usually present.

The history of 4 families each with more than one child affected by primary endocardial fibroelastosis was reviewed. The diagnosis was made at autopsies in 8 out of the 9 children. On the basis of these families and a review of reported familial incidence in the literature, it is suggested that this condition may be a dominant autosomal trait rather than a recessive autosomal as previously suggested.

REF. Hunter AS, Keay AJ.: Primary Endocardial Fibroelastosis. Archives of Disease in Childhood 48:1, 66-69, 1973.

218. Q. What are the cardiovascular responses to postural changes in the neonate?

A. In the newborn infant, passive head-up tilting has been shown to result in an increase in the heart rate. A small rise in systolic blood pressure, measured clinically, has been described in babies who were resting but awake at the time of investigation. Direct measurements of aortic blood pressure have shown an initial increase followed by a fall in both systolic and diastolic pressure. A rise in pulse rate of 15-40 beats per minute on tilting from the supine to the upright position in resting but awake newborns. In the sleeping newborn, the same tilting procedure gave a 10-20 beats per minute lower rate.

The relation found between respiratory slowing and heart rate may be explained by alterations in the efficiency of the "abdomino-thoracic" pump. Slower breaths in the upright position may be associated with larger intrathoracic pressure swings helping to augment venous return, thus masking or reducing cardiac acceleration on tilting. In the adult there is either no change or a slight increase in respiratory rate on tilting.

The reduction in forearm blood flow on tilting was comparable to the adult in whom a fall of 40% occurs. Systolic blood pressure fell a little, while most resting adults, despite a fall in cardiac output, experienced no change in blood pressure when tilted. Difference may have been in some way related to the fact that the babies were deeply asleep. Their vasoconstrictor response was none the less as active as in the adult. So, vasomotor inactivity or "immaturity" is unlikely to be the explanation for the slightly lower systolic blood pressure in the upright position. Perhaps the demands of cerebral blood flow in the infant are so great that pronounced vasoconstriction elsewhere does not compensate for the fall in cardiac output.

The responses of the newborn circulatory system to tilting were the same in the first three days as later. They were comparable to the adult from the earliest age. These observations provide good evidence of a well-developed control of peripheral circulation from birth.
REF. Picton-Warlow CG, Mayer FE.: Cardiovascular Responses to Postural Changes in the Neonate. Archives of Disease in Childhood 45:241, 354-359, 1970.

219. Q. How frequent is the problem of hypertension among children?

A. One to two percent of children and adolescents have high blood pressure, while 10-20% of adults have hypertension. Systemic hypertension is not uncommon in the pediatric population and blood pressure should be measured routinely as part of the physical exam in children of all ages. This may require some time with young children and the application of a proper sized cuff is important. The cuff should cover roughly two-thirds of the upper arm. Little interest has been shown in hypertension in children until recently and yet essential hypertension may have its etiology in the pediatric population.
REF. Loggie J, M.D., B.Ch.: Systemic Hypertension in Children and Adolescents. Pediatric Clinics of North America 18:4, 1273-1307, 1971.

220. Q. How can a nurse recognize some common skin infections in school age children?

A. The nurse practitioner, in trying to identify and diagnose common skin disorders in children needs to follow certain guidelines in her history and physical. For example, a complete history should include: how did the rash start, when, where and how has it been treated; are there drug allergies, photosensitivity, or history of hay fever, eczema, asthma, or any genetic disorder; has there been any change in living habits or environment? Physical findings should include a detailed cutaneous examination of the entire body, done in good light, using a magnifying glass and a Wood's lamp. The primary lesion should be identified, and described according to location on the body, distribution and arrangement of lesions, and presence of any secondary changes such as scaling, ulceration, pigmentation, or excoriation. Some common skin infections found in children include:

(1) Tinea capitis is a reddened, round, or oval-shaped scaling patch of alopecia. The noninflammatory form can be passed from person to person. Identification is by Wood's light (green fluorescence), and by microscopic examination and culture of hair and scales. The prognosis of this fungal infection is good. However, family members should also be checked so that treatment can be begun on them also.

(2) Body ringworm, tinea corporis and tinea cruris, begin with a reddened papule, followed by scales and vesicles with peripheral spreading and central clearing. The most common sites include the trunk, neck and hands. Tinea cruris, or "jock itch", is frequently seen in boys and men. It is easy to recognize because of scaling, pruritis and inflammation of intertrigenous areas of the thighs, examination and culture. Prognosis is good with treatment of griseofulvin.

(3) Tinea pedis, ringworm of the feet, is a scaly maceration and fissuring of the skin between the toes, particularly the fourth web space, and can extend to the soles of the feet as a patchy red eruption with deep seated vesicles. Identification is by culturing skin scrapings, and prognosis is good although it can become a benign chronic condition.

(4) Tinea unguium, ringworm of the nails, is usually secondary to tinea pedis, as the toenails are more often involved than the fingernails. There is a thickening and scaling under the nail plate, as well as lateral nail fold involvement. Diagnosis is made by microscopic examination of part of the infected nail and by culturing. Prognosis is poor for toenail involvement.

(5) Impetigo contagiosa is a highly contagious pruritic disorder, characterized by a papular, vesicular lesion most commonly found on the face and nares. The skin lesions are probably caused by certain strains of group A streptococcus, which may precede a glomerulonephritis. Diagnosis is aimed at isolating the bacteria

through a culture of the lesion and the throat. Treatment is prompt antibiotic therapy of patient and family members who are at risk.

(6) Scabies is an intensely pruritic contagious dermatosis character-ized by papules, vesicles and crusts between the fingers, on the heel of the palms, axillary and the buttock folds, male genitalia, and fe-male breasts but seldom on the face. It is caused by the female sar-coptes scabiei, which lays her eggs in linear burrows under the skin. Diagnosis is established by the presence of the female mite, her ova, and feces in the skin. Treatment is good with a scabicide such as Kwell (benzene hexachloride), and treatment of all family members to prevent reinfection.
REF. Rice A.: Common Skin Infections in School Children. Ameri-can Journal of Nursing 73:11, 1905-1909, Nov. 1973.

221. Q. What is toxic erythema of the newborn?

A. Toxic erythema of the newborn is also termed erythema toxicum neonatorum or flea bite dermatites. It is a benign self-limiting dermatites, occurring in the first week of life. The lesions first appear as blotchy macular erythema and within the area of erythema, one or more white papulo-vesicles or pustules may ap-pear. The lesion can be distinguished from infectious lesions of the neonate by taking a smear of the pustule infiltrate. Eosinophils are the predominant cell present in these smears. The sites most com-monly involved are the buttocks, trunk, face and proximal extremi-ties. The lesions of erythema toxicum almost always appear in the second 24 hours of life and are rarely present at birth. No treat-ment is required.
REF. Hodgman J, M.D., et al.: Neonatal Dermatology. Pediatric Clinics of North America 18:3, 713-756, 1971.

222. Q. What is atopic dermatitis?

A. Atopic dermatitis is one of the most common dermatologic-al problems of childhood and is one of the 10 most frequent skin con-ditions in the under 25 age group. The child is born with easily ir-ritated skin and suffers from pruritis and a tendency to develop der-matitis. The dermatitis is a persistent superficial inflammation which varies in duration and degree from patient to patient. Atopic dermatitis commonly begins in the first few months of life and usu-ally clears spontaneously by 2 years of age leaving unscarred skin. In most cases, treatment minimizes the problem greatly. Infants with atopic dermatitis frequently develop asthma in childhood and hay fever as adults, as the most common sequence of events.
REF. Norins A, M.D.: Atopic Dermatitis. Pediatric Clinics of North America 18:3, 801-837, 1971.

223. Q. What types of dermatologic lesions can occur due to birth trauma?

A. Some degree of trauma to the presenting part occurs in every vaginal delivery. The term Caput Succedaneum is applied to edema of the presenting part. This may occur in vertex and breech deliveries. Although the edema may cause a grotesque appearance, they resolve spontaneously in 24-48 hours. Intrauterine sucking blisters may appear on the hands of normal full term infants. They are differentiated from other bullous lesions of the newborn by their rapid resolution and failure to cause new lesions after birth. Pressure necrosis may be the most difficult to diagnose correctly at birth. These may be seen on one or both parietal lobes, in first-born term infants. When the infant is born, the overlying dermis appears normal, but within hours the affected area becomes red and swollen. A sterile abcess forms and drains with a resulting ulcer which exhibits undermined borders and is slow to heal. Antibiotics are not indicated in the treatment of pressure necrosis.
REF. Hodgeman J, M.D., et al.: Neonatal Dermatology. Pediatric Clinics of North America 18:3, 713-756, 1971.

224. Q. What is a "collodian baby"?

A. The collodian baby is a form of icthyosis congenita. These disorders are characterized by cutaneous scaling. The collodian baby may be a phenotypic expression of inheritance by X-linked dominant or recessive genes. The infant is born covered with a taut membrane that resembles collodian. The tightness of the membrane may cause temporary extropion, fish mouth, a claw-like appearance of the hands and immobility of the baby. Within 24 hours desquamation begins. As desquamation occurs, the infant's condition improves rapidly. These infants usually survive, but may show persistent signs of icthyosis. Infants who recover completely represent the so called collodian skin, which may be present in dysmature syndrome.
REF. Hodgeman J, M.D., et al.: Neonatal Dermatology. Pediatric Clinics of North America 18:3, 713-756, 1971.

225. Q. What is the cause of sore bottoms in the newborn?

A. The occurrence of a sore bottom is relatively common during the first 14 days of life. Sore bottom is defined as an area of erythema surrounding the anal region.

Factors which might influence a baby's susceptibility to this condition are: sex, skin and hair coloring, whether breast or bottle fed and birth weight.

Conclusion reached was that "fair" (blonde or red hair with white skin) babies seemed more prone to develop a sore bottom than "dark" (dark or brown hair and white skin).

Second significant factor was that bottle fed babies rather than breast fed babies developed sore bottoms. The breast feeding mothers might have given better "mothering care" to their babies but this is debatable.

A control group showed lower incidence of the condition due to change in type of feeding. Nurses spent more time with mothers on how to care for the babies. An improved diaper was used. Male babies fared no worse than female babies. Birth weight was not contributory.
REF. Grantham E.: Sore Bottoms in the Newborn. Archives of Disease in Childhood 48:7, 568-570, 1973.

226. Q. What are some causes of urinary tract infection in children?

A. Urinary tract infection is a general term which can be classified according to the anatomic location such as urethritis, cystitis, ureteritis, pyelitis, and pyelonephritis. This condition, which occurs frequently among children, is about 10 to 30 times more prevalent among females than males after one month of age. Several anatomic factors account for this. The longer male urethra and the antibacterial properties of prostatic secretion inhibit entry and growth of bacteria. In females, the short urethra and the close proximity of the urinary meatus to the anus favors the entry and presence of bacteria. The blood stream may also be a source of infection, such as from sepsis. Adjacent organs can be reservoirs of infection, such as the male prostate and the female para-urethral gland. An anatomic abnormality which favors the growth of bacteria is vesicoureteral reflux. Incomplete bladder emptying and stasis of urine in the bladder favor conditions for bacterial growth.
REF. Khan A, Pryles C.: Urinary Tract Infection in Children. American Journal of Nursing 73:8, 1340-1343, Aug. 1973.

227. Q. How should urinary tract infections in children be managed?

A. When a urinary tract infection has been detected, a urine culture should be taken and appropriate antibiotic therapy instituted. An intravenous urogram is recommended to detect the presence of upper urinary tract obstruction or other serious renal disorders. Most investigators feel that after an initial urinary tract infection in the male and an initial or secondary infection in the female, a complete investigation of the urinary tract should be made. A voiding cystourethrogram should be performed 6 weeks after the infection has subsided in order to detect reflux. Reflux due to infection will have subsided by this time in two thirds of the children. An abnormal voiding cystourethrogram is an indication for cystoscopy. If cystoscopy is abnormal, surgical correction of ureteral orifices may be indicated.
REF. Burke H, M.D., Rhamy R, M.D.: Lower Urinary Tract Problems Related to Infection: Diagnosis and Treatment. Pediatric Clinics of North America 17:2, 233-253, 1970.

228. Q. What is correct cleaning procedure for clean-catch urine specimens?

A. Proper technique for obtaining clean-catch urine specimens for identification of bacteria has always been a problem, since perineal contamination can significantly alter results. The authors of this study attempted to evaluate a cleansing procedure presently widely used to prepare the infant for this test. They cleansed the genitals of male and female low birth weight infants using a 3% hexachlorophene solution, and rinsed with tap water. In males, the preputial sac was then irrigated gently with 10 ml. of sterile saline. In females, the tip of the syringe was placed above the clitoris and the interlabial area was irrigated twice with 10 ml. of sterile saline. The area was then dried with sterile gauze and swabbed with 1:500 tincture of benzalkonium chloride. A plastic collection bag was then applied. If the voided specimen showed a colony count of 100,000 or more, a suprapubic aspiration was done.

To detect if the cleansing procedure altered the results, a dye was substituted for the saline as the irrigant of the preputial sac or vulva. Radiography showed dye present in the bladder of the males, but not of the females. When the cleansing procedure was changed, no reflux of dye was present.

These authors feel that the preputial sac should not be irrigated with a syringe, but rinsed by gently pouring the water over the penis, because pressure from the syringe can cause introduction of bacteria into the bladder.
REF. Thrupp L, et al.: Transurethral Reflux During Cleansing Procedure for Clean-Voided Urine Specimens in Low-Birth Weight Infants. Journal of Pediatrics 82:6, 1057-1059, June 1973.

229. Q. How is the nephrotic syndrome defined and classified?

A. The nephrotic syndrome, sometimes termed nephrosis, may be defined as a clinical entity in which gross proteinuria of high but varying selectivity is always present together with consequential selective hypoproteinemia. Edema, ascites, hypovolemia and hyperlipidemia are usually present. Systemic hypertension, erythrocyturia, azotemia and hypocomplementemia are seen occasionally. Nephrotic syndrome may be divided into 3 groups, as follows:

1. Congenital Nephrotic Syndrome - this is a lethal form of the disease due to autosomal recessive inheritance and is usually resistant to all forms of therapy.
2. Secondary Nephrotic Syndrome - in this group a primary cause is known or presumed to be known. The causes are malaria or other parasitic disease, collagen diseases e.g. lupus, disease following acute glomerulonephritis, toxic nephropathy due to heavy metals or drugs and diverse rare causes such as amyloidosis, renal thrombosis and sickle cell disease.

3. Idiopathic Nephrotic Syndrome - most cases of the disease fall into this category of unknown etiology. Insidious edema and proteinuria are the rule. Idiopathic nephrosis must not be considered as a single disease, but probably has several causes as well as several differing histological appearances.

REF. Arneil G, M.D., Ph.D.: The Nephrotic Syndrome. Pediatric Clinics of North America 18:2, 547-559, 1971.

230. Q. What is the treatment of nephrotic syndrome?

A. Treatment of children with nephrotic syndrome must cover at least 4 factors, namely general and dietetic management, diuretic therapy and corticosteroid therapy.

(1) General management involves the home supervision, schooling and psychological aspects of the illness. The child may have episodes of health intermittent with gross edema. During edematous episodes bed rest and comfort measures for edema are indicated.

(2) Dietetic management - edema cannot be removed by a low sodium diet, but it may be used to slow the rate of increase of edema. A high protein, sodium restricted diet is indicated when renal function is adequate.

(3) Diuretic therapy - the object of diuretic therapy is to overcome sodium and water retention. Optimal diuretic therapy for the majority of children is with adequate corticosteroids. Other diuretic therapy may be required when a viral infection exists or when steroids are contraindicated or gross steroid toxicity is present.

(4) Corticosteroid therapy - steroid therapy is used to hasten remission and prevent relapse, although the problems of steroid overdose and toxicity are always present. The International Cooperative Study of Kidney Disease in Children recommends oral prednisone in a dose of 60 mg per day per meter square for 28 days with a maximum daily dose of 80 mg. This is followed by 28 days of a dose of 40 mg per day per meter square for 3 days out of each 7, a maximum daily dose of 60 mg. Prednisone therapy is then stopped.

A 5 year study of nephrotic children shows that improvement in survival is related at least as much to the use of antibiotics as it is to the use of steroids. Elimination of death from acute infection with the use of antibiotics has greatly reduced the morbidity and mortality of nephrotic syndrome.

REF. Arneil G, M.D., Ph.D.: The Nephrotic Syndrome. Pediatric Clinics of North America 18:2, 547-559, 1971.

231. Q. Are pediatric patients good candidates for kidney transplants?

A. Some authors have expressed the opinion that children are prone to a more virulent form of rejection of renal homografts and are more susceptible to glomerulonephritis. In a study of 57 pedi-

atric renal transplants immunological control was found to be no
different in quality or quantity from adult patients. However, pediatric transplant patients may have special problems, such as surgical techniques required when transplanting adult size organs into a
small child. Also, proper electrolyte balance must be meticulously
maintained. After the immediate effects of transplant have been resolved, the problem skeletal deformities and failure to grow may be
major. Many growth and orthopedic problems are caused by preexisting uremia and the necessity of administering high doses of steroids for long periods post-operatively. Some patients experienced
emotional problems, but the authors feel that in spite of the special
physical and emotional problems pediatric transplant patients may
present, they should be considered prime candidates for renal transplant.

REF. Lilly JR, M.D., et al.: Renal Homotransplantation in Pediatric Patients. Pediatrics 47:3, 548-556, 1971.

232. Q. What are the psychological reactions of children and their
families to renal dialysis and kidney transplantation?

A. There are many emotional and social stresses on the child
with kidney disease and his parents. As kidney function deteriorates
to the point of renal failure there are depression and withdrawal responses from the child and parents. Families may not have time for
the resolution of grief because of the need for dramatic treatment.
Hemodialysis may represent renewed hope to both the patient and
family as the possibility of extended life is introduced. The possibility of kidney transplant is at first invested with hope and magic, although bilateral nephrectomy to prepare for transplantation may be
very hard for the child and the family. It implies a final negative
verdict about the child's own kidneys that parents may question to
be sure it is absolutely necessary. The child mourns the loss of
part of himself and the inability to urinate and complete dependence
on the dialysis machine. The transplant itself is a time of mixed
hope and doubt on the part of the parents. The child may be more
concerned with the more immediate anxieties and physical discom-
forts.

Some of the most severe emotional trials occur in the post transplant
period for the patient, the family and the staff. Surgical complications, rejection crises, infection and delay in onset or interruption
of urine production combine to torment the patient and staff. Parents tend to overprotect their children after transplant and fear injury or trauma to the new kidney. Children may feel that if they
try hard enough and are good enough their new kidney will function
longer. When a transplanted kidney is rejected and has to be removed and child is returned to dialysis the whole process of denial,
hope and doubt begins again.

REF. Korsch B, M.D., et al.: Experiences with Children and Their
Families During Extended Hemodialysis and Kidney Transplantation.
Pediatric Clinics of North America 18:2, 625-637, 1971.

233. Q. What are the long term psychological problems in children with exstrophy of the bladder?

A. This severe congenital anomaly, which affects both urinary and sexual functioning is being treated with new reconstructive urological techniques, designed to fit the requirements of each individual patient. However, substantial psychological support and guidance are needed in addition to surgical repairs. Many cases require urinary diversion with an ileal conduit or cutaneous ureterostomy, which change body image, as they necessitate a "bud" of everted mucous membrane on the abdomen. Penile size and functioning may also be affected. Work with patients and their families has shown that children who have exstrophy have many more psychologic problems, particularly during adolescence, than the average child.

The chief areas of conflict center around wetness and concern for sexual adequacy. Fears of inadequate penile size, ugliness of genitalia, inability to procreate and fear of being rejected by the opposite sex are paramount. An ongoing guidance team, which becomes acquainted with the patient and family at birth and extends its services into young adulthood, is felt to be an excellent method for providing guidance. Discussion groups to help parents and children ventilate their feelings and fantasies may aid in the resolution of some of their conflicts and allow for maximal growth.
REF. Feinberg T, et al.: Questions that Worry Children with Exstrophy. Pediatrics 53:2, 242-250, 1973.

234. Q. Is one operative procedure for urinary diversion in children better than another?

A. Diversion of the urinary stream plays an important role in the management of many congenital disorders of the urinary tract. Indications are urinary incontinence, severe damage to the drainage system from the kidneys, removing the lower urinary tract when it is the seat of malignant tumors.

There has been a high incidence of postoperative dilatation in normal urinary tracts to contraindicate ureteroileostomy to control urinary incontinence. Electrical sphincter pacemakers may help. Cutaneous ureterostomy has been used to prevent renal function deterioration. A pyeloileocutaneous diversion may produce more direct renal pelvis drainage. Intermittent stomal occlusion caused by diversion appliances, clothing, or body posture may be producing high pressure in the ileal conduit and will result in gradual upper and urinary tract dilatation.

The physiological characteristics of colonic motility as a urinary conduit instead of ileum appears more suitable. A length of colon becomes peristaltically inert.
REF. Scott JES.: Urinary Diversion in Children. Archives of Disease in Childhood 48:1, 199-206, 1973.

235. Q. What is reflux of the urinary bladder?

A. Vesicoureteral reflux is an abnormal condition in which urine from the bladder passes up into the ureter. The incidence of reflux in the general population is not known, but it has been found in 12-48% of children with urinary tract infections. The growing kidney is considerably more sensitive to infection than the adult kidney and the result of chronic or recurrent reflux of infected urine is the development of chronic pyelonephritis by route of ascending infection. In a series of patients with chronic reflux 12% developed an atrophic kidney. These changes usually started before the age of 5 and in most instances, prior to 2 years of age.
REF. Burko H, M.D., Rhamy R, M.D.: Lower Urinary Tract Problems Related to Infection: Diagnosis and Treatment. Pediatric Clinics of North America 17:2, 233-253, 1970.

236. Q. What is the cause of urinary reflux?

A. Several causes for reflux are known:

(1) The most common cause is lower urinary tract infection. The edema caused by bladder infection renders the ureterovesicular junction incompetent. Reflux disappears when infection subsides.
(2) Primary reflux of a congenital nature may be seen predominately in girls with thin walled bladder and congenitally deficient ureterovesicular junctions.
(3) Chronic obstruction causing bladder hypertrophy as in neurogenic bladder can produce reflux.
(4) Reflux may be neurogenic in origin following lumbar sympathectomy.
(5) Reflux may be iatrogenic following ureteral meatotomy and transurethral dissection.
REF. Burko H, M.D., Rhamy R, M.D.: Lower Urinary Tract Problems Related to Infection: Diagnosis and Treatment. Pediatric Clinics of North America 17:2, 233-253, 1970.

237. Q. What is the best age for surgical treatment of cryptorchidism (undescended testes)?

A. For multiple reasons cryptorchidism should be corrected by the fifth birthday. Many testes descend spontaneously during the first year. During the second year, the tissues are still very fragile and extensive dissection can be difficult. Also a factor is the anxiety experienced by the child when separated from his parents at this time. Hormone treatment in the form of human chorionic gonadotropin can be initiated at age four to help enlarge the scrotum or in cases of bilateral cryptorchidism. This treatment can be completed before the fifth birthday. The testes should be brought into the scrotum sometime before age five, or at the latest age six. If left in the abdomen longer, they may be damaged by body heat. Having both testes in the scrotum by this age may also prevent psychological problems related to body image.

REF. Lattimer J, et al.: The Optimum Time to Operate for Cryptorchidism. Pediatrics 53:1, 96-99, 1973.

238. Q. Should orchiopexy be done if the testes are not normal in size?

A. The undescended testes should be brought down into the scrotum despite the fact that it may often be inferior to its mate and that it is sometimes impossible to predict the adequacy of spermatic function. Undescended testes are usually regarded as worth saving because of their unimpaired capability of secreting testosterone, regardless of whether they produce sperm. Also, because of their increased propensity toward neoplastic changes, cryptorchid testes are better observed in the scrotal position.
REF. Lattimer J, et al.: The Optimum Time to Operate for Cryptorchidism. Pediatrics 53:1, 96-99, 1973.

239. Q. Are urinary problems the basis of adolescent enuresis?

A. In a study of 27 adolescent enuretics, 75% were found to have some form of organic abnormality. This high incidence would warrant urologic investigation of any adolescent with the problem of enuresis. However, the urological lesions were often minimal, such as urethral strictures and stenosis, discovered most easily by cystourethrogram and I.V.P. Correction of these lesions generally resulted in only temporary cessation or decrease of enuresis. The same group of enuretics were found to show considerable pathology of a social or psychological nature. Therefore, organic pathology, although frequently found, would rarely be considered the sole causative factor in enuresis.
REF. Murphy S, M.D., Chapman W, M.D.: Adolescent Enuresis: A Urologic Study. Pediatrics 45:3, 426-431, 1970.

240. Q. Is there a neurological basis for enuresis in adolescents?

A. The relationship between neurological dysfunction was explored as an etiologic factor in chronic enuresis with 27 adolescent patients. Twenty-two nonenuretic patients were studied as controls. The study indicates that the chronic enuretics had relatively normal prenatal, neonatal and childhood health histories. The adolescent enuretic showed no evidence of even minimal cerebral dysfunction, based on physical exam, EEG, or psychological testing. Deep sleep does not appear to be associated with the enuresis. It is felt that the causes of chronic enuresis extending into adolescence must be sought in areas other than the neurologic.
REF. Murphy S, et al.: Neurological Evaluation of Adolescent Enuretics. Pediatrics 45:2, 269-275, 1970.

241. Q. How is the diagnosis of acute otitis media made?

A. Acute otitis media or middle ear infection in the symptochild is confirmed by the otoscopic appearance of the tympanic membrane. Because of the frequency of middle ear disease, it should be

suspected even when specific symptoms are absent in the child with URI or respiratory manifestations of allergy. The diagnosis of suppurative otitis media can be definitively established only by examination and culture of middle ear fluid. Earache is not a reliable guide and may be absent in 75% of cases. Fever is noted in only 40-70% of cases. Symptoms are not consistently present with middle ear effusions. Because of the variability of symptoms, children presenting with otoscopic evidence of middle ear infection should be suspected of having suppurative otitis. Diminished or absent mobility and opacification of the eardrum are constant findings. Patients with a red tympanic membrane alone, do not have acute otitis media.
REF. Bluestone C, M.D., Shurin P, M.D.: Middle Ear Disease in Children. Pediatric Clinics of North America 21:2, 379-397, 1974.

242. Q. What is the treatment of otitis media?

A. Antibiotics are the mainstay of acute otitis media therapy. The drugs most widely used are the penicillins, erythromycin and sulfonamides. Ampicillin appears to be the singularly most effective drug in the treatment of acute otitis media. The usual duration of antibiotic therapy is 10 to 14 days. It is essential that no patient be considered cured until there is complete resolution of all signs of middle ear disease. Myringotomy (incision of the eardrum) may be indicated in cases of otitis media with: (1) unusually severe earache requiring immediate relief, (2) progression of symptoms in spite of adequate medical treatment, (3) suppurative complications. Tympanostomy tubes may be indicated when:(1) middle ear effusions are persistent despite adequate medical treatment, (2) they are recurrent attacks of otitis media, (3) tympanic membrane retraction pockets persist with impending cholesteatoma, (4) there is persistent negative pressure with significant hearing loss.
REF. Bluestone C, M.D., Shurin P, M.D.: Middle Ear Disease in Children. Pediatric Clinics of North America 21:2, 379-397, 1974.

243. Q. Is otitis media a problem in children with cleft palate?

A. Middle ear infection or suppurative otitis media is a universal complication in unrepaired cleft palate. If left untreated, chronic otitis media can lead to superimposed infection, adhesions and scarring and cholesteatoma. These changes are associated with significant hearing loss. Maintaining normal hearing acuity throughout early life helps assure optimal conditions for intellectual, language and emotional development in these children. Treatment may be accomplished with middle ear aeration by means of myringotomy, aspiration of middle ear liquid and insertion of tympanostomy tubes. Palate repair results in sharp improvement of middle ear status.
REF. Paradise J, Bluestone C.: Early Treatment of Universal Otitis Media in Infants with Cleft Palate. Pediatrics 53:1, 48-54, 1974.

244. Q. What is tympanometry?

A. Tympanometry is a new method of examining the middle ear with the use of an instrument called the electro-acoustic impedance bridge with which a tympanogram can be obtained. To perform tympanometry a small probe is inserted in the external auditory canal. A tone of fixed characteristics is presented via the probe and the compliance of the tympanic membrane is measured electronically while the external canal pressure is verified. Acoustic compliance is greatest when pressures are equal on both sides of the tympanic membrane. Less compliance is present in middle ear effusions. Tympanometry is a reliable, simple procedure which aids in diagnosis when otoscopy is difficult to perform, or when the results of otoscopy are equivocal and is equal to or superior to otoscopy in reliability in many cases.

REF. Bluestone C, M.D., Shurin P, M.D.: Middle Ear Disease in Children. Pediatric Clinics of North America 21:2, 379-397, 1974.

245. Q. What is bronchiolitis?

A. The clinical definition of bronchiolitis is of an acute respiratory disorder of infants and young children. It often occurs in epidemics and is characteristically preceded by an upper respiratory infection. The URI is followed by the symptoms of bronchiolitis, cough, rapid shallow respirations, expiratory wheeze, suprasternal and subcostal retractions and emphysema. The clinical and radiological picture may mimic asthma. The respiratory syncytial virus, RSV, appears to play a predominant role in the origin of bronchiolitis. Parainfluenza mycoplasma and adenovirus have also produced similar clinical and pathological pictures. Treatment is with humidified oxygen by mask or tent, antibiotics to prevent secondary bacterial infection and maintenance of hydration. Prognosis is good, the course of the disease is 4-10 days.

REF. Wittig H, M.D., Chang JCH, M.D.: Bronchiolitis or Asthma? Pediatric Clinics of North America 16:1, 55-66, 1969.

246. Q. How does bronchiolitis differ from bronchial asthma?

A. Differential diagnosis may be difficult in those instances where bronchiolitis recurs. Most attacks of bronchiolitis occur only once. The following points may be helpful in differentiating bronchiolitis from infantile bronchial asthma: (1) bronchiolitis most often occurs in epidemics, (2) viral studies should be obtained where possible, since RSV and other viruses cause bronchiolitis, (3) X-ray may be helpful, (4) a nasal smear may help identify the asthmatic child if more than 10% eosinophils are present, (5) concurrent allergic responses may help identify the asthmatic child, (6) bronchial asthma has been defined as recurrent paroxysmal dyspnea with expiratory wheezing, characteristically relieved by epinephrine, therefore the diagnosis of acute bronchiolitis decreases with the number of dyspneic episodes. The more recurrent the condition, the more likely it is to be asthma.

REF. Wittig H, M.D., Chang JCH, M.D.: Bronchiolitis or Asthma? Pediatric Clinics of North America 16:1, 55-66, 1969.

247. Q. What is acute epiglottitis?

A. Acute epiglottitis is a dramatic potentially lethal condition caused by hemophilus influenza infection. Patients are usually between the ages of 2 and 7 years and 60-70% are boys. There is history of rapidly developing sore throat with croup, fever and prostration. Within a matter of hours the respiratory distress may progress to complete obstruction, shock and death. The characteristic signs are fever, prostration and a large cherry-red, shiny epiglottis which tends to act as a ball-valve obstruction. Tracheostomy or a nasotracheal tube to establish an airway is urgent. After an airway is established, the exhausted child characteristically drops off to sleep. Parenteral antibiotics should be given and marked improvement can be noted in 12 to 24 hours. The epiglottis loses edema and shrinks, so that the airway can be removed in 3-4 days.
REF. Sell SHW, M.D.: The Clinical Importance of Hemophilus Influenzae Infections in Children. Pediatric Clinics of North America 17:2, 415-426, 1970.

248. Q. What types of infection can be caused by hemophilus influenzae in children?

A. Hemophilus influenzae is one of the important bacterial species which produces serious infection in children. The species can act as an etiological agent in septicemia, meningitis, obstructive epiglottitis, pneumonia, osteomyelitis, and cellulitis. Hemophilus influenza is a gram-negative, pleomorphic bacillus. Most of these serious infections have been attributed to encapsulated, typable strains, principally type B. The availability of antibiotic therapy has taken the panic out of treatment of these infections. However, the precise bacteriological diagnosis is essential in order to select the proper drug.
REF. Sell SHW, M.D.: The Clinical Importance of Hemophilus Influenzae Infections in Children. Pediatric Clinics of North America 17:2, 415-426, 1970.

249. Q. Can cytomegalovirus cause congenital defects?

A. It appears that the cytomegalovirus is the most common cause of fetal infection and that asymptomatic infection in utero may be responsible for subtle neurological damage which is not evident until childhood. In its most severe form, congenital infection may involve multiple organs causing hepatosplenomegaly, jaundice, petechia, microcephaly, cerebral calcifications, chorioretinitis and optic atrophy. Both these infants and those with less severe clinical manifestations, who survive, generally show brain damage of varying degrees. Visual and auditory defects may also be present. The occurrence and severity of infection depends on the stage of pregnancy at which maternal infection is acquired. Most infected babies with severe disease are born to mothers who were were infected in the first half of pregnancy. The incidence of cyto-

megalovirus infection is 1%. Ten percent of those babies show varying degrees of detectable brain damage. The incidence of more subtle damage remains undetermined.
REF. Kibrick S, M.D., Ph.D., Loria R, Ph.D.: Rubella and Cytomegalovirus. Pediatric Clinics of North America 21:2, 513-525, 1974.

250. Q. Can bacterial infection in the fetus and newborn be prevented or minimized?

A. Defense mechanisms developed in intrauterine life enable an infant to withstand the infective hazards of birth canal passage. Maternal bacteraemia can lead to fetal bacteraemia; bacilli may ascend from the vagina through ruptured membranes to the uterine cavity or be encountered in the vagina during delivery. If a male infant is born prematurely his defense mechanisms are less developed. The hands of nursing personnel and equipment used to resuscitate him at birth, clear his airways, maintain his temperature, or even artificially ventilate his lungs may be a source of infection.

Because of the proximity of umbilical wound and perineum, gram-negative organisms have always constituted a threat to the newborn. With the control of the streptococcus and staphylococcus they now assume greater importance and bowel organisms have been joined by those flourishing in the humidification units of equipment.

The environment is kept bacteriologically clean as possible by a high standard of household and hand cleanliness rather than widespread use of antibiotics, for these may alter the balance of flora and encourage resistant organisms.
REF. Davies PA.: Bacterial Infection in the Fetus and Newborn. Archives of Disease in Childhood 46:245, 1-20, 1971.

251. Q. What is the effect of steroids on the treatment of pertussis?

A. Pertussis and its complications remain a prominent cause of death in infancy. No specific treatment for this disease is available. Antibiotics and pertussis immune globulin both showed promise of affecting the mortality of pertussis, but both soon proved of dubious value in modifying the course of the disease.

In a controlled clinical trial, all the children were in the first week of paroxysmal stage. Seventy out of 135 were treated with hydrocortisone sodium succinate for 7 to 8 days. The rest were used as a control group. All children received erythromycin for 10 days. Illness and complications were shorter in babies under 1 year of age. Steroids may have a beneficial effect on the course of pertussis if given early in the paroxysmal stage.

Steroids are potentially dangerous drugs and their use must be limited to moderately severe or severe cases, especially in infants under 6 to 9 months of age where the mortality is highest.

REF. Zoumboulakis D, et al.: Steroids in Treatment of Pertussis. Archives of Disease in Childhood 48:1, 51-54, 1973.

252. Q. What are some causes of bacterial diarrhea?

A. In the United States, common causes of bacterial diarrhea include infection with such organisms as salmonella or shigella. Both are ordinarily self-limiting, mild, and require no hospitalization or antibiotic treatment, unless the dehydration in infants necessitates fluid replacement.

Salmonella is a rod-shaped, gram-negative organism which is capable of causing diarrhea, typhoid fever syndrome, septicemia, or osteomyelitis. The bacteria are widely distributed in nature meat, poultry, dried eggs, milk and can be transmitted by pet turtles, chicks, dogs or cats. Relatively large numbers must be ingested orally for infection to occur.

Shigella, also a rod-shaped, gram-negative organism, is less widely distributed in nature. Transmission is ordinarily from man to man. Infants and young children are most often affected because they are least immune and least careful of the oral fecal contamination. Although the illness is usually self-limiting, antibiotic therapy is effective in severe cases.

Escherichia coli is also a gram-negative rod, which normally makes up less than 1% of normal bowel flora. Various strains can cause a mild diarrhea, but which can be fatal in an infant.

Diarrhea can also be caused by the toxin of coagulase-positive Staphylococcus aureus or epidermitis. These organisms are found nearly everywhere, including human flora. The toxins are relatively heat stable, and can be found in improperly cooked or refrigerated foods, vomiting, mild cramps, and watery stools usually appear 2 to 6 hours after ingestion.

Clostridium perfringes, an anaerobic spore-forming organism, is a normal inhabitant of the human gastrointestinal tract and contaminates most uncooked meat and poultry. Its toxin, when ingested, produces symptoms of profound cramps and mild diarrhea in about 8 to 15 hours.
REF. Keusch G.: Bacterial Diarrhea. American Journal of Nursing 73:6, 1028-1032, June 1973.

253. Q. What is neonatal inclusion conjunctivitis?

A. Neonatal inclusion conjunctivitis is one of the specific inflammatory diseases of the external eye that affects young infants. It is caused by Chlamydia, obligate intracellular-parasites.

Characteristically, the disease has its onset 4 to 12 days after birth. The conjunctiva is red, swollen and there is a whitish yellow discharge from the eye. There are usually no systemic signs.

The treatment is 10-15% sulfacetamide eye drops for 3 weeks. Improvement will begin within 3 days or less after the institution of treatment.
REF. Kripke SS, Golden B.: Neonatal Inclusion Conjunctivitis. Clinical Pediatrics 11:261-263, May 1972.

254. Q. What is the status of gonorrhea among children?

A. Although it is well known that the incidence of gonorrhea has increased, the true incidence is unknown. Gonorrhea occurs in all age groups but is primarily a disease of the young.

Gonococcal infections among children and infants have also increased. Usually the disease is not transmitted by sexual contact, but by contaminated maternal hands. Gonococcus may be manifested in many forms such as conjunctivitis, arthritis, meningitis and endocarditis. The child should be promptly diagnosed and treated.

Standard of treatment consists of penicillin injections for 7 to 12 days. In addition, case finding, reporting of the disease to a public health facility and family counselling are an integral part of therapy.
REF. Allue X, et al.: Gonococcal Infections in Infants and Children. Clinical Pediatrics 12:584-588, Oct. 1973.

255. Q. How valuable are external ear cultures?

A. Culture of the external ear canal of the newborn can be used to identify neonatal sepsis. Since the external ear is a receptacle for amniotic fluid in utero and is in contact with vaginal secretions during labor and delivery, it will reflect this contamination. Also, the early canal is not exposed to antibiotics and is rarely washed with other prophylactic substances.

Infections such as gonorrhea, group-A and non-group-A beta hemolytic streptococci can be detected in mother and infant.
REF. Scanlon JW.: Diagnosis of Gonorrheal Infection by Culture of the External Ear Canal in the Newborn. Clinical Pediatrics 10:528-529, Sept. 1971.

256. Q. What are the symptoms of rabies?

A. The incubation period for rabies varies from 10 days to 8 months, the average time being 1-2 months. Generally this period is long enough to allow for the administration of vaccines to induce antibodies. The initial symptoms are chills, fever, malaise, nausea and vomiting, headache, anxiety, vertigo and dyspnea. These symptoms are non specific and vary in duration and intensity. Frequently, the initial complaint is pain of a neuritic nature at the site of the injury. After the onset of symptoms, death follows in a week or less.
REF. Cereghino J, et al.: Rabies: A Rare Disease but a Serious Pediatric Problem. Pediatrics 45:5, 839-843, 1970.

257. Q. What vaccines are available for rabies?

A. Two types of commercial vaccines are available, the Semple vaccine and the duck embryo vaccine. Hyperimmune serum is also available. With semple vaccine, actively induced serum neutralizing antibodies, with daily injections, may not be detectable for 10-15 days. DEV (duck embryo vaccine) is believed to produce an earlier production of antibodies than semple. For people severely exposed to rabies, anti rabies serum or gamma globulin is used to induce passive immunity.
REF. Cereghino J, et al.: Rabies: A Rare Disease but a Serious Pediatric Problem. Pediatrics 45:5, 839-843, 1970.

258. Q. What are some of the antimicrobial drug combinations currently being used in pediatrics?

A. Antimicrobial drugs may be used in combination for many valid reasons, including broad spectrum coverage and greater effectiveness. Three drug combinations of current interest in pediatrics are:

(1) Trimethoprim and sulfamethoxazole are synergistic against a wide range of microbes. The spectrum of activity of these drugs suggests a role in treating children with respiratory, genitourinary and alimentary tract infections.

(2) Combination of penicillinase-resistant penicillin and a hydrolyzable penicillin (benzylpenicillin or ampicillin) produces significant activity against some gram negative enteric bacillae. Penicillin when used alone is ineffective against these organisms. These combinations have been effective against some resistant urinary tract infections.

(3) Penicillins in combination with aminoglycosides are synergistic against some strains of enterococci and gram negative enteric bacilli. Because of their broad spectrum coverage these drugs are also used extensively for the treatment of serious infections such as sepsis in the newborn or the child with depressed normal host defenses.
REF. Klein JO, M.D.: Current Usage of Antimicrobial Combinations in Pediatrics. Pediatric Clinics of North America 21:2, 443-455, 1974.

259. Q. What are the adverse effects of orally administered ampicillin?

A. Ampicillin is one of the most frequently prescribed antimicrobial drugs in pediatrics. The common side effects of ampicillin are well known, particularly diarrhea, vomiting, or skin rashes. A study was done to establish if certain side effects were dose related, and what the severity and frequency of these side effects were.

Oral ampicillin was administered to four groups of children ages 2 months to 6 years, and a dose of 50, 100, 150, or 200 mg. per kilogram of body weight per day was prescribed.

Results showed that vomiting was not a significant problem. It rarely occurred, and if it did, it was mild and had no relationship to dosage. Mild to moderate diarrhea was commonly encountered in patients regardless of dose, and generally required no treatment. Typical ampicillin associated skin rashes, a generalized erythematous maculopapular eruption, occurred in about 5% of the patients, and was more common in those children receiving higher doses but the difference was not statistically significant. Urticarial skin rashes suggestive of true penicillin allergy occurred in less than 1% of all patients, and was not dose related. The only skin reaction observed to be significantly dose related was monilial diaper rash. It occurred exclusively in infants wearing diapers, and was usually associated with mild diarrhea.

REF. Bass CJ, et al.: Adverse Effects of Orally Administered Ampicillin. Journal of Pediatrics 83:1, 106-108, July 1973.

260. Q. When curare is used to treat tetanus, what nursing implications are involved?

A. Tetanus is a neurotoxic disease caused by the anaerobic organism, clostridium tetani. The toxin is thought to affect the nervous system by binding at the synapse of the anterior horn cells in the spinal cord, blocking the inhibiting impulses that follow muscle contraction thereby causing hypertonicity or spasm. The disease process begins at the level of the brainstem and proceeds downward. Frequently, the first sign is inability to close the mouth, followed by spasms in the back and extremities. Drug addicts are especially susceptible to this disease because of "skin popping" and use of street heroin which has been cut with quinine, a protoplasmic poison, both of which favor the growth of this anaerobic organism.

Medical treatment is aimed at controlling the severe spasms. Often, drugs such as valium and morphine sulfate fail, necessitating the use of curare. Curare (d-tubocurarine) is a neuromuscular blocking agent. It blocks the transmitter effect of acetylcholine. When curare is given intravenously, it acts rapidly to cause slight dizziness, a sensation of warmth, inability to keep eye lids open, difficulty in focusing, and heaviness of limbs. Gradually, paralysis is induced, although the patient is alert and conscious. Nursing implications of the curarized patient are many: maintenance of respiration (usually on a respirator), maintenance of muscle tone through daily range of motion and proper positioning, and prevention of infection (in any system, particularly respiratory and circulatory from intravenous lines). The patient needs complete physical care, including elimination with enemas and foley catheters. Nutrition needs to be maintained by methods such as hyperalimentation. Vital signs need to be monitored constantly. Besides these physical needs, the curarized patient who is alert and conscious, has no means of communicating. Therefore, his needs must be anticipated, and procedures must be carefully explained. As the dosage of curare is decreased, the patient regains eyelid movement and facial expression, which give him an opportunity to express likes and dislikes.

These patients need a most demanding and challenging kind of nursing care. Often, the physical care and recovery are complicated by the drug problem, which brought them to this life-threatening situation.

REF. Boyer C.: Caring for a Young Addict with Tetanus. American Journal of Nursing 74:2, 265-267, Feb. 1974.

261. Q. What is Reye's syndrome?

A. Reye's syndrome was first described in 1963. It is characterized by acute encephalopathy with fatty degeneration of the viscera. Typically this syndrome followed a minor prodromal illness. The fulminating encephalopathy which followed was usually fatal. Other characteristics are markedly elevated transaminase levels, hypoglycemia, hypoglycorrhachia, cerebral edema and fatty degeneration of the liver.

Several links have been suggested between Reye's syndrome and influenza virus B infection. This association of Reye's syndrome with common viral agents such as influenza B and varicella-zoster suggest a potential role for immuno or chemo-prophylaxis.

REF. Glick T, M.D., et al.: Reye's Syndrome: An Epidemiologic Approach. Pediatrics 46:3, 371-377, 1970.

262. Q. What do we know about Reye's syndrome?

A. Reye's syndrome was discovered in 1963 by Dr. Ralph D. Reye who thought it was caused by a combination of factors instead of a specific virus. Today, the cause and treatment of the disease are still unknown. The syndrome seems to follow an attack of influenza, beginning with persistent vomiting, followed by an altered state of consciousness. The disruption of the central nervous system is characterized by hyperexcitability, hyperactivity such as thrashing or shouting, generalized convulsions, depression, then coma and death. Internally, the liver is malfunctioning, causing enzymes and toxins to increase. One of the side effects is the building of ammonia in the bloodstream. Blood sugar decreased rapidly, cerebral damage occurs, and there is a fatty degeneration of the intestines. Laboratory tests for ammonia and blood glucose levels, as well as liver function are done if Reye's is suspected.

Treatment is aimed at reducing the toxins causing deterioration. Some techniques such as plasmaphoresis, peritoneal dialysis, and total blood exchanges have been tried with various degrees of success. Prognosis is still uncertain, and at best, poor.

REF. Simon R.: It Starts with a Child's Persistent Vomiting. Today's Health 52:6, 24-71, June 1974.

263.  Q. What are the clinical findings in childhood diabetes and ketoacidosis?

A. The onset of symptoms of diabetes may range from 1 to 2 days to as long as several months before the appearance of keto-acidosis.  Polyuria and polydipsia are common symptoms.  Also present may be polyphagia, nocturia and weight loss.  In some instances diabetic coma is precipitated by infection or emotional upset.  The rapidity of progression from carbohydrate intolerance to ketoacidosis is very unpredictable and warrants continuous medical surveillance once the diagnosis of diabetes has been made.  The diagnosis of diabetes mellitus is confirmed by glucosuria and ketonuria in the presence of blood sugar above 150 mg/100 ml.  Vomiting is an ominous sign which signals rapid deterioration and progression into acidosis and coma.  In moderate acidosis changes in respiratory rate occur with increase in the rate and depth of respirations.  In severe acidosis the characteristic Kussmaul breathing becomes obvious.  Serum Ph is lowered and blood sugar may range from 150 mg to as high as 2,000 mg/100 ml.  Signs of dehydration may be present and the state of consciousness may vary from drowsiness to coma.
REF. Schwartz R, M. D.:  The Critically Ill Child:  Diabetic Keto-acidosis and Coma.  Pediatrics 47:5, 902-909, 1971.

264.  Q. What are some important differences between adult and juvenile diabetes that can influence nursing care?

A. Although 95% of the diabetics are adults, the 5% who are children require some special considerations because of differences in the disease.  The first major difference is the rapid onset of juvenile diabetes.  Polyuria, polydipsia, and weight loss are acute signs of diabetes in about 90% of the children.  In fact, some of the children are diagnosed because of diabetic acidosis, rather than from less critical signs.  This fact necessitates a different kind of teaching, stressing early recognition of signs, rather than only urine screening tests, which can give false security to a parent whose child may be pre-diabetic.

Another large difference in terms of management and teaching are nutritional needs.  Unlike adult diabetics who are frequently overweight, these children tend to be thin at onset.  Their nutritional intake cannot be severely restricted, and must include added calories and protein for growth spurts.  Their diet needs to be well balanced in all essential nutrients but minimal in artificial food stuff, to be acceptable to the whole family, and to include snacks between regularly scheduled meals.

The third difference is the control of glycosuria.  Insulin regulation is based on the spillage of sugar in the urine.  At one time, physicians thought that insulin doses should be regulated to produce consistently negative results.  Now they feel that some glucose spillage is desirable, especially in highly active age groups.

REF. McFarlane J.: Children with Diabetes, Special Needs During Growth Years. American Journal of Nursing 73:8, 1360-1363, Aug. 1973.

265. Q. What are signs of ketoacidosis in a diabetic child?

A. Diabetes mellitus results from the body's inability to produce insulin needed for carbohydrate metabolism. Since glucose cannot be used as the source for cellular energy, fat is broken down, causing the production of ketone bodies faster than cells can oxidize and use them. As a result the ketones (beta-hydroxybutyric acid, acetoacetic acid, and acetone) accumulate in body tissues and fluids leading to ketosis. The kidney attempts to compensate by increasing its production of ammonia and exchanges some hydrogen ions for sodium ions. When the $CO_2$ combining power of the blood is lowered, metabolic acidosis results. Evidence of ketoacidosis includes:

(1) polyuria, polydipsia, and dehydration
(2) nausea and vomiting, which increase electrolyte imbalance (loss of chloride, potassium and bicarbonate)
(3) hypotension and rapid pulse from hypovolemia
(4) abdominal pain and tenderness, possibly from sodium loss
(5) kussmaul breathing (deep, rapid respirations)
(6) acetone breath
(7) weakness, paralysis, or parasthesia, and
(8) drowsiness, stupor, and finally coma.

Treatment includes reversal of metabolism from a fat to a carbohydrate substrate by administration of insulin. Fluid and electrolytes are given to reverse electrolyte imbalance and correct dehydration. Blood volume expanders are given if hypovolemia is severe enough to result in circulatory collapse. Glucose is given if glycogen stores have been depleted to prevent hypoglycemia.
REF. Carozza V.: Ketoacidotic Crisis: Mechanism and Management. Nursing '73 3:5, 13-14, May 1973.

266. Q. What is the treatment of diabetic acidosis in children?

A. Treatment in diabetic acidosis is always urgent and is based on the principles involved in other derangements of electrolyte physiology. That is, the fluid replacement is calculated from (1)previous deficit, (2) maintenance needs, (3) continuing abnormal losses. Correction of the ketoacidosis and hyperglycemia is dependent on the reversal of the pathophysiological mechanisms by the administration of insulin. Initial insulin is regular insulin in a dosage of from 1 unit to 3-4 units per kilogram of body weight. Parenteral fluids are continued until the patient is free of ketones and aglycosuric for at least the first 12 hours. Amounts of fluids and dosages of insulin for the second 24 hours are dependent upon the rate of repair of the estimated deficit and continuing losses. By the third day a planned dietary regime with long acting insulin may be introduced.
REF. Schwartz R, M.D.: The Critically Ill Child: Diabetic Ketoacidosis and Coma. Pediatrics 47:5, 902-909, 1971.

267. Q. How can nurses avoid complications of repeated insulin injections?

   A. Insulin, when injected into tissues, causes two major problems: hypertrophy and atrophy of the site. In hypertrophy, there is a thickening of subcutaneous tissues, which may appear as lumpy hard areas or as spongy areas. Atrophy is a loss of subcutaneous fat, evidenced by a depression or concavity at the site of injection. Unsightly scars and absent sensation occurs from the destruction of tissue. The cause of these problems is unknown but evidence suggests that repeated injection in the same site, biological activity of insulin, injection into the fatty layer, or use of cold insulin increases the probability of such complications.

Two principles can help prevent or lessen the possibilities of tissue damage. The first is selection of several sites, such as the thigh, abdomen, upper back, and upper arms. Each site is then mapped on a piece of paper with dots or X's to outline rows of possible injection sites. Depending on the person's size, a definite number of sites can be systematically located at one-inch intervals. The patient can then use the muscle area in the legs for several weeks without ever injecting the exact same site twice.

The second principle is correct injection technique, by injecting the insulin between the layer of fat and muscle. This is done by picking up the layer of skin and fat, and injecting a long enough needle at about an angle of 20-45 degrees. The best way to determine needle length is to measure the distance across the base of the fold. For children, a five-eighths needle is usually adequate. However, the thicker the layer of fat, the longer the needle that is necessary. Also, insulin should be allowed to warm up at room temperature before it is given.
REF. Burke E.: Insulin Injection: The Site and the Technique. American Journal of Nursing 72:12, 2194-2196, Dec. 1972.

268. Q. How can we help patients learn the use of the U-100 insulin and syringe?

   A. Recently, the Committee on the Use of Therapeutic Agents of the American Diabetes Association has recommended that the U-40 and U-80 strengths of insulin be replaced by U-100 insulin. Because of the confusion between U-40 and U-80 insulin in terms of strength and dosage, the U-100 insulin was selected because of its compatibility with the decimal system. Since U-100 insulin means that each cc equals 100 units, then any dosage of insulin is the corresponding number in volume. For example 35 units of U-100 insulin is 0.35 cc of medication. Some suggestions in teaching this new system includes:

(1) When you are explaining the new preparation, watch patients draw up the medication in the new syringe. Also, evaluate the procedure they use and the understanding they have in drawing

up their old insulin as well. This is a good time to pick up long-term errors and misconceptions.

(2) Persuade patients to discard old syringes and vials and adopt only this new method.

(3) Be sure that patients understand that the new syringe makes the adjustment in volume for them. For example, 28 units of U-40 insulin is still 28 units of U-100 insulin in the U-100 syringe.

(4) Be careful to evaluate all patients' performance because education and intelligence need not prevent errors from occurring.

REF. Lawrence P.: U-100 Insulin: Let's Make the Transition Trouble Free. American Journal of Nursing 73:9, 1539, Sept. 1973.

269. Q. What are the consequences of neonatal diabetes?

A. The author suggests that neonatal diabetic infants were born small for gestational age (S. G. A.) because of insulin deficiency in utero. He states:

(1) No reason to suspect S. G. A. neonatal diabetic becomes insulin-openic right at birth, he is probably insulinopenic in utero.

(2) Level of circulating insulin in the normal fetus is low, it must be performing a necessary growth-promoting function.

(3) Insulin is known to be, extra uterine protein-sparing and growth-promoting.

(4) It is unlikely that intrauterine growth retardation (I. G. R.) causes neonatal diabetes because S. G. A. infants usually have normal or high insulin levels.

The large size of the infant of the diabetic mother may be caused by exposure of the fetus to super-normal levels of its own insulin. It seems logical to conclude that insulin is an important intrauterine growth hormone. If there is excess insulin in utero, the fetus will be large. If there is subnormal insulin in utero, the fetus will be born small.

REF. MacDonald MJ.: Neonatal Diabetes. The Lancet 1:7860, 737, 1974.

270. Q. How is the physical growth affected in diabetic children?

A. Controlling blood sugar levels within physiological range should be attempted. There is clinical, anatomical, and biochemical evidence that vascular complications of diabetes are related to high blood-glucose and low serum-insulin level i.e., the degree of regulation of diabetes.

Evidence suggests that a fall in growth rate and delayed maturation occur only in diabetic children who receive inappropriate insulin therapy and/or suboptimal dietary supervision. There are varying degrees of glycosuria most of the time. This will lead to diabetic retinopathy about 15 years after onset of disease.

The key to excellent regulation of diabetes is early recognition of the disease, prompt institution of appropriate insulin therapy, proper meal planning using high-quality foods and intensive education of the parents and child.
REF. Murthy DYN, Jackson RL.: Growth in Diabetic Children. The Lancet 1:7860, 736-737, 1974.

271. Q. What are some causes of hypoglycemia in infancy and childhood?

A. The causes are best thought of according to the age of onset of symptoms.

(1) 1 year of age:
    Glycogen disease of the liver
    Reye's syndrome (fatty liver, encephalopathy, hypoglycemia)
    Gastroenteritis
    Central nervous system disease
    Islet cell tumor of pancreas
    Idiopathic hypoglycemia of infancy
(2) 1-3 years of age:
    Ketotic hypoglycemia
    Reye's syndrome
    Gastroenteritis
    Hypopituitarism
    Adrenal Insufficiency
(3) 3 years of age:
    Islet cell tumor of pancreas
    Ketotic hypoglycemia
    Hypopituitarism
    Adrenal insufficiency
REF. Ehrlich RM.: Hypoglycemia in Infancy and Childhood. Archives of Disease in Childhood 46:249, 716-719, 1971.

272. Q. How can hypoglycemia be recognized in infancy and childhood?

A. Hypoglycemia is only a symptom of some underlying disease process. Lack of glucose, the essential nutrient in the developing nervous system, may result in permanent alteration of brain structure and function.

Convulsions are the most common symptom under 1 year with pallor, weakness, profuse perspiration, and limp spells. In older children, weakness, fatigue, headache, drowsiness, and irritability may be present. If symptoms occur before meals or after prolonged fasting (early morning) hypoglycemia should be suspected. Small infants eat frequently but still may have hypoglycemic convulsions.

Physical examination may reveal hepatomegaly suggesting glycogen disease of Reye's syndrome. Short stature may be due to an endocrine cause.

Causes in infancy and childhood are best thought of according to the age of onset of symptoms. Hypoglycemia is a medical emergency to be treated promptly. Then, treatment is directed against a specific cause when found, for example, administration of growth hormone, or cortisone, or surgery.
REF. Ehrlich RM.: Hypoglycemia in Infancy and Childhood. Archives of Disease in Childhood 46:249, 716-719, 1971.

273. Q. What three groups of children with hypoglycemia may pose special problems?

A. (1) The child with symptoms suggestive of hypoglycemia such as episodes of pallor, drowsiness, headache, irritability relieved by food but in whom blood sugar values are normal. Epilepsy, migraine, anxiety, behavior disorders, pheochromocytoma, may mimic hypoglycemia.

(2) The child with symptoms appropriate to hypoglycemia in whom a low blood sugar is found only once. A history and physical examination is done, a 6 hour glucose tolerance test with insulin and growth hormone values, intravenous tolbutamide test with insulin levels, diurnal blood cortisol levels, and serum electrolyte determinations should be made. The skull X-rayed and skeletal maturation estimated. If ketotic hypoglycemia is suspected, a provocative ketotic diet should be tried before other tests.

(3) The symptom-free child in whom a low blood sugar (often 40-50 mg/100 ml.) is found only once. This child is a diagnostic challenge. If a careful history and physical examination offer no clue, further investigation beyond repeating the blood sugar determination periodically is unnecessary.
REF. Ehrlich RM.: Hypoglycaemia in Infancy and Childhood. Archives of Disease in Childhood 46:249, 716-719, 1971.

274. Q. What is cystic fibrosis?

A. Cystic fibrosis is an autosomal recessive hereditary disease affecting the exocrine glands of the body. The chief manifestations of C.F. are tenacious secretions of the tracheo-bronchial tree leading to bronchial plugging and repeated respiratory infections. Pancreatic enzymes are abnormal, leading to pancreatic insufficiency. The electrolyte content of the sweat is also abnormally increased.
REF. Kraus L, M.D., et al.: Metachromasia and Assay for Lysosomal Enzymes in Skin Fibroblasts Cultured from Patients with Cystic Fibrosis and Controls. Pediatrics 47:6, 1010-1018, 1971.

275. Q. What is maple syrup urine disease and how is it treated?

A. Maple syrup urine disease is a result of a genetic error in the metabolism of the branch chain amino acids, leucine, isoleucine and valine. Affected infants appear healthy at birth, but during the first week of life develop increasing spasticity, opisthotonus,

high pitched cry and irregular breathing. A maple syrup odor to the urine is noted by the second week of life. These children have neurological deterioration which results in intractable seizures, coma, and death within a few months. The treatment is with diets low in leucine, isoleucine and valine. Dietary treatment must be begun in the first 2 weeks of life if permanent brain damage is to be prevented. Unfortunately, early diagnosis and treatment does not solve the problems of this disease and even treated children may die of minor illnesses which increase the metabolic demands.
REF. Fenichel G, M.D.: Recent Clinical Advances in the Treatment of Neurological Diseases. Pediatric Clinics of North America 17:2, 323-335, 1970.

276. Q. What is the cause of congenital adrenal hyperplasia?

A. Congenital virilizing adrenal hyperplasia (adreno-genital syndrome) is caused by a defect in the biosynthesis of cortisol as a result of deficiency in one of the essential enzymes, most commonly 21-hydroxylase. The effect of the enzyme deficiency is a reduction in the secretion of cortisol. The plasma level falls and by a negative feedback mechanism there is a compensatory rise is ACTH secretion. The resulting over-stimulation of the suprarenal cortex causes an excessive production of androgens with consequent virilization. In the fetus, this is the cause of the incomplete differentiation of the external genitalia in the females and, after birth, of the progressive virilization in both sexes, together with rapid growth and advance in development of the epiphyses - leading eventually to premature fusion and stunted growth. In about one-third of patients with 21-hydroxylase deficiency a severe salt-losing syndrome develops soon after birth, which if untreated may prove fatal.
REF. Annotation.: Congenital Adrenal Hyperplasia. Archives of Disease in Childhood 49:1, 1-3, 1974.

277. Q. What can be done to improve growth and skeletal maturation in congenital adrenal hyperplasia?

A. In 20 children with the salt-losing variety of congenital adrenal hyperplasia there was a significant degree of stunting and their skeletal maturation was delayed. Fourteen children were treated in the first year of life with long-acting steroid preparations and 13 of this group achieved normal height velocities during this period. Treatment thereafter was with prednisone and 9-OC-fludrocortisone, and it is concluded that the growth retardation of the children was due to a specific effect of these drugs, or the drug overdosage. Those children receiving a long-lasting prednisone analogue in the first year of life show evidence that such compounds cause more growth retardation than hydrocortisone. One child who did not achieve a normal velocity was given higher dosages and this suggests that, like most of the steroid drugs, the stunting effect of PTMA (Prednisone trimethyl acetate) is dose related. This regimen proved an easily regulated reliable method of treating the children and does not appear to cause significant stunting.

PTMA in the first year of life provides a convenient method of control for children with this condition and appears not to influence rate of growth in the first year. Subsequent therapy with prednisone appears to have stunted growth in this group, due either to an effect of the drug itself or to too strict control leading to unnecessarily high dosage.

Consideration is being given to using hydrocortisone to control these children and placing greater emphasis on maintaining the rate of skeletal maturation parallel to chronological age.
REF. Bailey CC, Komrower GM.: Growth and Skeletal Maturation in Congenital Adrenal Hyperplasia. Archives of Disease in Childhood 49:1, 4-7, 1974.

278. Q. Can routine screening tests in phenylketonuria produce negative results?

A. The routine screening of babies for phenylketonuria is now widely practiced, using either a blood sample (Guthrie test) or a urine sample (paper chromatography or ferric chloride methods).

The validity of the test depends on an adequate dietary protein intake, a false negative may result if the infant is tested too early in life, is feeding poorly, or if the infant is vomiting. Sampling for routine screening tests should not be performed unless there has been an adequate protein intake for a minimum of 4 days. Vomiting is a particular problem, as infants with PKU tend to vomit more frequently than normal infants. Testing should be repeated several weeks later.

In children with neurological or developmental problems, no reliance should be placed on the fact that a screening test has been performed or on its presumed normality.
REF. Yu JS, et al.: False Negative Screening Tests in Phenylketonuria. Archives of Disease in Children 46:1, 124-125, 1971.

279. Q. What are the basic genetic principles in determining hereditary risk?

A. The simple types of inheritance are autosomal dominant and recessive and X-linked dominant and recessive.

Autosomal Recessive Inheritance - in order to be affected by a disease the individual must receive 2 genes, one from each parent, i.e. he must be homozygous. Both parents contribute a gene and may be normal i.e., heterozygous, or affected themselves i.e. homozygous. At each conception there is a constant 25% risk of the offspring being homozygous and affected if both parents are heterozygous. The risk is 50% at each conception for heterozygous offspring and 25% for normal offspring.

Autosomal Dominant Inheritance - in order to be affected an individual has only to be heterozygous. He need receive the disease producing gene from only one parent. One parent will be affected and the risk of producing the disease in an offspring is 50% for each conception. Diseases produced by autosomal dominance are rare.

X-Linked Inheritance - genes located on the X-chromosome cause X-linked conditions. Since males have only one X-chromosome, they are neither heterozygous nor homozygous. Since females have 2 X-chromosomes, they can be homozygous or heterozygous carriers. A male therefore cannot transmit X-linked genes to his sons, but can transmit them to all of his daughters. Females can transmit X-linked genes to sons or daughters.

X-Linked Recessive Inheritance - this is a rare type of inheritance in which only males in the maternal line are affected. Since males have only one X-chromosome, a single disease producing X-linked gene will produce the disease. The X-linked gene of an affected male must come from his mother. Since the father does not carry the X-linked disease no daughters will be affected, but the risk is 50% that they will be carriers.
REF. Watson W, M.D., Cann H, M.D.: Genetic Counseling in Dermatology. Pediatric Clinics of North America 18:3, 757-771, 1971.

280. Q. What is the significance of an XYY complement in males?

A. According to studies that have been carried out, the XYY complement increases the risk of a male engaging in anti-social behavior.

In infancy these children appear normal; many exceed the norm in length and/or height. Intelligence ranges from normal to retarded; most have subnormal intelligence.

Later in childhood and into adulthood these males are irresponsible, and unaware of the future consequences of their behavior. They are unable to tolerate frustration and have few constructive or realistic goals.

It appears that the XYY chromosome complement, which is inborn and permanent, may cause permanent and inborn behavior disorders.
REF. Valetine GH.: The YY Chromosome Complement--What Does It Mean? Clinical Pediatrics 8:350-355, June 1969.

281. Q. How can one detect Klinefelter's syndrome (XXY)?

A. Klinefelter's syndrome (XXY) is second in frequency to Down's syndrome occurring in about 1.7 per 1000 newborn males. However, because of its characteristic findings it is usually not detected until adolescence. Since these individuals generally do not produce sufficient androgens, it would be desirable to diagnoses them during childhood to begin testosterone replacement. Clinical clues to detection fall into three general categories:

(1) Psychosocial problems - dull mentality (I.Q. above 50) and behavioral and personality problems are common. Problems noted in these children are usually aggravated by school entrance and may include nervousness, excessive shyness, immaturity, lack of self-confidence, intermittent aggressiveness, and antisocial acts. Such situations in addition to learning difficulties should lead to the consideration of XXY syndrome.

(2) Body habitus - these boys tend to be slim, underweight for height, with relatively long extremities in proportion to the trunk.

(3) External genitalia - the testes and phallus tend to be small, and do not mature during puberty. The phallus, in addition to its small size, may also be incompletely formed with some degree of hypospadias. Cryptorchidism is not unusual. Infertility is common due to the testosterone deficiency.

Early diagnosis is essential in order to provide age appropriate hormone replacement, which should insure more normative adolescent growth, prevent gynecomastia, and retard behavioral maladjustment.

REF. Caldwell P, Smith D.: The XXY (Klinefelter's) Syndrome in Childhood: Detection and Treatment. Journal of Pediatrics 80:2, 250-258, Feb. 1972.

282. Q. What anomalies characterize Turner's (XO) syndrome?

A. Turner's syndrome is a chromosomal anomaly of absence of one chromosome, the remaining one always being an X, so that the total chromosome number is 45 (44+XO). There are many variants of this disorder such as mosaicism of XX/XO. Two outstanding symptoms of Turner's syndrome are absence of the ovaries (gonadal dysgenesis or agenesis) and short stature. These may be associated with other anomalies such as webbed neck, webbed fingers and toes, small receding chin, pigmented moles, epicanthal folds, heart or kidney defects, or hearing loss. Although mental functioning is ordinarily normal, there are usually deficits in space-form perception, directional sense, and motor coordination. One unusual characteristic of this syndrome is the females' unusual capacity to deal with stress and adversity, often leaving them well adjusted to their physical condition. They tend to be very feminine and maternal in their play.

One special problem arises with these girls - the problem of sterility. The author strongly believes that the child should know early about her inability to become pregnant, and the importance placed on other means of having a family, such as adoption. He feels that if the disclosure is made in a positive manner that the ideal of parenthood and normalcy is left intact.

REF. Money J.: Sex Errors of the Body. Johns Hopkins Press, Baltimore, 1968, pp. 19-21.

283.  Q. What is the significance of a single palmar crease?

A. The single palmar crease is frequently found among prematures, stillborns, dying neonates, infants with congenital anomalies and babies whose mothers have had complicated pregnancies.

Palmar crease studies were done on 276 children who attended a Child Development Clinic. Notes were made of the occurrence of single palmar lines. Among the experimental group, 31 had a palmar crease. Sixteen of them had borderline or low intellectual ability, sixteen of the 31 also had congenital anomalies.

The author postulates that "palmar hand creases suggest some insult to fetus during the first trimester." Thus the insult might have also caused the intellectual impairment and congenital anomaly. REF. Johnson CF, Opitz E.: The Single Palmar Crease and Its Clinical Significance in Child Development. Clinical Pediatrics 10:392-403, July 1971.

284.  Q. What role does heredity play in families with allergy?

A. Because of the high prevalence rates of allergic disorders such as asthma, eczema, hay fever or contact dermatitis, the prevailing opinion is that heredity is a significant factor in the etiology of allergic disease. The results of this study indicate that the hereditary component may be less pronounced than has been generally stated, but occurs with sufficient frequency to warrant genetic counseling. Results included the following:

(1) individuals with asthma or eczema have a 2 to 3.5 times greater chance of developing an additional allergy,
(2) first degree relatives have a 3.3 fold increased risk of having asthma if the patient has asthma and either eczema or hay fever; the risk is decreased to 1.5 to 2 times if only one allergy is present,
(3) if a parent has a severe allergy, the chance of the siblings developing an allergy is about half the risk of a recessively inherited disorder.
REF. Lubs M.: Empiric Risks for Genetic Counseling in Families with Allergy. Journal of Pediatrics 80:1, 26-31, Jan. 1972.

285.  Q. What is Cornelia deLange syndrome?

A. This syndrome is characterized by (1) pre and post natal growth retardation with mental impairment, (2) a characteristic appearance of the facies, (3) hypoplastic limbs with syndactyly, oligodactyly or phocomelia, (4) congenital malformations of the heart, usually septal defects and the G.I. tract, stenosis, malrotation, atresia, especially of the small bowels. These anomalies often lead to an early death. The etiology of the disorder is obscure and has not proven to arise from any currently detectable chromosomal anomaly. The characteristic features of CdL syndrome may be difficult to diagnose at birth.

REF. Passarge E, et al.: Cornelia deLange Syndrome: Evolution of the Phenotype. Pediatrics 48:5, 833-836, 1971.

286. Q. What are the causes of increased intracranial pressure in children?

A. There are many disorders that can cause increased intracranial pressure in childhood, however the most frequent causes are hydrocephalus and intracranial lesions such as tumors, brain abcess or chronic subdural hematoma. In the newborn increased intracranial pressure is usually the result of congenital hydrocephalus or a traumatic birth complication resulting in intracranial hemorrhage. In early infancy the most common causes of increased intracranial pressure include hydrocephalus, subdural hematoma, brain tumor and central nervous system infection such as meningitis or encephalitis. In later childhood head trauma or vascular disorders can account for increased intracranial pressure and in adolescence additional causes include infections and brain tumors.

REF. Rosman PN, M.D.: Increased Intracranial Pressure in Childhood. Pediatric Clinics of North America 21:2, 483-499, 1974.

287. Q. What are the signs and symptoms of increased intracranial pressure?

A. Headache is present in most children with increased intracranial pressure, although toddlers may express only increased irritability or anorexia. It is frequently most pronounced in the morning and tends to become worse upon coughing, sneezing, straining at stool or sudden changes in head position.

Vomiting often associated with nausea is frequently a sign and may occur at first in the mornings and then later at any time of day.

Personality changes are frequently a sign of increased intracranial pressure. Irritability, argumentativeness, apathy or depression may be apparent. Mood changes are common and children may be drowsy, fatigued and have memory loss.

Head circumference may increase and excessive head growth can be seen up to 3 years of age. Closure of the anterior fontanel may be delayed beyond 18 months and separation of cranial sutures can be seen in children up to 10 years of age.

Double vision may be noted by the child or may be manifested by the sudden appearance of strabismus.

Papilledema which is usually bilateral is probably the most reliable sign of increased intracranial pressure. Visual acuity may be normal.

Vital signs are altered with slowing of respirations, decrease in pulse rate and increase in systolic pressure.

If intracranial pressure increase progresses, herniation of intracranial structures, specifically temporal lobe herniation into the tentorial notch. This herniation can cause a sudden worsening of symptoms and result in coma and fatal hemorrhages with respiratory or cardiac arrest.
REF. Rosman PN, M.D.: Increased Intracranial Pressure in Childhood. Pediatric Clinics of North America 21:2, 483-499, 1974.

288. Q. What is the treatment of increased intracranial pressure?

A. If possible the cause of the increased intracranial pressure should be treated directly. An adequate airway should be maintained and respirations assisted if necessary. Medical treatment with such agents as mannitol and urea is indicated because of rapid action, however, on a long term basis they disturb fluid and electrolyte balance. For longer treatment corticosteroids may be effective. Hypothermia is helpful as a therapeutic adjunct as is passive hyperventilation, in all cases of increased intracranial pressure. Occasionally lumbar puncture is of value and ventricular drainage can dramatically relieve marked elevations of pressure. Seizures if present should be treated with anticonvulsants.
REF. Rosman PN, M.D.: Increased Intracranial Pressure in Childhood. Pediatric Clinics of North America 21:2, 483-499, 1974.

289. Q. What is benign intracranial hypertension?

A. This is a syndrome of raised intracranial pressure in the absence of space-occupying lesion or obstruction to the cerebrospinal fluid pathways. It is manifested by headache, papilledema, sixth nerve palsies, sometimes vomiting and absence of other neurologic signs, earache, blurred or double vision. Though most common in young adult women, it occurs in childhood.

Some patients have been identified as having "silent lateral or longitudinal sinus thrombosis". Infections or slight head injuries have been blamed.

Otitis media was the most common single etiological factor to be associated with the syndrome. Other factors incriminated in producing the symptom are:

(1) Drugs: tetracycline, chlortetracycline, nalidixic acid, steroid hormones when withdrawn or diminished, vitamin A in excess or deficiency
(2) Addison's disease

(3) Iron deficiency anemia
(4) Pernicious anemia
(5) Hypocalcemia
REF. Grant DN.: Benign Intracranial Hypertension. Archives of Disease in Childhood 46:249, 651-655, 1971.

290. Q. What is the importance of benign intracranial hypertension?

A. (1) In establishing the diagnosis, concern with ruling out a space-occupying lesion which is more likely to be the explanation of the signs of raised intracranial pressure in a child even in the absence of localizing neurological signs. Diagnosis must still be made by exclusion.

(2) Concern appears to be to ensure that long-continued raised intracranial pressure does not damage the eyesight. There is the risk of permanent damage to vision from persistent papilloedema.

(3) The condition is of theoretical interest in that there is presumably some underlying process common to the various etiological types of benign intracranial hypertension.
REF. Grant DN.: Benign Intracranial Hypertension. Archives of Disease in Childhood 46:249, 651-655, 1971.

291. Q. What observations should be made following head injuries in children?

A. Since accidents are the leading cause of death in children over one year of age, it is imperative that nurses know what signs should alert them to cerebral damage from a head injury. Because cerebral edema usually does not develop early, clinical signs may become evident during the 24 hour period following the injury, necessitating frequent assessment of the patient's behavior and vital signs.

The single most important observation is level of consciousness. Arousing a child from sleep, looking for signs of drowsiness, and assessing degree of alertness are part of the evaluation for level of consciousness. Increasing irritability, as well as lethargy, is a sign of increasing intracranial pressure in children.

Headache, vertigo, or vomiting may suggest cerebral damage. Young children may demonstrate a headache through restless irritability, or fussiness interspersed with periods of comfort. Vertigo is observed when a child assumes one position and vigorously opposes being moved. If forcibly repositioned, he may vomit and show spontaneous nystagmus of the eyes. Vomiting is usually projectile and not associated with feeding.

Vital signs may also change depending on the area of the brain involved. If pressure is placed upon the brainstem, vital signs will be irregular, and respiratory-cardiac arrest could occur. Pressure on the hypothalamus will cause temperation variations, usually elevations.

Pupil size, reaction to light, and accommodation are valuable indices of increasing intracranial pressure. The appearance of a unilateral dilated pupil later in the course of recovery could represent a space-consuming lesion which is causing the brain to shift across the midline and herniate through the tentorium.

Observation for hemiplegia, hemiparesis, seizures, sensory or proprioceptive loss and altered reflexes such as the Babinski can alert a nurse to impending danger from head injury.
REF. Reeves K.: Children's Reactions to Head Injuries. American Journal of Nursing 70:1, Jan. 1970.

292. Q. What is the present prognosis for a child with myelomeningocele?

A. With the advent of comprehensive care of the child with spina bifida with meningomyelocele, the mortality rate has decreased from 90% to 30%. Many factors have contributed to this improved prognosis.

Early surgery on the neonate with meningomyelocele has been a contributory factor. In addition, general management of these children has improved.

The most common complication of meningomyelocele is hydrocephalus. With the introduction of the Holter valve bypass system, the survival of the spina bifida child has improved.

In addition, improved bladder function tests have contributed to a decrease in renal complications. Many deaths that occur are caused by progressive renal damage.

Equally as important, attention has been paid to guiding the child to utilize his innate resources. This has contributed significantly to better use of his functions physically and emotionally.
REF. Zachary RB.: The Improving Prognosis in Spina Bifida. Clinical Pediatrics 11:11-14, Jan. 1972.

293. Q. What guidelines can nurses offer parents of a neurologically handicapped child?

A. The author of this article offers suggestions for nurses on how to help parents of a neurologically handicapped child based on her own experiences with a minimally brain damaged son. Some of her suggestions include:

(1) The hyperactive child needs plenty of rest and sleep, overstimulation during rest periods such as toys or brightly colored objects, even wallpaper should be avoided.

(2) Discipline is usually a problem because these children are easily frustrated, angered, and subject to temper tantrums. Firmness and consistency are essential in limit setting. Avoid giving choices such as "What do you want for lunch?" Rather, give a choice between two foods.

(3) These children lose control easily, especially when overstimulated. Therefore, group play is better avoided in favor of play with one or two other children.

(4) Teaching is best done through play and should emphasize coordination, especially fine motor and hand-eye coordination, perceptual abilities, and his self-image.

(5) Balance and coordination can be improved by using a walking board. The concept of right and left, backwards and forwards, up and down can be developed through games such as "Simon says". Hand-eye coordination can be improved by picking up popcorn one at a time and putting them in a narrow top container, by shuffling cards and fanning them out, and by coloring, cutting out, and pasting.

(6) Mathematical concepts can be learned by cutting an orange in half and putting it back together to demonstrate fractions. Following a recipe can teach concept of measurement and give the satisfaction of achievement.

(7) These children need the feeling of success. Parents should try to keep failures at a minimum. This may mean curtailing involvement in competitive sports.
REF. Bierbauer E.: Tips for Parents of a Neurologically Handicapped Child. American Journal of Nursing 72:10, 1873-1874, Oct. 1972.

294. Q. What type of shunts may be done to help alleviate hydrocephalus in a child?

A. Hydrocephalus is a pathological condition of increased cerebral spinal fluid because of failure of reabsorption of the fluid from the cerebral subarachnoid space (communicating type) or because of blockage of fluid somewhere within the ventricular system (non-communicating type). Congenital hydrocephalus causes the ventricles to enlarge, as well as the skull because the sutures are still open. Signs of increased intracranial pressure include bulging fontanels, dilated scalp veins, "sunset eyes" (sclera is visible above the iris), internal rotation and bulging of the eyes, papilledema, and lethargy and irritability. The infant may also have projectile vomiting that is not associated with feeding.

Several procedures can be done to treat hydrocephalus. If a subdural hematoma or brain tumor is present, surgery is aimed at removing the cause. In congenital hydrocephalus where no treatable cause is evident, shunting procedures are done to alleviate the build-up of fluid. The most common shunts are the ventriculo-atrial and the ventriculo-peritoneal, although ventriculo-ureteral, lumbo-ureteral, and lumbo-peritoneal shunts may also be done. In a ureteral type shunt, a kidney is removed and cerebrospinal fluid is drained into the bladder via the ureter. Since cerebrospinal fluid is excreted rather than reabsorbed, electrolyte imbalance can result. (Normally, 350-500 cc. of fluid are produced every 24 hours and reabsorbed into the circulation).

In the ventriculo-atrial shunt, a catheter is inserted through a burr hole over the occipital-parietal area of the skull, threaded through a facial vein, into the internal jugular veins to the superior vena cava, and into the right atrium. A one-way valve presents backflow of blood and spinal fluid into the ventricles.

In the ventriculo-peritoneal shunt, a catheter is threaded from the lateral ventricle, subcutaneously to the peritoneal cavity where it is sutured in place. In the last two shunting procedures, fluid is reabsorbed rather than excreted.

Long-term prognosis is still doubtful because of the relative newness of the procedure. Often, as the child grows shunting revisions are necessary to elongate the tubing or repair a valve.
REF. Braney ML.: The Child with Hydrocephalus. American Journal of Nursing 73:5, 828-831, May 1973.

295. Q. What nursing intervention is involved in the care of a child with hydrocephalus?

A. When a child has hydrocephalus, frequently the head is enlarged and the skin taut and friable. Prevention of infection and damage to the spinal cord necessitate careful handling with support to the neck and head, frequent positioning to prevent decubiti, and good skin care to maintain integrity. Both after and before surgery, the child needs to be watched for signs of increasing intracranial pressure. Analgesics and sedatives are usually avoided because they can mask signs of lethargy and irritability.

Immediately post-operatively, the child is kept flat in bed for up to two to four days to prevent a subdural hematoma and sudden loss of cerebral spinal fluid. He is kept quiet, and handling is kept to a minimum. The valve is checked frequently, and pumped by the nurse to relieve pressure. Since infection of the nervous system can occur, the nurse needs to carefully observe for signs of meningitis, increased temperature, and local swelling, tenderness and redness along the shunt tract.

One big area of nursing intervention aside from the physical care is preparation of the parents for the surgery and care at home. Parents are usually frightened and need information about the nervous system and effects on the brain. They need to understand the mechanics of the shunt and valve, and how to check for potency at home. Awareness of the signs of increased intracranial pressure are essential in order to prevent brain damage. Most important, emphasis needs to be placed on the normal growth, development, and behavior of children. Often, the degree of brain damage is unknown until the child is older, but parents need to encourage learning and skills in light of the child's potential.

REF. Braney M.: The Child with Hydrocephalus. American Journal of Nursing 73:5, 828-831, May 1973.

296. Q. What are the long term effects of neonatal jaundice on brain function?

A. Neonatal icterus may not be fatal but may leave neurological sequelae. A continuum of damage ranging from serious sequelae, such as cerebral palsy, to minor intellectual impairment has been demonstrated. These sequelae are most likely to occur in hemolytic jaundice when the serum bilirubin levels have risen to high values. Kernicterus may also occur at quite low levels of serum bilirubin in low birth weight infants. Thirty children of low birth weight and bilirubin levels above 20 mg/100 ml were followed for periods of from 4 to 11 years. I.Q. scores were found to be lower in the more severely jaundiced group, but the differences were not significant. The group also had a significantly higher incidence of mental retardation (I.Q. below 70). The authors concluded that nonhemolytic jaundice per se had probably small effect on the ultimate I.Q. of low birth weight babies.

REF. Chrichton J, et al.: Long Term Effects of Neonatal Jaundice on Brain Function in Children of Low Birth Weight. Pediatrics 49:5, 656-668, 1972.

297. Q. Is there any relationship between the motor development of children with congenital rubella and gestational age of maternal rubella?

A. In a study of 43 children ages 3-4 1/2 years with hearing loss as a result of maternal rubella, eleven categories of motor skills were tested. The most significant finding was between the severity of motor deficit and the gestational age at which the rubella infection had occurred. Infection during the first four weeks of pregnancy produced the most severe multiple defects and serious motor deficits. These are considerably reduced if infection occurs after the eighth week. A frequent finding in children whose mother had rubella between the 5th and 8th weeks of gestation was defects in equilibrium. These children were also deaf, and the study suggests that damage to structures of the inner ear, also affects equilibrium.

The relationships between motor abilities and gestational age of maternal infection, supports the hypothesis that motor defects in children with congenital rubella can be attributed to damage at specific stages of embryologic development. This damage occurs when the most important structures involved in a particular motor activity are in the most crucial stages of organization and differentiation.
REF. Zausmer E, M.D.: Congenital Rubella: Pathogenesis of Motor Defecits. Pediatrics 47:1, 16-25, 1971.

298. Q. Can diazepam be safely used in the treatment of status epilepticus in infants and children?

A. Status epilepticus, meaning either continuous convulsions with unconsciousness or serial epileptic attacks, between which there is no return to consciousness, is always a serious and potentially fatal emergency. Infants and young children have a lower convulsive threshold than adults. There is a possible relation between infantile status epilepticus and the subsequent development of temporal lobe epilepsy.

In a study of 37 infants and children prompt and lasting control of the seizures in 18 cases followed a single usually intramuscular injection of diazepam. In 9 cases more than one injection was required. In 8 cases other anticonvulsants had been given, often before admission to hospital.

Eight patients died, 2 of whom had diabetes mellitus, though there was no evidence that diazepam was responsible, but caution is urged regarding the use of the drug in similar circumstances. One case of reversible respiratory depression occurred after the use of the drug in a hypoxic infant.

Based on the above observations parenteral diazepam is an effective and safe anticonvulsant for the treatment of status epilepticus in infants and young children, and the view that this is a "first choice" drug is supported.
REF. McMorris C, McWilliam PKA.: Status Epilepticus in Infants and Young Children Treated with Parenteral Diazepam. Archives of Disease in Childhood 44:237, 604-611, 1969.

299. Q. What is the method used in rehabilitative "patterning"?

A. "Patterning" is a method advanced by Doman and Delacato for the rehabilitation of children with neuromuscular disorders, behavior abnormalities, learning disabilities and subnormal mentality.

Treatment Program 1 - recommended for non-walking children, requires that the patient spend most of the day on the floor in prone position, where creeping and crawling are encouraged.

Treatment Program 2 - is for patients unable to actively engage in the specific patterns of activity. In these patients the patterns are imposed by passive manipulation of the limbs by others. This passive manipulation is regarded as imposing "patterning" on the CNS. The procedure requires 3-5 adults who manipulate the right arm and leg, left arm and leg and the head in a precise smooth and rhythmic sequence. This is done for at least 5 minutes, 4 times a day, 7 days a week. After instruction by therapists these procedures can be carried out by family and friends. The patterning procedures are supplemented by sensory stimulation, breathing exercises, and a plan of restriction and facilitation designed to foster hemispheric dominance. Although great success has been claimed for the method, further data are required to justify affirmative conclusions about this system of treatment.

REF. Cohen H, M.D., et al.: Some Considerations for Evaluating the Doman-Delacata "Patterning" Method. Pediatrics 45:2, 302-313, 1970.

300. Q. What is Tay-Sachs disease?

A. Tay-Sachs disease is a neurodegenerative disorder caused by progressive lipid-storage in neurons. The child begins to show reversed motion and mental development at four to six months of age. This is associated with progressive muscle weakness, a pronounced "startle reaction" to sound, gradual onset of cranial enlargement with blindness and seizure activity and finally death. The disease itself is recessive genetic in nature.

A fluorometric assay can be used to detect heterozygous carriers among healthy non-pregnant persons and affected fetuses.

REF. Jackson LG.: Heterozygote Detection for Autosomal Recessive Genetic Diseases. Clinical Pediatrics 13:307-309, April 1974.

301. Q. Of what importance is the finding of the defect called "asymmetric crying facies"?

A. "Asymmetric crying facies" is a defect resulting from partial paralysis on the contralateral side of the seventh nerve. It is only evident when the infant cries, not when he is smiling or suckling. Drooling is absent because the muscles affected act only to depress the lower lip margin. Because of these factors, this sign can go unnoticed, and if observed, can be given little importance.

However, several investigators have called attention to the relationship between this relatively benign defect and other more severe defects, namely congenital heart anomalies, hence the term "cardiofacial syndrome". These authors have found that other defects of the musculoskeletal, genitourinary, and respiratory system are common. Some of the cardiac defects included ventricular septal defect, atrial septal defect, patent ductus arteriosus, tetralogy of Fallot, aortic insufficiency, preductal coarctation, and others. Low-set and malformed ears, and cleft lip or palate of varying degrees were present. Musculoskeletal defects included abnormalities of toes, hip and vertebrae. Gastrointestinal abnormalities were imperforate anus, anal stenosis and pharyngoesophageal dyskinesia. Genitourinary anomalies included hydrocele, undescended testes, and hypoplastic kidney. The respiratory system was affected by absent lobes, abnormal vessels, and stenosis of bronchus. Central nervous system problems included some degree of retardation and convulsion.

The above is not a complete list, but it does serve to emphasize the need for excellent physical assessment. One other outstanding finding was the marked tendency for one-sided defects to occur predominately on the side of the partial facial paralysis.
REF. Pape K, Pickering D.: Asymmetric Crying Facies: An Index of Other Congenital Anomalies. Journal of Pediatrics 81:1, 21-30, July 1972.

302. Q. How does one learn to live with multiple sclerosis?

A. Multiple sclerosis is a progressively crippling, and incapacitating disease which affects the central nervous system. It affects both sexes, who are between the ages of 20 and 40 years. The progressive demyelination of the nerve fibers of the brain and spinal cord inhibits impulses from reaching brain centers. Progressive paralysis can occur anywhere, such as in the extremities, respiratory muscles, or facial and speech muscles. The disease is one of exarcerbations and remissions.

The author of the article speaks of her acceptance and adjustment to M.S. Her first reaction was denial of the diagnosis. As reality took hold, pessimism set in. She felt sorry for herself, blamed everything that went wrong on the disease, and was immobilized by fear. Gradually, she began to live with the disturbing symptoms of tremors of the hands and visual problems and to accept a daily routine of activity and sufficient, frequent rest periods. She learned to avoid hurried or anxiety-producing situations, which could cause an exacerbation of symptoms. One of her concerns was marriage and pregnancy, but her physician assured her that she could plan for both. Considering the age group for M.S., it is no wonder that a young man or woman would have such concerns about their future. The author feels that the goal for every patient should be to live life to its fullest potential.
REF. Jontz DL.: Prescription for Living with M.S. American Journal of Nursing 73:5, 817-818, May 1973.

303. Q. What is narcolepsy, and what are its implications for nurses?

A. Narcolepsy is a disorder characterized by an uncontrollable desire to sleep. This somnolence may occur at any time, even while standing or talking. Physical abnormalities are lacking in primary narcolepsy and laboratory studies on blood (e.g. blood gases and blood sugar), endocrine system, and sleep pattern are normal. Cataplexic attacks may occur with strong emotion or excessive fatigue. Diagnosis is made solely on symptoms and response to medications (agrypnotic drugs such as amphetamine, methylphenidate (Ritalin), or pipradol (Meratram).

Nurses play a unique role here, because this disorder can frequently go undetected when the parents' complaints about their child are such terms as "day-dreamer", "lazy and unambitious", "poor performance in school". A health assessment on patterns of sleep is essential, with such questions as "Do you fall asleep in spite of interesting activities?", "Do you have an irresistible urge to sleep, such as when standing up?", etc. Physical assessment can include a pupillogram; for example, alert persons have large stable pupils in total darkness, whereas narcoleptics will have small pupils when they appear awake, but are asleep. Another very important aspect of this disorder is helping parents and the child understand the illness, particularly since it sounds like "epilepsy", but has no association with it. Often, parents viewed the sleepiness as an "escape mechanism" and now need to realize this is an illness. Because the treatment of narcolepsy is a definite medication regime, parents and child need to understand the need for the drugs, especially since this disorder continues throughout most of adult life, the correct time schedule for drugs so that nocturnal sleep patterns are uninterrupted, and the side effects of the various medications. Often, the agrypnotics cause weight loss which necessitates a recalculation of dosage per body weight.

REF. Leidig R.: Narcolepsy: Jody's Story. American Journal of Nursing 73:3, 491-493, March 1973.

304. Q. What steps can be taken when carrying out a pediatric nutritional assessment?

A. Good nutrition during infancy and childhood is vital for normal growth and development. Determination of nutritional status among children and infants can be assessed. Utilization of background medical history which includes any variables that would interfere with assimilation and/or utilization of nutrients is essential information. Anthropometric data are important indices of nutritional status. This should be serially plotted on a graph on the basis of information obtained from the available data, the following steps can be taken in carrying out a nutritional assessment:

(1) State the questions which relate to the nutritional assessment.
(2) Decide upon the level of approach to be employed in asking questions.
(3) Employ necessary team for meeting objectives.
(4) Evaluate sub-samples of groups when appropriate and everyone when necessary.
(5) Develop practical solutions based upon the evaluation.
(6) Plan procedures for collecting specific data.

REF. Nutritional Status of the Infant and Child. American Journal of Public Health-Supplement 63:38, Nov. 1973.

305. Q. Can nutritional inadequacy be evaluated by laboratory tests?

A. Evaluation of nutritional status by laboratory methods utilize biochemical tests to measure levels of nutrients in blood or urine. In addition, certain biochemical functions which are dependent upon adequate supply of adequate nutrients can be evaluated. Laboratory tests can determine deficiencies in:

(1) Serum protein
(2) Blood forming nutrients: iron, folacin
(3) Water-soluble vitamins: thiamine, riboflavin, niacin, and vitamin $B_{12}$
(4) Fat-soluble vitamins: A, D, E, K
(5) Minerals: iron, iodine, and other trace elements
(6) Blood lipid levels: cholesterol and triglycerides, glucose and various enzymes.

REF. Laboratory Assessment of Nutritional Status. American Journal of Public Health Supplement 63:28, Nov. 1973.

306. Q. What are the caloric and water requirements of newborn infants?

A. The caloric requirements of infants is based on the number of calories available to the infant on breast milk and is set at 110 to 130 calories per kg. The minimal daily water requirement necessary to protect a full term infant from dehydration is 75-90 ml. per kg. Most infants greatly exceed this requirement. Mother's milk, cow's milk and formulas contain 20 calories per ounce (0.67 calories per ml ) and to approximate the caloric requirement of 110-130 calories per kg, most infants take in fluid levels of 150-200 ml per kg. per day.

REF. Davidson M, M.D.: Formula Feeding of Normal Term and Low Birth Weight Infants. Pediatric Clinics of North America 17:4, 913-927, 1970.

307. Q. Are caloric and water requirements for low birth weight infants different from normal term infants?

A. Low birth weight infants require a caloric intake of 120-130 calories per kg. in order to have sufficient calories for resting metabolic needs, physical activity expenditure, losses occurring during feedings and for growth requirements. The suggested daily water intake is 130-150 ml. per kg. In order to meet caloric requirements with these fluid volumes formulas with greater caloric concentrations than for normal newborns are necessary. A level of 24 calories per ounce (0.8 calories per ml.) is used in many nurseries. Concentrations as high as 1.1 calories per ml. are tolerated satisfactorily, but beyond these levels infants may develop fever, anorexia, diarrhea and dehydration.

REF. Davidson M, M.D.: Formula Feeding of Normal Term and Low Birth Weight Infants. Pediatric Clinics of North America 17:4, 913-927, 1970.

308. Q. What is the current feeling in regard to feeding infants commercial formulas fortified with iron?

A. The Committee on Nutrition of the American Academy of Pediatrics strongly recommends that when commercial formulas are prescribed, that iron-supplemented formulas be the standard rather than the exception. The use of these formulas is advocated to prevent iron deficiency anemia. The Committee is aware that only a small percentage of American babies are fed formulas after 6 months of age. Whole milk is usually substituted at this time. Whole and evaporated milks are not fortified with iron and therefore the infant receives less iron when his iron needs are greatest. It is recommended that a program of public education should be launched to convince American parents of the infants need for dietary iron. The Committee recommends that iron-fortified formulas be continued for as long as an infant is bottle fed. Thereafter the same iron-fortified formula should be used from the cup along with solid foods until the infant is at least 12 months of age. It is further recommended that iron-fortified whole and evaporated milk should be made available for infant feeding. The Committee on Nutrition feels that the problem of iron deficiency anemia can be combatted by the use of iron-fortified formulas.
REF. Committee on Nutrition: Iron Fortified Formulas. Pediatrics 47:4, 786, 1971.

309. Q. What factors should be considered in determining when to introduce solid food to infants?

A. The factors to consider in introducing solid foods to infants are physiological, developmental, nutritional, practical and psychological.

Physiologic - the digestive enzymes of the stomach are present from the 5th month of fetal life, however liver enzymes, especially lipase and amylase may be inadequate until the 4th or 5th postnatal month and complex carbohydrate digestion may be inefficient until that time. Proteins are absorbed more easily than fats for the first 3 weeks of life.

Developmental - the average age for acceptance of solid foods may be as follows: 2 1/2-3 1/2 months - cereal, 2 1/2-3 months - fruit, 4-4 1/2 months - vegetable, 5 1/2-6 months - meat. At 6-7 months "finger foods" which can be chewed can be introduced, and between 9-12 months the child is ready for transition from "junior" food to table food.

Nutritional - some researchers are questioning the desirability of too early feeding of solid foods. Solids with inferior nutritional content may satiate the infant causing refusal of milk. Sodium in prepared infant foods may predispose to later hypertension. There may be a relationship between early feeding of solids and the development of obesity. Also, food allergies are greatest in infancy.

Practical - baby food is more expensive than formula and extra time is required to feed solids to young infants.

Psychological - the mother's attitude affects the infant's acceptance of various foods. Fat may be associated with healthy and parents encourage babies to finish the bottle or clean the plate. Infants show a readiness to feed themselves in the first year of life and this should be encouraged.

REF. Ishida M, M.S., et al.: Introducing Solid Foods to Infants. Journal of Obstetric, Gynecologic and Neonatal Nursing 2:5, 27-32, 1973.

310. Q. What guidelines can be followed concerning the introduction of solid foods in an infant's diet?

A. At birth and for the first couple of months the infant is fed formula or breastmilk. Although both contain nutrients vital to the infant's survival, they lack vitamin C and iron. Orange juice or a vitamin C supplement is usually begun early, about two weeks of age. Cereals are introduced by two to four months to help supply iron. Initially, one teaspoon of cereal mixed with formula is sufficient. At about half a year, the infant may be eating up to five tablespoons. Fruit can also be given with cereal. These foods are specially prepared for infants so that carbohydrates are broken down into simpler forms such as disaccharide or monosaccharide for easier digestion. Egg yolk is usually begun about three to five months, but egg white is delayed until about one year because of the difficulty in digesting albumin and the possibility of developing a hypersensitivity to the protein. At six months vegetables and meats are introduced; fish is usually added near the end of the first year as a substitute for egg or meat. Solid foods such as toast, zwiebach, or crackers are usually added at about six months. Some suggestions for adding new foods to the diet include:

(1) introduce one food at a time (usually one teaspoon) at intervals of 4 to 7 days to allow time for detection of an allergic response,
(2) introduce the new food when the baby is hungry, after a few sucks of milk, not after the complete formula feeding,
(3) never introduce new foods through a bottle since infants need to develop taste preferences,
(4) reduce the quantity of formula as the amount of solid foods increases to prevent too rapid weight gain.

REF. Marlow D.: Textbook of Pediatric Nursing. W.B. Saunders Company, Philadelphia, 1973, p. 309

311. Q. What are the effects of prolonged bottle feeding?

A. Dental caries in children under three are unusual. However, "baby-bottle caries" do occur among children 18 months to 4 years of age.

Typically, the child has indulged in prolonged bottle-feeding beyond the first year of life or the child still takes a bottle in order to fall asleep. When the child does fall asleep while sucking, carbohydrates in the milk or juice, pool around the teeth and stimulate caries formation. The maxillary incisors are the teeth most greatly affected. Side effects such as viral and bacterial susceptibility, decreased food intake and immature speech patterns can occur with prolonged bottle feeding.

As a preventive measure, dental care and tooth-brushing should begin at 18 months rather than 3 years. Parents must be warned about the risks involved in prolonged bottle feeding for the child.
REF. Bernick SM.: What the Pediatrician Should Know about Children's Teeth. Clinical Pediatrics 10:243-244, April 1971.

312. Q. Do children malnourished in infancy suffer from irreversible intellectual impairment?

A. A single, severe nutritional stress, such as kwashiorkor does not appear to permanently affect mental development. The hypothesis that malnutrition during infancy and childhood inhibits brain growth and subsequent intellectual development remains to be proven and further defined. Some studies have shown that nutritional retardation of brain growth can occur in the first six months of life. In the meantime, it can be postulated that severe malnutrition after 6 months of age does not in itself cause retardation, but a whole complex of environmental circumstances associated with it may produce a combined retarding effect. The authors of this study feel that in the prepubertal period permanent damage need not necessarily have been done to the growth and intellectual capacity of the malnourished child. However, fundamental to the recovery of these children is improved nutrition, as well as health maintenance and improvement of the environmental and educational situations.
REF. Hansen JDL, et al.: What Does Nutritional Growth Retardation Imply? Pediatrics 47:1, 299-311, 1971.

313. Q. Does television advertising shape children's eating habits?

A. During one week's viewing of 29 hours of children's television, 388 network commercials were run, 82% were for ingestible items. In general, the food commercials were found to be anti-nutrition. Specifically, the four food groups were poorly represented. Forty percent of the commercials were for sweetened cereals. Many commercials carried the message that only sweet foods or food products taste good. The vitamin commercials told children that vitamins will make up for poor eating habits. Even though television gives messages about food, they do not promote nutrition or healthy food habits.
REF. Gussow J.: It Makes Even Milk a Dessert. Clinical Pediatrics 12:68-71, Feb. 1973.

314. Q. Is pica in children ever considered normal behavior?

A. Pica in children as an expression of personality disturbance
is a widely held view. However, such views may be questioned in
light of observations in West Africa, which make some forms of pica
appear to be normal, or even desirable behavior. The term pica
refers to the habit of chewing, with or without swallowing, non-edible
materials. A great variety of materials may be used, but chiefly
they are woods, clay or related substances such as plaster. Pica in
West Africa, particularly the chewing of pieces of wood, appears to
be the expression of an instinctual need for something hard to chew
on. Excellent decay resistant teeth prevail wherever children are
allowed to indulge in this type of pica. The need to chew on hard substances is tolerated only during the short period of teething in our
culture. It is suggested that the need for hard chewing may extend
over long periods and not just the teething stage. This instinct may
have value in the development of sound primary and secondary den-
tition. As it becomes rudimentary or suppressed, inappropriate
materials no longer serving the original purpose may be substituted
by the child. This author feels that the answer to the pica problem
may lie in supplying suitable material, such as hickory or birch
woods, that would satisfy the need for hard chewing in early childhood.
REF. Neumann H, M.D.: Pica-Symptom or Vestigial Instinct. Pediatrics 46:3, 441-444, 1970.

315. Q. What is the optimal age for treatment of PKU with diet?

A. A study of 19 patients with PKU indicated that treatment of
PKU patients with a low phenylalanine diet after the age of 8 months
does not result in the development of normal intelligence. An additional 27 patients who were treated within the first 3 weeks of life
developed I.Q.'s that compared favorably with their siblings. Those
treated within 3-6 weeks performed slightly less well on I.Q. testing. The children who were treated at 8 months or later did not
differ in their mean I.Q. from children with PKU who had never
been treated. Treatment by 3 weeks of life is indicated.
REF. Kang ES, M.D., et al.: Results of Treatment and Termina-
tion of the Diet in Phenylketonuria. Pediatrics 46:6, 881-890, 1970.

316. Q. Is there a way to tell if a baby needs to be "burped"?

A. A simple test to determine if an air bubble is trapped in an
infant's stomach involves gentle vertical bouncing, with the infant in
a sitting position, on your knee. If the stomach is distended by an
air bubble, the oscillation of the liquid produces a thumping sound
when it compresses the air bubble. The sound is similar to the
sloshing of water in a partially filled rubber bag. The sound can be
heard, or felt with the hands on the baby's abdomen. After eructation the stomach contracts and the sound disappears. Bouncing can
detect the presence of an air bubble before it causes pain and has
the additional advantage of causing the baby to "burp" up the air bubble.

REF. Penchina C, Ph.D.: On Testing to Predict the Need for Eructation. Pediatrics 47:2, 475-476, 1971.

317. Q. What is intravenous alimentation?

A. Insufficient caloric intake may cause death in a variety of illnesses in children. In 1968, it was first demonstrated that a fat free, amino acid and glucose solution, given intravenously, could support normal growth and development. Since that time the technique has been used widely, even with very small infants. The success of I.V. alimentation depends on the use of glucose for calories and protein hydrolysate as the source of nitrogen. Special equipment is required and the infusion of this hypertonic solution is at a uniform rate into the vena cava.
REF. Filler R, M.D., Eraklis A, M.D.: Care of the Critically Ill Child: Intravenous Alimentation. Pediatrics 46:3, 456-460, 1970.

318. Q. In what instances is intravenous alimentation indicated?

A. Total I.V. alimentation is reserved for those infants and children in whom feeding via the G.I. tract is impossible, hazardous or inadequate. The lives of these children are in jeopardy due to malnutrition and dehydration. Some conditions which may require I.V. alimentation are chronic intestinal obstruction, bowel fistulae, chronic nonremitting severe diarrhea, extensive burns and abdominal tumors. The method has also been used in premature infants, uremia and hyperkalemia of acute renal failure. In some instances, such as infants with chronic intractable diarrhea, putting the G.I. tract at rest is curative and the child can be nutritionally maintained.
REF. Filler R, M.D., Eraklis A, M.D.: Care of the Critically Ill Child: Intravenous Alimentation. Pediatrics 46:3, 456-460, 1970.

319. Q. What potential complications can occur in central venous alimentation?

A. Central venous alimentation is a parenteral form of administering sufficient calories and protein to sustain life when oral or gastric feedings are contraindicated. Solutions contain hypertonic dextrose, protein hydrolysate, or amino acids, vitamins, and minerals. The solution is administered through a catheter threaded into the subclavian or internal jugular vein, and advanced into the superior vena cava. Introduction of the catheter into a large vein allows for adequate hemodilution of the hypertonic solution.

Although the advantages of central venous alimentation are life-saving, several complications can pose potential risks:

(1) The hypertonic dextrose solution can cause hyperglycemia and metabolic acidosis from too rapid infusion rate. Signs of this complication include polyuria, increased temperature, decreased blood pressure, and disorientation. Sometimes the first indication is a

frontal headache, which may be followed by convulsions. Treatment consists of lowering the infusion rate and administering insulin.

(2) Hypoglycemic reactions can occur if insulin has been administered regularly, and suddenly the infusion is stopped. This can be prevented by gradually decreasing insulin and the hypertonic solution.

(3) Nausea, diarrhea, and vomiting can occur when excess of tolerance has been reached. Pure amino acid solutions rather than protein hydrolysate cause less gastric upset.

(4) Sepsis from contamination of the solution and catheter lines is a severe risk, especially since the preparation provides a rich culture media for organisms. Excellent sterile technique is needed to prevent contamination. Piggyback set ups should not be used for administering medications or for central venous pressure.

(5) Air emboli is a potential risk whenever the tubing is disconnected. Air should be removed by milking the bubble back toward the bottle, rather than by disconnecting the tubing.

(6) Pneumothorax can result from puncturing the apex of the lung while attempting to locate the subclavian vein. In small children, diminished breath sounds on the affected side may be the only sign of pneumothorax. Other symptoms present include severe back and chest pain, dyspnea, and cough.

(7) Hypervolemia is always a complication in small children whose fluid requirement must be accurately calculated. Cardiac and renal problems may further enhance the risk of fluid overload.
REF. Parsa M, et al.: Central Venous Alimentation. American Journal of Nursing 72:11, 2042-2047, Nov. 1972.

320. Q. What can be done to minimize systemic infection during complete parenteral alimentation of small infants?

A. Using intravenous alimentation increases the risk of septicemia greatly. Under general anesthesia in the operating room venous silastic catheters were introduced into the right atrium over an internal jugular vein and exited 5 cm. or more away onto the scalp behind the ear.

The basic solution in a plastic administration set was used without a connected venting tube. A 0.22mm milk pore filter was inserted immediately proximal to the central venous catheter, to act as a final barrier to particulate matter and micro-organisms before the solution entered patient's blood stream.

A constant rate infusion pump is essential to control within narrow limits the volume of fluid administered. Over-transfusion of such hypertonic solutions carries a very great risk from osmotic overload. Using fat-free parenteral feeding reduces catheter interconnections to a minimum. Junctions within the present feeding regimen were sprayed with antibiotic aerosols containing neomycin, polymycin, and bacitracin whenever they were used.

Prophylactic antibiotics cannot be added to the packs of solution because of incompatibility with protein hydrolysates. Their use probably increases the risk of infection by Candida albicans - this organism is most frequently associated with intravenous feeding. C. albicans is the most frequent cause of septicemia and such systemic candidiasis has carried a 45-50% mortality rate.

In the present parenteral feeding regimen indwelling central venous catheters were maintained in site for up to 7 weeks and for a mean duration of 24 days. The overall infection rate was 9%, which is lower than previously reported.

In the two cases of septicemia experienced, the causative organism was a coagulase negative staphylococcus, the organism which most frequently colonizes ventriculoatrial shunts.

No case of C. albicans septicemia occurred. It was possible to feed a malnourished infant who had a severe deficiency of both cellular and humoral immunity for 26 days by the parenteral route without developing a systemic infection.

REF. Nelson R.: Minimizing Systemic Infection during Complete Parenteral Alimentation of Small Infants. Archives of Disease in Childhood 49:1, 16-19, 1974.

321. Q. What are the advantages of nasojejunal feeding?

A. Nasojejunal feeding is a type of nutritional replacement which bypasses the esophagus and stomach, where malabsorption might be a problem, and avoids the hazards of parenteral alimentation. In nasojejunal intubation, feedings are deposited beyond the pyloric sphincter, which prevents regurgitation of food, and into the jejunum, where rapid absorption of fluids and nutrients takes place.

The equipment required for intubation consists of a weight (usually gold) which helps direct the soft, pliable feeding tube pass the pyloric sphincter. After the tube is passed, the child is positioned on his right side for about four hours to allow the catheter to pass the pylorus. The child can be repositioned on his back or abdomen, but not on the left side. Small frequent feedings of fluids as nearly isotonic to plasma are given; hypertonic fluids can theoretically cause a "dumping syndrome".

Some advantages to this method of feeding as opposed to gavage feeding or hyperalimentation include:

(1) less chance of aspiration as compared to gavage feeding,
(2) less chance of infection because no new portal of entry is created,
(3) less trauma to the patient, immobilization not needed and repeated intubations unnecessary,

(4) presentation of greater quantity of calories without danger of gastric distention,
(5) less danger of vagal stimulation, and resulting bradycardia and arrhythmia,
(6) elimination of chance of osmotic or volume overload as seen in parenteral hyperalimentation,
(7) economic feasibility of lower formula cost as compared to intravenous preparation.
REF. Rhea J, et al.: Nasojejunal Feeding: An Improved Device and Intubation Technique. Journal of Pediatrics 82:6, 951-954, June 1973; Cheek JA, et al.: Nasojejunal Alimentation for Full-Term Newborn Infants. Journal of Pediatrics 82:6, 955-962, June 1973.

322. Q. Should nurses screen for the orthopedic problem of scoliosis in schools or clinics?

A. According to a study done on 17,000 preadolescent and adolescent males and females, undetected scoliosis is prevalent among these children. A school nurse and physical education teacher screened the students during regular physical education classes. Boys were stripped to the waist, and girls to the bra. Students were observed standing erect from the back, side, and front to detect any obvious malalignment or curvature. They were also observed bending forward, with the spine flexed to approximately 60° to detect asymmetry of the rib cage.

The overall prevalence of scoliosis in this study was 1.6%, with 1.1% among boys, and 2.1% among girls. This prevalence is consistent with reports elsewhere in the literature (.07 and 4 percent, with 80 to 90 percent of the cases occurring in preadolescent and adolescent girls).

According to these authors, this type of screening test which takes about one-half minute per student is a practical and effective way for early detecting of scoliosis.
REF. Sells C, May E.: Scoliosis Screening in Public Schools. American Journal of Nursing 74:1, 60-62, Jan. 1974.

323. Q. How can nurses help prepare parents for the home care of their child after scoliosis surgery?

A. Nurses at the Alfred I. du Pont Institute have instituted a 3 day live-in program to teach parents how to give adequate care at home, the importance of routines and detail, the effects of immobilization and bedrest on body systems, and how to make adaptations in the home for the patient. The surgery for scoliosis is a spinal fusion, with a full body cast left on for six months, followed by a plaster jacket or brace for another six months.

The actual parent teaching begins after surgery, when the cast is dry. During the first day, the mother observes the nurse, the second day, she works under supervision with the nurse, and the third day, she assumes total responsibility. The teaching program includes several phases. The mother is given written materials describing procedures, schedules, positioning, diet, and equipment. She is shown pictures of bedsores to help her understand the need for prevention. Fundamental orthopedic procedures are taught such as cast "petalling" (a method of using adhesive tape on cast edges to preserve integrity), covering the cast with plastic sheeting during elimination or shampooing, preventing small objects from becoming trapped under the cast, frequent turning, and proper positioning. Emphasis is also placed on nutrition because weight gain means discomfort, pressure sores, and interference with breathing. The effects of immobilization on the body are discussed - the need for lung expansion through deep breathing exercises, maintenance of good blood circulation especially to pressure areas through frequent turning, prevention of constipation, and the need for passive and active exercise as tolerated. The mother is also helped to understand the child's, often an adolescent female's, psychological needs. Although she should not become the center of attention, she also should be included in family activities, allowed privacy with peers, and encouraged in self-care and independency.

REF. Raynolds N.: Teaching Parents Home Care After Surgery for Scoliosis. American Journal of Nursing 74:6, 1090-1092, June 1974.

324. Q. What care is necessary for a toddler who is in a spica cast?

A. The author cites some of her own personal problems with a toddler son in a spica cast and offers these clues:

(1) The cast can be lined with disposable cotton to allow for adequate cleaning under the cast and some degree of cleaning of urine and feces.
(2) An antiseptic such as zephiran chloride 1:1000 can be used to clean the cast and prevent bacteria from urine and feces causing a foul odor.
(3) Children may not need turning on schedule because of their own creative mobility, but may need restraint from crawling out of bed. This might necessitate keeping the child in a crib covered with a protective net while he is in a spica cast.
(4) Bringing the child outdoors presents hazards such as insects crawling under the cast. Positioning in the shade is necessary to prevent sunburn. A folding nylon cot, which is portable and washable, is a good bed for the child while outdoors.

REF. Lane P.: A Mother's Confession - Home Care of a Toddler in a Spica Cast: What It's Really Like. American Journal of Nursing 71:11, 2141-2143, Nov. 1971.

325. Q. What are some reasons for the complication of fat emboli following bone fractures?

A. Fat emboli following bone fracture is not common, and their cause is unknown. Two theories are that (1) biochemical changes in the plasma caused by shock results in a breakdown of

fatty acids in the pulmonary capillaries, or (2) fat droplets enter the circulation by means of lacerated vessels in the marrow of crushed bone. These fat droplets form emboli and circulate in the blood stream until they lodge in the capillary of the lungs or brain.
REF. Patterson T, et al.: Traumatic Amputation. Nursing '72 2:11, 40-45, Nov. 1972.

326. Q. What signs can alert a nurse to the possible complication of fat emboli?

A. Usually the sumptoms of fat emboli appear within 72 hours following the trauma. A fat embolus in the lungs produces severe constant chest pain, tachycardia, dyspnea, and anxiety. Sometimes, petechiae will develop over the chest. In the brain, a fat embolus causes delirium, muscle twitches, fever, and eventually coma.
REF. Patterson T, et al.: Traumatic Amputation. Nursing '72 2:11, 40-45, Nov. 1972.

327. Q. What are some varieties of bone disease?

A. The following are "chondrodystrophies" in which there is a disturbance of endochondral ossification.

(1) Achondroplasia - an abnormality of conversion of cartilage into bone predominantly affecting the epiphyses of long bones. Epiphyseal growth is retarded and ceases early, resulting in dwarfism with short extremities but normal trunk; the head is frequently enlarged, with flattened nose; usually dominant in inheritance, but an autosomal recessive type also exists.*

(2) Thanatophoric Dwarfism - the condition is a congenital chondrodystrophy characterized by very short limbs, a relatively large head, and narrow thorax. Death occurs within a few hours.

(3) Chondro-Ectodermal Dysplasia (Ellis-VanCreveld syndrome)- dwarfism with short limbs especially distally, polydactyly, and dysplastic hair, fingernails, and teeth. Also partial harelip, congenital heart disease, and a small thorax.
*Stedman's Medical Dictionary, 22nd ed. The Williams & Wilkins Company, Baltimore, 1972.
REF. Hull D, Barnes ND.: Children with Small Chests. Archives of Disease in Childhood 47:251, 12-19, 1972.

328. Q. What is osteogenesis imperfecta?

A. Osteogenesis imperfecta is a disease which manifests itself clinically by osteoporosis, fragility of the bones often leading to skeletal deformities, lax ligaments, recurrent dislocation of joints, dental abnormalities, deafness, blue sclera and blue tympanic membranes. Most investigators have considered osteogenesis imperfecta to be a disease primarily of connective tissue. However, more recent observations suggest that many metabolic processes

may be disturbed as indicated by abnormal platelet function, increased BMR, and increased oxygen consumption of white blood cells. Clinical signs of excess sweating, hyperpyrexia, small body size and hyperkinetic circulation have also been noted. These clinical and physiological observations suggest that osteogenesis imperfecta is a disease which affects most or all tissues of the body during the prepubertal phase of life, that its progression becomes arrested at puberty and that it may be reactivated in women after menopause.
REF. Cropp G, Myers D.: Physiological Evidence of Hypermetabolism in Osteogenesis Imperfects. Pediatrics 49:3, 375-391, 1972.

329. Q. What is the etiology of slipped epiphysis of the femur?

A. In a slipped capital femoral epiphysis the actual separation between the epiphysis and the metaphysis usually takes place through the layer of hypertrophied cartilage cells adjacent to the zone of calcifying cartilage of the epiphyseal plate. The likelihood of a slipped epiphysis occurring would thus appear to depend on the strength of this layer of the epiphyseal plate and on the shearing stress to which it is exposed.

Factors which increase the risk for slipped epiphysis can be related to their tendency to weaken the layer of hypertrophied cartilage or increase shearing stress. The average age at onset is 13-14 years in boys, and 11-12 years in girls. Males are more frequently affected and there is a greater incidence among Blacks. Many children with slipped epiphysis are overweight and have slower than average skeletal maturation. Trauma is at most only a minor contributing factor. Adolescent growth spurt is felt to be a contributing factor. Though considerable progress has been made in understanding the roles of factors such as sex, age, body build and rate of skeletal maturation, more research is needed for unexplained and as yet unknown factors influencing this condition.
REF. Kelsey J, Ph.D.: Epidemiology of Slipped Capital Femoral Epiphysis: A Review of the Literature. Pediatrics 51:6, 1042-1049, 1973.

330. Q. What is arthrogryposis?

A. Arthrogryposis multiplex congenita or AMC is a syndrome characterized by contractures of joints present at birth which are persistent. Some authorities have demonstrated a hereditary factor in which the disease is inherited as an autosomal recessive. Flexion contractures of more than one joint are characteristic and AMC is sometimes associated with severe congenital heart malformations.
REF. Lebenthal E, M.D., et al.: Arthrogryposis Multiplex Congenita: 23 cases in an Arab Kindred. Pediatrics 46:6, 891-899, 1970.

331. Q. What is endemic skeletal fluorosis?

A. Skeletal fluorosis is common in children and can occur between 11-14 years of age. Clinical features are manifested by mottled dental enamel pigmentation and diffuse osteosclerosis of the skeleton. Vague pains, restricted joint movements, backache, stiffness and rigidity of spine, inability to close fists, constipation. There are grossly limited movements of spine, thoracic kyphosis, and flexion deformities at the hips and knees.

It is recommended that all children living in endemic zones regardless of symptoms and dental mottling should be screened for skeletal disease, since its early diagnosis will help in preventing the crippling state of the disease.
REF. Teotia M, et al.: Endemic Skeletal Fluorosis. Archives of Disease in Childhood 46:249, 686-691, 1971.

332. Q. What is the respiratory distress syndrome?

A. Labored or distressed breathing with pulmonary atelectasis, persisting beyond the immediate newborn period with laboratory evidence of hypoxia, $CO_2$ retention and metabolic acidosis, represents the clinical entity known as respiratory distress syndrome or RDS. This diagnosis is made when respiratory distress due to congenital anomalies, asphyxia, pneumonia, pneumothorax, aspiration and congestive heart failure have been ruled out. RDS is the clinical counterpart of the disease characterized by pathologists as hyaline membrane disease.
REF. Brumley G, M.D.: The Critically Ill Child: The Respiratory Distress Syndrome of the Newborn. Pediatrics 47:4, 758-767, 1971.

333. Q. What is the clinical picture of RDS?

A. Almost all infants who develop RDS are born before 38 weeks' gestation and have Apgar scores below 7 at 1 and 5 minutes. The abnormal respirations persist beyond 20 minutes of age. Many have a maternal Hx which includes anemia, bleeding and delivery by cesarean section before the onset of labor. The infant with RDS is tachypneic, has retractions, flaring of nares, sternal rocking, grunting and decreased ventilation on auscultation. The infant is often cyanotic and shows temperature instability, poor peripheral circulation and edema. Frequently these signs worsen over the first 12 to 24 hours.
REF. Brumley G, M.D.: The Critically Ill Child: The Respiratory Distress Syndrome of the Newborn. Pediatrics 47:4, 758-767, 1971.

334. Q. How is RDS treated?

A. The treatment of RDS has many components and care must be taken that therapy does not become an iatrogenic source of further respiratory insult. Treatment includes maintenance of body temperature with an environmental temperature of $90^o$ to $94^o$ F, administration of alkali therapy (sodium bicarbonate) if blood Ph, $CO_2$ and $O_2$ levels so indicate, oxygen therapy with humidified $O_2$

and parenteral fluids and glucose. These infants should be carefully monitored in a facility equipped for cardiorespiratory, temperature, blood pressure and inspired oxygen monitoring. Expert laboratory support is essential as is well trained nursing personnel in an Intensive Care nursery.

REF. Brumley G, M.D.: The Critically Ill Child: The Respiratory Distress Syndrome of the Newborn. Pediatrics 47:4, 758-767, 1971.

335. Q. What care is needed when a neonate has respiratory distress syndrome?

A. Respiratory distress syndrome (RDS), also called idiopathic respiratory distress or hyaline membrane disease, is the major cause of death in the neonatal period. It is a disease primarily of premature infants; incidence is also increased by: delivery by cesarean section, maternal bleeding, asphyxia during delivery, maternal diabetes, or a history of RDS in previous siblings.

The infant may appear normal at birth but in a short time have tachypnea and labored respirations, followed by intercostal and abdominal retraction. The infant assumes a frog-like position, has edema of the extremities, and has generalized cyanosis. The hypoxemia is accompanied by metabolic and respiratory acidosis. Several principles are essential for survival of the infant:

(1) Body temperature must be kept as close to normal as possible. If hypothermia is present, the body will try to produce heat by increasing tissue metabolism, requiring increased oxygen. A too warm environment can also increase metabolic activity, as well as trigger apneic spells. Humidity may also be provided to decrease heat loss by evaporation. Nursing becomes involved with keeping the environment warm and dry, but the infant quiet and undisturbed, changing the infant's positions frequently while arranging all the monitoring leads; and maintaining optimal environmental temperature while doing all the above.

(2) Intravenous feeding is essential to maintain weight and prevent dehydration. Nursing challenges involve protecting the fragile I.V. lines while repositioning, frequently checking infusion rate and any signs of infiltration, preventing infection at the infusion site, keeping accurate intake and output records, and weighing the infant to assess caloric efficiency.

(3) Oxygen therapy is essential, and treatment usually involves endotracheal intubation, assisted ventilation, administration of high oxygen concentrations (up to 100%). Nursing intervention consists of careful monitoring of vital signs, analyzing $O_2$ concentration frequently, suctioning the endotracheal tube as needed, and observing for signs of oxygen toxicity.

Caring for these high risk infants is challenging from purely a physical standpoint. The mother also needs emotional support at a time when she is separated from her infant. Parents need to see the infant and be kept informed of his progress.
REF. Kumpe M, Klunman L.: Care of the Infant with Respiratory Distress Syndrome. Nursing Clinics of North America 6:1, 25-37, March 1971.

336. Q. Is mechanical ventilation of any value in infants with hyaline membrane disease?

A. One hundred and four infants with hyaline membrane disease were studied over a period of 3 years. Seventy-two infants survived without mechanical ventilation (endotracheal intubation and Bennett respirator). Thirty-two infants were mechanically ventilated; of these 7 survived. This study concludes that mechanical ventilation is unlikely to increase survival of infants severely affected with hyaline membrane disease. Many infants with severe abnormalities of gas exchange survived without mechanical ventilation and it is felt that relying on blood gas criteria may subject infants unnecessarily to a potentially hazardous procedure.
REF. Reynolds EOR, M.D.: Implications for Mechanical Ventilation in Infants with Hyaline Membrane Disease. Pediatrics 46:2, 193-202, 1970.

337. Q. What is the pathophysiology present in asthma?

A. Respiratory function is basically altered in asthma by an increase in airway resistance. This resistance is brought about by 3 mechanisms: (1) bronchospasm, (2) mucosal edema, (3) accumulation of secretions. Since the tracheobronchial tree elongates and dilates on inspiration, but shortens and narrows on expiration, the increased resistance of the airway is more pronounced during expiration. However, both phases of respiration are affected. Expiratory obstruction produces lung hyperinflation which advances to produce increased dead space in the lung which leads to a reduced alveolar ventilation. The increased work of breathing produces greater oxygen consumption and $CO_2$ build up. As more and more airways become obstructed, the total ventilation becomes insufficient to maintain a normal $PCO_2$ and hypercapnia occurs. Both hypoxia and hypercapnia may result in acidosis. Hypercapnia produces respiratory acidosis due to the conversion of carbon dioxide to carbonic acid. Hypoxia produces metabolic acidosis due to interference in the conversion of lactic acid to carbon dioxide and water with the resultant accumulation of lactic acid. Unless corrected acidosis can lead to cardiac failure and death.
REF. Richards W, M.D., Siegel S, M.D.: Status Asthmaticus. Pediatric Clinics of North America 16:1, 9-27, 1969.

338. Q. What factors involved in the pathophysiology of asthma relate to nursing care?

A. Asthma is one of the more common respiratory disorders affecting children. An asthmatic attack often constitutes a medical emergency, and is extremely frightening to the patient, family, and staff. Asthma is not a disease but rather a reversible syndrome characterized by bronchoconstriction, spasm, edema, and excess mucus. An attack usually begins with coughing, expiratory resistance characterized by wheezing, diaphoresis, and flaring of the nares. Accessory muscles of the abdomen and pectus are used to increase pace of expiration. Breathing is rapid and shallow; pulse is rapid.

Besides these physical signs, nurses need to be familiar with blood gas values, which become a guideline for therapy. Initially, respiratory alkalosis (arterial pH above 7.45 and $pCO_2$ below 35 mm. Hg) may result from hyperventilation. Hypercapnia is more likely to result from severe airway obstruction. In respiratory acidosis $CO_2$ rises above 45 mm. Hg. Rising $pCO_2$ levels can cause respiratory center depression. Oxygen is then given in controlled flow to stimulate breathing. The administration of oxygen requires careful observation of blood gases and the patient's condition. The nurse should also be alert to signs of hypokalemia resulting from the recovery phase of hypercapnia.

Bronchodilators, such as epinephrine and aminophylline, are given to relieve bronchospasm and constriction. Nurses must be alert to the side effects of tachycardia, arrhythmias, and increased blood pressure.

Reducing anxiety and teaching breathing exercises which emphasize slowed respiratory rate with improved depth can help the patients prevent further attacks, and minimize present ones.
REF. Moody L.: Asthma Physiology and Patient Care. American Journal of Nursing 73:7, 1212-1217, July 1973.

339. Q. What causes status asthmaticus?

A. Status asthmaticus is that state of severe asthma which fails to respond to treatment with epinephrine. The reasons for the failure to respond to epinephrine in status asthmaticus are not fully understood. One of the factors which may play a role in causing status asthmaticus is infection, which is frequently present in children who present with this condition. Other factors which may be contributory are dehydration, leading to the formation of mucus plugs, sedation and narcotics, failure to administer large doses of steroids, and acidosis. The presence of severe hypoxemia may also be a factor in the failure of these patients to respond to epinephrine.
REF. Richards W, M.D., Siegel S, M.D.: Status Asthmaticus. Pediatric Clinics of North America 16:1, 9-27, 1969.

340. Q. What is the treatment of status asthmaticus?

A. The management of status asthmaticus has three components: (1) therapy of the asthma itself, that is bronchospasm, mucosal edema and mucus plugs, (2) correction of blood gas and acid base abnormalities, (3) treatment of the complications of asthma particularly infection.

(1) Therapy of the asthma involves hydration, mist therapy, administration of expectorants, epinephrine, isoproterenol, aminophylline, and corticosteroids.

(2) Therapy of blood gas and acid-base abnormalities requires the correction of hypoxemia by the administration of oxygen, the administration of sodium bicarbonate or hydroxymethyl aminothane (THAM) to correct acidosis, and artificial ventilation and if necessary with intubation and IPPB.

(3) Therapy of complications of status asthmaticus involves the administration of antibiotics to patients with signs of infection, usually pneumonitis.

Sedatives and tranquilizers are contraindicated in the treatment of status asthmaticus because of their CNS depressant effects. Anithistamines are contraindicated because of their drying effects.
REF. Richards W, M.D., Siegel S, M.D.: Status Asthmaticus. Pediatric Clinics of North America 16:1, 9-27, 1969.

341. Q. How can a nurse recognize oxygen toxicity in a patient?

A. Oxygen, a gas that normally constitutes about 20% atmospheric air, is essential to life. However, current evidence suggests that prolonged exposure to high oxygen tensions can cause damage to cell membranes and cellular contents. The human lung can withstand 100% oxygen for approximately 24 hours before lung damage occurs. In infants oxygen levels over 40% can cause retinal detachment (retrolental fibroplasia).

The symptoms of oxygen toxicity are nonspecific: tightness of the chest, a dry non-productive cough, and progressive dyspnea. The most reliable sign, however, is blood gas values. Arterial oxygen tension or $O_2$ saturation decreases despite an increase in the inspired oxygen concentration. This is known as "refractory hypoxemia".

Oxygen toxicity is due to both concentration and duration of excessive oxygenation. Forty percent oxygen can be tolerated for weeks or a few months, but the lowest flow rate of this gas should be used to provide adequate arterial oxygenation without risking lung damage.
REF. Nett L, Petty T.: Oxygen Toxicity. American Journal of Nursing 73:9, 1556-1558, Sept. 1973.

342. Q. What is cromolyn sodium?

A. Cromolyn sodium (disodium cromoglycate) is an antiasthma drug that has two unique features:

(1) It is given prophylactically
(2) It is directly inhaled into the bronchial tree

The medication interferes with the release of chemical mediators of allergic responses at the mast cells of the lung. In order for cromolyn to act prophylactically, it must be at the mast cell membrane before an antigen/antibody reaction takes place.
REF. Crawford LV.: Experiences with Cromolyn Sodium in Asthma in Children. Clinical Pediatrics 12:519, Sept. 1973.

343. Q. Is cromolyn an effective treatment for asthma?

A. In a double-blend crossover study 30 chronic asthmatic children who wheezed 80% of the time on either cromolyn sodium four times a day or a placebo, were studied. After four weeks, the group was reversed. Sixty-three percent (N=19) of the children had a 50% reduction in wheezing when on cromolyn.

The investigators state that "cromolyn sodium can bring about a definite reduction in asthma symptoms and a reduced need for bronchodilators and corticosteroids". However, they also recommend that each child have a total comprehensive anti-allergic program.
REF. Crawford LV.: Experiences with Cromolyn Sodium in Asthma in Children. Clinical Pediatrics 12:519, Sept. 1973.

344. Q. What are the long term effects of cromolyn sodium?

A. Twenty-seven children with asthma, who had not been responsive to routine treatment were studied. Forty-five percent took cromolyn sodium for periods ranging from 11 months to over 20 months.

Of the twenty-seven subjects, 74% had a decrease in all asthma symptoms, need for bronchodilators, fewer school absences, fewer hospitalizations and less need for corticosteroids. Thirteen children were able to stop taking corticosteroids and thirteen were able to reduce their dosage.

A positive dimension of the study was that the families of the children felt more hopeful. In addition, the children seemed to develop more self-confidence.
REF. Mascia AV.: Review and Assessment of the Efficacy of Cromolyn Sodium, Particularly After Long-Term Administration. Clinical Pediatrics 9:523-524, Sept. 1973.

345. Q. What are the principles in suctioning a child with a tracheostomy?

A. An obvious danger in suctioning a tracheostomized child is infection. Bacteria can be carried into the trachea and bronchi, unless the strictest sterile technique is employed. Of special importance in infants and children is the size of the suction catheter. To avoid the rapid aspiration of oxygen from the airway system with subsequent hypoxia, a catheter size should be in a 1:3 proportion to tube lumen. Catheters should have a "T" or side arm opening and suction should not be applied until the catheter, properly inserted in the tracheostomy tube, is being withdrawn. Prolonged suctioning, suctioning with too large a catheter or failure to allow the patient time to ventilate between suction attempts can lead to hypoxia, predisposing the patient to cardiac arrest. At the first sign of any respiratory distress, interrupt suctioning and provide humidified oxygen. The left main stem bronchus may be entered by positioning the head to the right and vice versa. When a patient also requires oral and nasopharyngeal suctioning, separate clean equipment should be used.

REF. Crocker D, M.D.: The Critically Ill Child: Management of Tracheostomy. Pediatrics 46:2, 286-296, 1970.

346. Q. Are there special problems in the care of cuffed tracheostomy tubes?

A. In patients who have tracheostomy tubes with inflated cuffs secretions accumulate above the cuff of the tube and, upon deflation, immediately descend into the lungs. To prevent this problem, the cuff of the tube should be deflated and positive pressure should be applied to the airway via the tracheostomy tube. This causes secretions to be ejected over the vocal cords where they may be swallowed or suctioned from the oropharynx.

REF. Crocker D, M.D.: The Critically Ill Child: Management of Tracheostomy. Pediatrics 46:2, 286-296, 1970.

347. Q. What are the major complications of tracheostomies?

A. The 2 complications causing the most difficulty in the first weeks following tracheostomy are mechanical problems and infection. Mechanical problems which are the most common cause of airway obstruction, can be prevented. The child should be well positioned at all times, never be allowed to sleep in a prone position and have coverings carefully placed. In infants restraints may be necessary to prevent pulling out of the tracheostomy tube. Respirators should never be attached to tracheostomy tubes unless constantly monitored by a nurse.

Infection probably occurs in all tracheostomies at some time. The most important problem is preventing lung involvement. Culture and sensitivity tests should be done routinely and if positive treatment begun with the proper antibiotic. Eventually patients develop immunity and a symbiotic relationship with common bacteria; however, every attempt must be made not to introduce pathogens into the tracheostomy.

REF. Crocker D, M.D.: The Critically Ill Child: Management of Tracheostomy. Pediatrics 46:2, 286-296, 1970.

348. Q. What is meant by children with small chests?

A. When the process of growth in length of the ribs at the costo-chondral junctions is disturbed, the thorax is small and bell shaped, narrow at the upper part with slight flaring at the lower ribs. Circumference is reduced. The upper ribs lie horizontally and clavicles appear high. Ribs are short and may be expanded and irregular. Chest X-ray demonstrates small lung fields also suggesting collapse consolidation. Normal sized heart appears enlarged. Abdomen appears distended. Liver and spleen are of normal size.

Breathing is rapid, shallow and abdominal with virtually no movement of the chest. Rales may be present over the lung fields in absence of overt infection.

There are a variety of bone diseases which affect the skeleton which may delay or disturb rib growth.
REF. Hull D, Barnes ND.: Children with Small Chests. Archives of Disease in Childhood 47:251, 12-19, 1972.

349. Q. What are the consequences of small chests or thoracic dystrophy?

A. There is a serious impairment of pulmonary function. Respiratory failure is due to underventilation caused by the restrictive defect. The most useful index is probably the partial $CO_2$ in arterial or "arterialized" capillary blood. Progressive $CO_2$ retention occurs followed by hypoxia.
REF. Hull D, Barnes ND.: Children with Small Chests. Archives of Disease in Childhood 47:251, 12-19, 1972.

350. Q. What is the prognosis for thoracic dystrophy?

A. The prognosis for respiratory function depends on the capacity of the ribs for growth and of the lungs for expansion to an adequate volume. Respiratory problems are most severe in the first few months; if the children survive the first year, the respiratory problems will resolve. In infants where the associated abnormalities are not crippling, early recognition and treatment of the respiratory problem are vital.
REF. Hull D, Barnes ND.: Children with Small Chests. Archives of Disease in Childhood 47:251, 12-19, 1972.

351. Q. What treatments can be done to alleviate the distress of thoracic dystrophy?

A. General measures such as administration of oxygen, correcting acidosis, physiotherapy. Antibiotic therapy at first sign of infection. Artificial ventilation is used as a temporary supportive

measure. Surgical operation: splitting and fixation of the sternum can provide a considerable increase in thoracic volume.
REF. Hull D, Barnes ND.: Children with Small Chests. Archives of Disease in Childhood 47:251, 12-19, 1972.

352. Q. How can a nurse mechanically stimulate coughing?

A. Coughing serves several important functions, mainly expulsion of pulmonary secretions and stimulation of deep breathing. If coughing is not forceful enough, deep endotracheal suctioning may be necessary, but it can lead to vagal stimulation or hypoxia. Before attempting to stimulate a patient to cough, you should position him from side to side or in any position facilitating the flow of secretions. During coughing a semi-Fowler's to high Fowler's position is best.

Children usually have weak cough reflexes, and refuse to cough if there is pain. However, the nurse can use direct external mechanical stimulation of the trachea to induce coughing. She should place her index finger on the trachea, exerting firm pressure while moving the finger up and down. This causes an irritation sensation in the trachea triggering coughing.

A second procedure to induce coughing requires the cooperation of the child. Stimulation is achieved through forceful prolonged expiration of all inhaled air. This drying effect of the continuous flow of air over the trachea and the slight build-up of carbon dioxide produce a paroxysm of coughing. Children can be taught this procedure by blowing bubbles or balloons, but it usually takes practice and concentration for this method to be successful.

If the above two procedures fail, then a sterile catheter can be introduced through the nose or mouth into the trachea to stimulate coughing. Suction must always be ready if thick tenacious secretions cannot be expectorated easily.
REF. Ungvarski P.: Mechanical Stimulation of Coughing. American Journal of Nursing 71:12, 2358-2361, Dec. 1971.

## III. EXCEPTIONAL CHILDREN

353. Q. Can a workable definition of learning disabilities be formulated?

A. Several definitions now in common use are based on the concept of discrepancy between the child's measured level of achievement and his measured level of intelligence.

For Bateman (1965) and Myklebust and Johnson (1967) the discrepancy between achievement and potential is a basic criterion for the diagnosis of a learning disability.

Definitions which do not specifically mention the term discrepancy often imply a deficient relationship with the use of terms such as specific retardation, disorder, defects in learning, and delayed development (Kirk, 1962)
REF. Salvia J, Clark J.: Use of Deficits to Identify the Learning Disabled. Exceptional Children 39:4, 305-308, 1973.

354. Q. What is dyslexia?

A. Most researchers believe that dyslexia is a syndrome caused by delayed maturation of the area of the brain that coordinates vision, reading, and writing and speech. Thus the child with dyslexia has normal intelligence, vision,and learning but cannot learn to read well utilizing the traditional methods.

Children who cannot read begin to develop low self-esteem. They may become bored and disruptive in school. As written work increases, the child's school achievement decreases because of the amount of reading required.

Once the problem has been recognized, special educational techniques are designed to improve reading and spelling. Classroom work should be done and graded orally. The child must be helped to understand his problem. Support, guidance, and encouragement must be given in order to help the child move forward.
REF. Faigel HG.: When Children Can't Read. Clinical Pediatrics 8:11-15, Jan. 1969.

355. Q. What is the psychosocial adjustment of children with dyslexia?

A. Dyslexia is defined as an inability to read normally because of minimal neurological dysfunction. The dyslexic child possesses the essential integrities for learning: average intelligence or better, adequate sensory acuity, no debilitating emotional disorders, no severe motor deficiency, and sufficient educational opportunity and instruction - yet he is unable to read properly.

This research was designed to explore the dyslexic child's psychosocial reaction to his reading disability and to evaluate this reaction in terms of its effect on the child's functioning.

The dyslexic child's psychosocial adjustment does not seem to be characterized by emotional disturbance, although certain personality traits were found to be associated with this disorder. He appears to have compensated for his disability, in some way, so that his interaction with the environment is not qualitatively different from non-dyslexic children.

This conclusion is an example, perhaps, of the flexibility of the psyche and the capacity of the human organism to successfully adapt to adverse circumstances.
REF. Connolly C.: The Psychosocial Development of Children with Dyslexia. Exceptional Children 36:2, 126-127, 1969.

356. Q. How can the linguistically different child be helped?

A. The educational practice of grouping children on the basis of ability can be viewed as a method of removing deviant children from the mainstream of our schools. Also, this practice has been charged as discriminatory because the tests used for educational placement may be linguistically and culturally biased and may serve to place disproportionate numbers of minority group children (especially nonstandard English speakers) into special classes.

Because of this indictment, the linguistic deficit and the linguistic difference models are explored as possible explanation of the verbal behavior of linguistically different children. The educational implications of each model are discussed.
REF. Bryen DN.: Special Education and the Linguistically Different Child. Exceptional Children 40:8, 589-599, 1974.

357. Q. What are the behavior patterns of learning in disabled, emotionally disturbed, and average children?

A. The assumption that children with learning disabilities can be differentiated from emotionally disturbed children in terms of observable social behaviors was systematically explored by means of the behavior problem checklist. The findings have implications for the management of emotionally disturbed and learning disabled children. The findings are:

(1) Ratings of the child's problem behavior may be an additional criterion to be considered in diagnosis and placement of these children. The more problems present and/or the greater the degree of severity, the more likely it is that the child's behavior resembles that of the emotionally disturbed group.

(2) The main problem is conduct. Provisions should be made to deal with acting out behavior, overt aggressiveness, hostility, negativism, and hyperactivity in classes of both emotionally

disturbed and learning disabled children. A provision such as a crisis room or teacher's aide should be considered in planning such programs.

(3) The second order behavior problem for the typical emotionally disturbed child appears to be immaturity, inadequacy, withdrawal, inattentiveness, dislike for school, etc. The third order problem is neuroticism, self-consciousness, lack of self confidence, fearfulness, depression, etc. For the learning disability group, both immaturity - inadequacy and neuroticism are of equal importance.

Priorities in terms of time, resources, or methods for dealing with behavior problems of these children, immaturity will have a higher priority than neuroticism in emotionally disturbed children but will have the same priority in learning disabled children.
REF. McCarthy JM, Paraskevopoulos J.: Behavior Patterns of Learning Disabled, Emotionally Disturbed, and Average Children. Exceptional Children 36:2, 69-74, 1969.

358. Q. Is the mildly retarded child's language cognitive deficit or cultural difference?

A. Speech is the most telling stereotypic clues to an individual's social class membership. Individual worth is often based on grammatical and syntactic conformity. A majority of functionally retarded persons come from the lower socioeconomic areas of the community. Language defects are judged by middle class standards, and defects found in the lower classes may merely represent deviations from these standards rather than retarded development. There also is the factor of educational deprivation and social isolation. Some causes of speech defects are:

(1) Maladjustment: Associated with reactions to environmental pressures than with congenital or organic predisposition. Linguistic inadequacy rather than speech deficiency causes lack of intelligence and may result in development of feelings of inferiority which may be manifested in defective speech. Hearing loss, emotional disturbance, and language disorders may also be responsible.

(2) Social class: Assigning inferior status to people is an arbitrary decision by the dominant class. The question of whether speech and language of the mildly retarded reflects cultural difference and/or cognitive deficit cannot be answered at this time. The interaction of environment/intelligence points to not so much from cognitive deficit as cultural difference.

Beginning language is primarily a matter of establishing associations for arbitrary symbols which name common objects and people, actions, and qualities.

Oral and written language involves 4 linguistic systems each of which contributes to the development of acceptable words, phrases, and sentences:

(1) Phonological (sound features);
(2) Semantic (meaning);
(3) Syntactic (word order);
(4) Morphologic (tense, person, number, case).

Language remediation should improve cognition. In reality, mild mental retardation among the poor may be the result, in part, of cognitive confusion resulting from illogical deviant language patterns. Irretrievable time must not be wasted in correcting benign dialectical differences which clash with prevailing speech patterns.
REF. Valletutti P.: Language of the Mildly Mentally Retarded: Cognitive Deficit or Cultural Difference? Exceptional Children 37:6, 455-459, 1971.

359. Q. Does background music have an effect on learning?

A. This study investigated the effects of calming background music on task relevant and task irrelevant learning of educable mentally retarded students. The independent variables were:

(1) Calming background music
(2) Distractors during a learning task
(3) Age level of the subjects.

The dependent variables were:

(1) Task relevant learning scores
(2) Task irrelevant learning scores.

The population consisted of all pupils within the chronological age range of 120 to 173 months and within an I.Q. range of 50 to 87. The findings seem to indicate that music may be an aid in enabling students to attend to relevant stimuli. Music does not appear to reduce the performance of subjects on processing extraneous visual stimuli since the scores on the irrelevant task were not significantly affected, either positively or negatively, by the music.

It appears that music enables institutionalized educable retarded children to process more information since relevant learning was increased without reducing irrelevant learning.
REF. Stainback SB, Stainback WC.: Effect of Background Music on Learning. Exceptional Children 40:2, 109-110, 1973.

360. Q. Can a special child be taught in a regular classroom?

A. During the past several years many educators have expressed concern about the efficacy of the traditional special education approach of self contained classrooms in the education of children with a variety of exceptionalities. The North Sacramento Model Program described here is suggested as one of these possible alternatives in the development of more effective programs in the education of exceptional children.

Three educable mentally retarded children who had previously been placed in special self-contained classrooms were integrated with 22 nonhandicapped children in a third grade classroom during the first year of the North Sacramento Model Program. A similar number were integrated into a fourth grade classroom during the second year of the project. A precision teaching procedure was used with both experimental groups. Control groups of educable mentally retarded and educationally handicapped children in regular classrooms were maintained.

Results indicate that the handicapped and nonhandicapped children in the integrated setting improved as much or more than did their controls in academic skills, social behavior, and attitude change.
REF. Bradfield RH, et al.: The Special Child in the Regular Classroom. Exceptional Children 39:5, 384-390, 1973.

361. Q. Can a child benefit more from tutorial instruction rather than small groups in resource rooms?

A. In the study each child was taught both by a cross-age tutor individually and by a resource teacher in a small group. Results suggested that children learned more from a tutor than in a small group. The effect was observed for word recognition, spelling, oral reading and multiplication.

Tutorial instruction was also superior to self instruction, and tutors appeared to benefit academically from the experience.

Small group instruction permits the teacher to individualize instruction more than is possible in larger groups. Children learn at different rates and progress differently through a sequence of instruction, mastering various skills at their unique paces. The groups' pace in the curriculum will only imperfectly represent the optimal pace for an individual group member.

In a tutorial setting, the learner controls his progress through an instructional sequence by his rate of mastery. Thus one of the significant values of tutoring is the modification of instructional pace.

Resource teachers may be required, in terms of individualizing instruction, to change their role from instructor to that of instructional manager.
REF. Jenkins JR, et al.: Comparing Small Groups and Tutorial Instruction in Resource Rooms. Exceptional Children 40:4, 245-250, 1974.

362. Q. What are the attitudes of children toward their special class placement?

A. The purpose of this study was to determine and analyze the expressed attitudes of children in special classes for the educable mentally retarded.

It appears that children in special classes are capable of clearly communicating their feelings regarding their educational placement. The findings do not support the assumption that most retarded children resent their special class placement with accompanying feelings of rejection and stigmatization. Some of them disliked being in a special class because of the fighting and antisocial behavior of their retarded peers. Children of elementary school age are more apt than those of high school age to be satisfied with their placement. Most mildly retarded children are fairly realistic in terms of their academic deficiencies. They show a degree of maturity in that many view their special class placement as representing an opportunity for them to learn, catch up, or improve themselves.

Overall impression is that the special class is a generally stimulating and comfortable placement for children who have had difficulty in adjusting to other placements within the educational system.
REF. Warner F, et al.: Attitudes of Children Toward Their Special Class Placement. Exceptional Children 40:1, 37-38, 1973.

363. Q. Can zone planning be used for accelerating adaptive behavior in the retarded?

A. This study describes an approach to habilitating developmentally disabled children who do not function well in most classroom settings in order that they may return to their normal classrooms. An initial one to one relationship is necessary in addition to specific training in groups. Benefits are:

(1) Early establishment of self control necessary for any type of viable group training.
(2) Maintenance of self control in therapy zones which consist of small, physically separable group situations for special education, speech, socialization, or motor training.
(3) An economically feasible treatment program for returning children to group instructional situations where they may benefit from a normal special education classroom environment.

The normalization principle (Nirje 1969) uses college students, parents, family members where the child is exposed to a variety of behavioral expectations, and is constantly challenged to adapt and meet these expectations. The habilitation of retarded children is seen as a cooperative parent-professional-community venture where normal behavior is reinforced by its most powerful consequences, the natural ones.
REF. Stabler B, et al.: Zone Planning for Accelerating Adaptive Behavior in the Retarded. Exceptional Children 40:4, 252-257, 1974.

364. Q. Can the home be used as a career education center?

A. As a result of the increasing sophistication of our communication technology, a new role for the home as a learning center is developing. The home as a learning center can serve the purposes of developing children's concepts of work and leisure; training young persons and adults for occupational competency, preparing older workers for new careers; developing competencies of men and women for their homemaking and family life responsibilities; serving in unique ways the career education needs of exceptional children; and promoting personal development and a sense of worth for persons of all ages. Career education in the home is a way to provide for increased learning opportunity for many people for an entire lifetime. It may also enhance home and family life.

In the field of education it offers an increasing array of possibilities for responding to the needs of exceptional children.
REF. Simpson EJ.: The Home as a Career Education Center. Exceptional Children 39:8, 626-630, 1973.

365.   Q. Should exceptional children be punished in the classroom?

A. Teachers of exceptional children are often faced with the problem of eliminating or weakening certain behaviors that are either interfering with a child's learning or hindering his social adjustment. The learning principles which one can select to weaken or eliminate a particular behavior are:

(a) Extinction
(b) Satiation or negative practice
(c) Counterconditioning
(d) One of two forms of punishment

While all such procedures serve to weaken behavior, the most efficacious technique depends on the nature of the behavior, characteristics of the child, context of the situation. In every instance possible positive reinforcement procedures must be used. Some conclusions form the study are:

(1) A prior-positive relationship with the recipient renders punishment more effective.
(2) Punishment should be, if it must be used, in the sequence of misbehavior and consistently applied.
(3) A relatively intense aversive at the onset may be more effective than having to gradually escalate the intensive. One must guard against "punishment overkill".
(4) Punishment should be paired with cognitive structure, i.e., specification of the behavior being punished.
(5) Punishment is more effective if alternative is available to the punished behavior and if incompatible behavior is positively reinforced.
(6) The same aversive should not be used over and over, e.g., wording of the reprimand should be changed.
(7) Soft reprimands, i.e., reprimands directly only at the recipient, are probably more effective.

Specific guidelines need to be formulated in their respective settings. Also guidelines should be based on individual differences between and among groups of exceptional children. Even if such guidelines ultimately do nothing more than preclude the use of punishment, they should at least be the product of serious consideration of the above issues.
REF. Macmillan DL, et al.: The Role of Punishment in the Classroom. Exceptional Children 40:2, 85-96, 1973.

366. Q. What are the effects of loud and soft reprimands on the behavior of disruptive students?

A. In this study two children in each of five classes were selected for a 4 month study of their high rates of disruptive behavior. During a baseline condition the frequency of disruptive behaviors and teacher reprimands was assessed. Almost all teacher reprimands were found to be of a loud nature and could be heard by many other children in the class.

During the second phase of the study, teachers were asked to use primarily soft reprimands which were audible only to the child being reprimanded. With the institution of the soft reprimands, the frequency of disruptive behavior declined in most children. Then the teachers were asked to return to the loud reprimand and a consequent increase in disruptive behavior was observed. Finally, the teachers were asked to again use soft reprimands, and again disruptive behavior declined.

The authors do not recommend soft reprimands as an alternative to praise. An ideal combination would probably be frequent praise, some soft reprimands, and very occasional loud reprimands.

The study concludes that soft reprimands can be a useful method of dealing with disruptive children in a classroom. Combined with praise, soft reprimands might be helpful in reducing disruptive behavior. In contrast, it appears that loud reprimands lead one into a vicious cycle of more and more reprimands resulting in even more disruptive behavior.
REF. O'Leary K, et al.: The Effects of Loud and Soft Reprimands on the Behavior of Disruptive Students. Exceptional Children 37:2, 145-155, 1970.

367. Q. What is the delayed development project?

A. The delayed development project, in San Joaquin, California is a program offering comprehensive services for handicapped children from birth through three years of age and their families. The program is funded under Title VI-B of the Education for the Handicapped Act. The program is for the city's children, up to three years of age, who have evidenced significant delays in growth and development, regardless of the cause. The project is specifically designed to promote motor skills, language development and self-help skills. At the age of three, each child is transferred to a program for the handicapped or other appropriate agency. Parent participation is encouraged in order to foster positive attitudes toward the child.

The approach to the child and family is inter-disciplinary and provides stimulation, education, counselling, health care and physical therapy where necessary. Children below 18 months of age are visited in their homes twice weekly by a teacher and/or physical therapist and a public health nurse. Supportive help and training designed to foster the child's development is given to the parents. After the age of 18 months, the child is bussed to a relocatable nursery where he receives individual therapy and participates in small group activities. Each parent is asked to spend one morning per month in the school. Other family members are involved as possible and feasible.

Studies done on some of the children at the end of three years demonstrates that consistently great gains in developmental skills were made.
REF. Jew W.: Helping Handicapped Infants and Their Families: The Delayed Development Project. Children Today 3:7-10, May-June 1974.

368. Q. What is minimal brain dysfunction?

A. Minimal brain dysfunction (MBD) may be known as hyperkinetic reaction of childhood or hyperkinetic syndrome. The diagnosis depends on clinical findings since there are no pathognomic findings. The syndrome is characterized by motor restlessness, short attention span, poor muscle control, learning difficulties and emotional lability. Usually these children come to medical attention because of school problems, both behavioral and academic. The diagnosis is made on the basis of treatment and symptoms, rather than testing, since both physical and psychological testing may be formal.
REF. Eisenberg L, M.D.: The Clinical Use of Stimulant Drugs in Children. Pediatrics 49:5, 709-715, 1972.

369. Q. What is the cause of minimal brain dysfunction?

A. The cause of MBD is unknown, although some evidence indicates that it may run in families. The pathophysiology of this condition is also unknown. The treatment of childhood hyperkinesis is with the stimulant drugs dextroamphetamine and methylphenidate. These agents suppress overactivity and lengthen attention span in these children. This allows the child to become amenable to learning. Treatment with stimulant drugs may be from 6 months to 3 years.
REF. Eisenberg L, M.D.: The Clinical Use of Stimulant Drugs in Children. Pediatrics 49:5, 709-715, 1972.

370. Q. What is the hyperactive form (Pattern I) of the general disorder "Hyperkinesis"?

A. It is proposed that this is one of two patterns which accounts for confusion and inconsistency in the literature. This distinction is based on clinical observation and experience with the hyperkinetic child.

(a) Appears constantly stimulated, regardless of time, place or context.
(b) Virtually no capacity for sustained effort.
(c) Unstable peer relationships.
(d) Lack of "common sense".
(e) Awkwardness and clumsiness.
(f) Perceptual motor problems.
(g) Specific learning disabilities.

Most consistent etiological factors are:
(1) Organic brain damage criteria are:
    (a) observable hyperkinesis from birth
    (b) repeated neurological and psychological signs
    (c) aimless perseverative tendencies
(2) Matural lag criteria are:
    (a) absence of significant evidence of brain damage
    (b) slowness in progressing through developmental stages
    (c) generally immature behavior
    (d) hyperlunesis observable from early infancy
(3) Constitutional or "pure hyperkinesis". Occurrence of Pattern I behavior in the absence of brain damage, maturational lag, emotional disturbance, or anxiety.

Factors in diagnosing Pattern I child are complete lack of self control and the innate or inherent nature of his hyperkinetic behavior. The child's behavior does not appear to be affected by the surrounding elements of his environment.
REF. Marwit SJ, Stenner AJ.: Hyperkinesis: Delineation of Two Patterns. Exceptional Children 38:5, 401-406, 1972.

371. Q. What is the treatment for hyperactive (Pattern I) form of the hyperkinetic child?

A. The main treatment objective is the modulation of the child's energy level and the subsequent directing of excess energy into socially appropriate behaviors. The child's need to express his energy is almost as natural as breathing. Both are, for the most part, biologically based.

Through pharmacological means his energy output is reduced to a manageable level and then the child is taught when and where the expression of his energy will be tolerated.

It must be realized that the child's heightened activity level is not a learned response and for that reason cannot be unlearned or extinguished. New learning can only take place when there is a reduction of hyperkinetic activity.

REF. Marwit SJ, Stenner AJ.: Hyperkinesis: Delineation of Two Patterns. Exceptional Children 38:5, 401-406, 1972.

372. Q. What is the hyperreactive form (Pattern II) of the general disorder "Hyperkinesis"?

A. It is proposed that this is one of two patterns which accounts for confusion and inconsistency in the literature. This distinction is based on clinical observation and experience with the hyperkinetic child. The child appears:

(a) to be periodically and selectively stimulated
(b) to be able to control himself when he deems it beneficial
(c) to be capable, if properly motivated, of sustained effort comparable to that of the normal child of similar age and ability
(d) to show leadership potential

Most consistent etiological factors are:

(1) Emotional disturbance: A sudden onset of hyperkinetic tendencies in later childhood. No evidence of maturational lag or organicity. Pattern II is a learned response, i.e., a hyperreaction to an unstructured, unorganized environment characterized by instability and by inconsistent and inappropriate handling. It is, in essence, a life style developed by the child to cope with his environment.
(2) Anxiety: The occurrence of hyperkinetic behavior in the presence of an anxiety provoking situation and the subsequent disappearance of this behavior following the removal of (or from) the precipitating stimulus.

REF. Marwit SJ, Stenner AJ.: Hyperkinesis: Delineation of Two Patterns. Exceptional Children 38:5, 401-406, 1972.

373. Q. What is the treatment for hyperreactive (Pattern II) form of the hyperkinetic child?

A. The hyperreactive hyperkinetic child is exhibiting a learned response acquired by the child to help him cope with his environment. The degree to which the individual behavior was learned is the same degree to which it can be unlearned by the substitution of more appropriate responses and/or by the modification or elimination of the previously supporting environment.

The use of behavioral and environmental modification techniques the Pattern II child's hyperreactivity can be reduced and eventually eliminated. Drugs, if used at all, are ancillary.

The more successful results have been obtained with those therapies based on the principles of learning theory.

REF. Marwit SJ, Stenner AJ.: Hyperkinesis: Delineation of Two Patterns. Exceptional Children 38:5, 401-406, 1972.

374. Q. Can hyperkinetic children have an organic etiology based on academic deficiencies?

A. Some authors point to low achievement scores in arithmetic. Educational histories are generally below average. It has also been shown that their tested overall I.Q.'s are quite often normal or above normal.

For purposes of attributing hyperkinesis to an organic etiology, the psychological battery appears to be of limited use. There appears to be no clinical signs, or physiological or psychological test results that unequivocally demonstrate a causal relationship between brain damage and the "Hyperkinetic syndrome". In a certain percentage of cases, depending on the nature of the sample employed, there does exist an association between organicity and hyperkinesis. Whether this is a coincidental relationship or one that reliably constitutes a particular subgroup has yet to be systematically explored. REF. Marwit SJ, Stenner AJ.: Hyperkinesis: Delineation of Two Patterns. Exceptional Children 38:5, 401-406, 1972.

375. Q. What are some neurological signs in hyperkinetic children?

A. (1) Deficiency in fine motor control.
(2) Slight coordination and balance disturbances.
(3) Slight choreoathetotic movements.
(4) Schilder's phenomenon of arms convergence.
(5) Disturbance in eye convergence.
(6) Abnormal EEG recordings - difficult to read and that different abnormal conditions involving the brain may produce similar wave patterns.
REF. Marwit SJ, Stenner AJ.: Hyperkinesis: Delineation of Two Patterns. Exceptional Children 38:5, 401-406, 1972.

376. Q. What kind of behavior is most often associated with hyperkinesis?

A. (1) Overactivity: Constant motor activity in excess of normal child. The child is "motor precocious", having crawled, walked, and run earlier than normal.
(2) Impulsivity: Does things without thinking. An inability to tolerate delays of gratification.
(3) Low frustration tolerance: Reacts with explosive fits of anger, and not easily controlled and anger becomes heightened when reasoned with.
(4) Short attention span: Powers of concentration are limited. He seldom completes a task and shifts from one activity to another.

(5) Distractability: Easily distracted by extraneous movements and noises.

(6) Overly aggressive: Often destructive, bullies younger children, is rebellious, resentful of authority, angered by set limits.

In addition boys manifest the syndrome more than girls, first born children more than latterborn, children aged 6 to 10 more than those who are younger or older.

REF. Marwit SJ, Stenner AJ.: Hyperkinesis: Delineation of Two Patterns. Exceptional Children 38:5, 401-406, 1972.

377. Q. What other characteristics have been associated with hyperkinesis?

A. Most of these symptoms are associated with difficulties in motor functioning and are unlike those manifested by nonhyperkinetic brain injured children:

(1) Awkwardness in locomotion
(2) Poor fine and gross motor coordination
(3) Motor speech difficulties in the form of poor articulation and rhythm disturbances
(4) Dyslexia, dyscalchia, and dysgraphia
(5) Perceptual motor problems

These symptoms have been shown to be present in a number of cases, they have been conspicuously absent in others, therefore it is questionable whether they are truly pathognomonic to hyperkinesis.

REF. Marwit SJ, Stenner AJ.: Hyperkinesis: Delineation of Two Patterns. Exceptional Children 38:5, 401-406, 1972.

378. Q. What treatment can be employed in modifying the hyperkinetic child's behavior?

A. The three possible treatment orientations are:

(1) Pharmacological manipulation
(2) Environmental modification
(3) A combination of both

The treatment chosen will depend on the diagnosed behavior pattern and its corresponding etiological factor.

REF. Marwit SJ, Stenner AJ.: Hyperkinesis: Delineation of Two Patterns. Exceptional Children 38:5, 401-406, 1972.

379. Q. What are the practical advantages of maintaining a macroscopic and microscopic examination of the hyperkinetic child?

A. Macroscopically all hyperkinesis is associated with high activity levels, impulsivity, distractability, low frustration tolerance, short attention span and overaggressiveness.

Microscopically, hyperkinesis reveals two separate patterns, each with its own associated behaviors and etiological factors.

The advantages of maintaining this delineation are:

(1) It increases our understanding of the disorder and clarifies certain ambiguities in the traditional literature.
(2) It allows the practitioner increased precision in diagnosing the disorder and consequently aids in his choice of appropriate treatment procedures.
(3) It provides the researcher with a new conceptual framework from which to conduct future investigations.

At present, the distinction between hyperactive and hyperreactive patterns is theoretical and needs empirical validation.
REF. Marwit SJ, Stenner AJ.: Hyperkinesis: Delineation of Two Patterns. Exceptional Children 38:5, 401-406, 1972.

380. Q. How can the infant and toddler with hyperkinesis be identified?

A. Most of the data about hyperkenetic children have focused on the preschool and school age child. At the same time, little attention has been given to the infant and/or toddler with hyperkinesis; groups in whom atypical behavior traits may be manifested.

The person who is familiar with normal growth and development during the year should, with alertness, be able to recognize aberrant abnormalities. One deviant behavioral sign may be a fluctuation from the norm. However, when viewed over time and interacting with other behaviors, these deviations may point to hyperkinesis.

Beginning with the neonate, minimal brain dysfunction may be manifested by lethargy, hyperactivity and feeding problems. During infancy, activity is excessive and the baby is rarely relaxed or placid. Crying may continue for weeks or months. The crying cannot be controlled by soothing methods, feeding changes or medication. In fact, phenobarbital or other anti-spasmodic drugs tend to aggravate crying and hyperactivity. Sleeping patterns are unpredictable. With the onset of walking, motor activity and purposeless movements continue. Toward the end of the first year, most toddlers begin to talk. By contrast these children may not speak until the second or third year and the speech is usually defective.

The impulsive, destructive and aggressive activities of these children make them particularly vulnerable to accidents and injury. Violent temper tantrums above average and frequency is another deviation. These are not controlled by any intervening methods, They are attributed to the child's low frustration threshold.

The expressions of minimal brain dysfunction are often interspersed with periods of nearly normal behavior. More mature, acceptable

behavior is usually observed in one-to-one interactions with little distracting stimuli. The crucial factors which distinguish the hyperkinetic child from the normal child are the degree and intensity of behaviors manifested.
REF. Nichamin SJ.: Recognizing Minimal Cerebral Dysfunction in the Infant and Toddler. Clinical Pediatrics 11:255-257, May 1972.

381. Q. How can the hyperkinetic child be managed?

A. In any treatment program for hyperkinesis, the cooperation of the child is essential. Thus, his cooperation should be cultivated by direct interaction with him. This can be done either in the parents' presence or with their knowledge. All persons involved in his care, must convey to the child that he is respected and considered a person.

The school should be informed of the child's problem and mode of management. Regular reports from the school, particularly the child's teacher, are excellent means of learning more about the child's behavior and whether or not treatment has resulted in any changes.

Follow-up is a vital facet of treatment. Its importance must be understood by the parents. This is especially true if the child is taking stimulant drugs. The child should also report how he feels several times during the year.

The family should be aware of the side effects of stimulants in order to be assured and assuring to the child should they occur. Counselling is a vital adjunct to treatment.
REF. Arnold LE.: The Art of Medicating Children. Clinical Pediatrics 12:35-41, Jan. 1973.

382. Q. What is the self-concept of hyperactive adolescents?

A. The subjects in the study were 83 children ages 12-16 who had been diagnosed as hyperactive. Each child was interviewed regarding the symptoms of hyperactivity, school performance, self-esteem and their social life.

Most of the children reported that they were restless, impulsive, and easily upset. Almost half said they had difficulty concentrating and finishing tasks. Many felt they had symptoms of the hyperactive syndrome. Most had social problems at home and school due to their behavior. Some admitted to truancy and petty stealing. Many children held themselves in low esteem.
REF. Stewart MA, et al.: Hyperactive Children as Adolescents, How They Describe Themselves. Child Psychiatry and Human Development 4:3-11, Fall 1973.

383. Q. What is the medical-neurological syndrome explaining the learning problems of hyperactive children?

A. Research done on hyperactive children shows agreement on maladaptive social and behavioral characteristics associated with hyperactivity, findings specifying the nature of educational deficits are inconsistent and inconclusive.

One hypothesis proposed to explain the medical-neurological syndrome is: learning problems, distractibility, perceptual problems, and motor activity are perceived as caused by neurological impairment. A significant number of children with signs of neurological dysfunction are found in a typical group. Symptom patterns are variable, and the relationships of symptomatology to learning and behavior are unclear.

Treatment of hyperactivity with medication is common and provides a kind of indirect support for the neurological hypothesis. Functions that improved under one medication (dextroamphetamine) were attention, new learning, school and home behavior, and an ability to "plan" rather than to respond hastily or impulsively. Measures of visual and auditory perception, motor inhibition, general intelligence, and short term memory were not significantly affected by the medication.

The neurological hypothesis may reasonably be called upon to explain the behavior of hyperactive children. Evidence does not allow acceptance of this hypothesis as a definitive and broadly encompassing explanation for the learning problems of hyperactive children.
REF. Keogh BK.: Hyperactivity and Learning Disorders: Review and Speculation. Exceptional Children 30:2, 101-109, 1971.

384. Q. What is the information acquisition hypothesis explaining the learning problems of hyperactive children?

A. One hypothesis proposed concerns information acquisition: It is assumed that the child is neurally intact. Motor activity is seen as interfering with attention to task, failure to learn - in part at least, a function of disruptive activity in the information acquisition stages of problem solving. Much information seeking is done to learn a new task. Interference with the seeking process limits the amount of information acquired; heightened and/or inappropriate motor activity may be a powerful interference. The successful problem solver "modulates, or regulates, his activity, so that expressive activity is inhibited during crucial points of problem solving where it might constitute an interference." Extraneous movement, of head and eyes, appear associated with learning difficulties. New learning has been shown to be negatively affected in high activity retarded subjects; new learning is sometimes benefited by medication.

Regardless of the particular therapeutic agent, i.e., medication or behavior management, decrease in motor activity allows more accurate intake of information and increases the probability of successful learning.

REF. Keogh BK.: Hyperactivity and Learning Disorders: Review and Speculation. Exceptional Children 30:2, 101-109, 1971.

385. Q. How do hasty and impulsive decisions explain the learning problems of hyperactive children?

A. One hypothesis proposed states that hyperactive children have disturbed and speeded up decision making processes. These children make decisions too rapidly. They are considered to lack thoughtfulness, to respond too quickly, to lack ability to think things through, and to be unable to delay response.

If impulsivity is heightened in situations of high response uncertainty, he may be caught in a circular situation: his hyperactivity disrupts the development of consistent and stable precepts and concepts; lack of stability of precepts and concepts leads to heightened motor activity; and heightened motor activity increases the disruption of stability of precepts and concepts. Much of the touching, manipulating behavior may be efforts to achieve perceptual confirmation or constancy and thus reduce ambiguity.

REF. Keogh BK.: Hyperactivity and Learning Disorders: Review and Speculation. Exceptional Children 30:2, 101-109, 1971.

386. Q. How is mental retardation classified?

A. Mental retardation is generally defined as a low intelligence quotient. Legally most states use an I.Q. score of 70 or lower as qualification for special education. The American Association of Mental Deficiency (AAMD) defines retardation as, "subaverage general intellectual functioning originating during the developmental period and associated with impairment in adaptive behavior." This statement has important implications:

(1) Subaverage is defined as one standard deviation below the mean; since mean I.Q. is generally 100, one SD below the Wechsler scales is 84, and below the Stanford-Binet scale is 83. That definition represents about 16% of the population, while the scores of 70 represents only 2-3%.

(2) The second implication is that the definition does not refer to etiology but rather to impairment in adaptive behavior. If through environmental or sensory stimulation or psychotherapy the individual functions in an adaptive manner, he may no longer be considered retarded.

Mental retardation is further classified into categories:
    (1) Educable - I.Q. score approximately 50 to 70
    (2) Trainable - I.Q. score approximately 30 to 49
    (3) Custodial - I.Q. score below 30

Educable children can generally learn to read, write, and do arithmetic at an achievement level from second to the fifth grade. These people can learn limited vocational skills and usually can function in society. Trainable children generally learn activities of daily living and social skills. Their academic achievements are very limited. They can be trained to work in a sheltered workshop. Custodial children require constant, almost total physical care and are usually, institutionalized or kept at home.
REF. Chinn P.: <u>Child Health Maintenance</u>. C. V. Mosby Company, St. Louis, 1974, pp. 464-466

387. Q. What are some guidelines that can be followed when working with a child who is mentally retarded?

    A. When a nurse is caring for a child with any physical or mental handicap, her first step in planning care is assessment. She must know what his level of functioning is, not only his chronological age, as well as what the environment is like that he is used to. Then some general principles can be followed:

(1) Retarded children generally respond to concrete ideas and objects rather than to abstractions. For example, demonstration is much more effective than just talking about how to do something.

(2) Retarded children respond better to learning step by step rather than one whole process at once. For example, if he is to learn to tie a shoe, the nurse needs to practice the skill several times herself, breaking down the process into simple steps. Each step should be fully learned by the child before attempting to teach him the next step.

(3) Routines that are part of the child's normal daily life should be maintained as much as possible, especially if he is hospitalized. Disruption of routine and ritualistic behavior is extremely difficult for the retarded child.

(4) Appropriate goals should be set for these children based on their developmental age. Behavior modification techniques are very effective methods of reinforcing wanted behavior and skills. Maintaining feelings of success in these children is important in development of their self-esteem.

(5) Parents need to be encouraged and assisted in working with their retarded child, especially in helping him reach his potential functioning.
REF. Chinn P.: <u>Child Health Maintenance</u>. C. V. Mosby Company, St. Louis, 1974, pp. 476-477

388. Q. What are the fundamental principles in teaching motor skills to mentally retarded children?

A. (1) Evaluate the mentally retarded student carefully and attempt to learn as much as possible before training begins. Establish the student's present level of skill and readiness to learn.

(2) Keep learning situations pleasant, the mentally retarded learn much faster when their efforts lead to enjoyable activity.

(3) Repetition, practice, and imitation are necessary.

(4) Use play situations in place of drill where possible.

(5) Employ equipment in a manner that is profitable to individuals specifically.

(6) Be versatile and ready for anything. Have a variety of activities available for implementation, and be able to present each a number of different ways.

(7) Be sensitive to students' needs, desires, and safety. They are more dependent upon you than normal children would be under similar circumstances.

(8) Be involved with each student not in the emotional sense, but in the sense that you are completely and totally dedicated to his growth, improvement, and well being.

REF. Dunham Jr., P.: Teaching Motor Skills to the Mentally Retarded. Exceptional Children 35:9, 739-744, 1969.

389. Q. Is past experience helpful in teaching motor skills to mentally retarded children?

A. In situations in which experimental research is either lacking or not applicable, past experience is most helpful. The following actions, cautions, and principles are found to be invaluable:

(1) Use the same tone of voice each time you speak to the student (patient). Your voice may well be his major clue to your feelings toward him.

(2) Use the same gestures, for the same reasons as above, this will present a consistency and help prevent confusion.

(3) Be firm. Make sure the child does what you say.

(4) Use the same words each time in reinforcing the child. He may have considerable difficulty understanding you.

(5) Reward the student while he is still performing the desired act; he may not otherwise associate his reward with the action performed. Put a delay between an undesirable act of behavior and a situation for which you plan to reward him.

(6) Watch off guard actions. Much teaching will be informal and may well communicate unintended attitudes or feelings.

(7) Share and discuss your progress and procedures with other teachers (nurses), benefiting from their past experiences.

(8) Be patient! Teach simple, easy tasks first, gradually moving on to the more difficult as the students' performances dictate. Progress is sometimes slow.

REF. Dunham Jr., P.: Teaching Motor Skills to the Mentally Retarded. Exceptional Children 35:9, 739-744, 1969.

390.  Q. What is the language comprehension in the moderately retarded child?

A. It is widely accepted that many mentally retarded children
have problems in language development.  Retardation is in part defined as below average functioning or language related tasks ( as on
the Peabody Picture Vocabulary Test and vocabulary subtests or the
Binet and the Wechsler tests).  It is a matter of concern in view of
the importance of communication skills in the overall functioning of
retarded persons.

In this study the Carrow Auditory Test of Language Comprehension
was administered to retarded trainable pupils attending public school
special education classes:  (a) to evaluate the appropriateness of the
Carrow test for use with trainable retarded children, (b) to compare
the development of linguistic comprehension of children with normal
I.Q.'s with that of trainable retarded children.  The results suggest
that the Carrow Test can provide useful information concerning the
language comprehension development of trainable retarded children.

Results further demonstrate systematic language growth in children
with I.Q.'s as low as 20 and 30.  These children acquired mastery
of vocabulary terms and aspects of morphology and syntax.  When
matched on mental age, the retarded children's use of lexical items
did not differ from nonretarded children to a great extent; however,
retarded children's use of grammatical categories was inferior to
that of nonretarded children.
REF. Bartel NR, et al.: Language Comprehension in the Moderately
Retarded Child. Exceptional Children 39:5, 375-382, 1973.

391.  Q. Can mentally retarded children learn language by means
of visual imagery?

A. Several reasons are suggested to account for the effectiveness of visual imagery in this experiment:

(1) The use of imagery requires that the subject become completely
    involved in the learning task.  This means, that greater atten-
    tion is given to the words to be learned.
(2) Learning situations which employ imagery are more meaning-
    ful to the individual.  Essentially, such situations represent a
    form of concrete learning, thus permitting the learner to more
    easily form a connection between the symbol and the object it
    represents.
(3) Images may operate as associational aids and mediate the easy
    recall of the verbal symbols the subject has learned.

When the individual thinks in terms of images, the result is a somewhat continuous review of the details of an object.  Indirectly, this
helps develop in the subject a habit of thinking of objects in descriptive terms.

REF. Christiansen T.: Visual Imagery as a Factor in Teaching Elaborative Language to Mentally Retarded Children. Exceptional Children 35:7, 539-541, 1969.

392. Q. What are some tentative conclusions on self concept and the retarded?

A. (1) The existence of the "self concept of the retarded" as a unique and generalizable construct is questionable.

(2) Segregated placement patterns are not ordinarily conducive to overall positive concepts of self and cannot be justified on that basis.

(3) Retarded children with I.Q.'s from 50 to 80 are educable. Studies of trainable retarded children are rare. Information on self concept development in the trainable population could prove useful.

(4) The referent group by which the retarded child judges himself may change with the particular aspect of self concept being measured at any given moment, i.e., academic, self identity, social, etc. Such changes do not visibly manifest themselves in global scores, and these scores may be of less value in placement, treatment, or program development.

(5) Studies using placement age, comparing segregated versus partially segregated placements while ignoring the self concepts of teachers, or curricular emphasis of a program are incomplete.

(6) Higher scores on self concept scales have been found to correlate positively with higher achievement.

(7) Psychotherapy or counseling in improving self concept have been characterized by the brevity of treatment.

(8) The validity and standardization of many of the measuring instruments can be questioned.
REF. Lawrence EA, Winschel JF.: Self Concept and the Retarded: Research and Issues. Exceptional Children 39:4, 310-317, 1973.

393. Q. Do mentally retarded children have a negative self-concept?

A. There is a great deal of psychological and educational controversy surrounding this topic. The accepted position of Snygg and Combs (1949) states: "What a person does and how he behaves are determined by the concept he has of himself and his abilities".

The relationship of self concept and academic achievement is that the more positive the self concept, higher the achievement level. The self esteem of girls exceeded that of boys with exceptions in performance with arithmetic, sports, and games in comparison with boys.

The effect of age has received scant attention in the literature on retardation. Although 6 year old retarded subjects have been tested increase in chronological age led to increased personal adjustment.

Little attempt has been made to study the relationship of race and self concept among the retarded.

Ideal self attitudes were found to be independent of the effects of age, length of institutionalization, or intelligence. It is felt that ideal self is conceptualized rather early in the history of these individuals. REF. Lawrence EA, Winschel JF.: Self Concept and the Retarded: Research and Issues. Exceptional Children 39:4, 310-317, 1973.

394. Q. Can the mentally retarded benefit from psychotherapeutic relationships?

A. In one study to improve the self concept maternal group counseling was used. Thirty-six educable retarded black preadolescents were divided into an experimental and a control group. The experimental group engaged in a 6 week systematic parent counseling program including home visits, classroom visitations, and discussions. No significant difference in self concepts was found between the two groups of subjects following the parent counseling program.

In a similar study, Wechsler (1971) found that an experimental group of underachieving (rather than mentally retarded) boys whose mothers had engaged in 4 extended encounter group counseling sessions disclosed a significantly higher level of self acceptance than a control group.

Encounter group counseling with mothers employed by Wechsler might also prove effective in modifying the self concepts of retarded children.

Interaction by men had a favorable effect upon the self concepts of institutionalized boys. Similar results were obtained with retarded girls following a planned program of physical fitness training. REF. Lawrence EA, Winschel JF.: Self Concept and the Retarded: Research and Issues. Exceptional Children 39:4, 310-317, 1973.

395. Q. What is color blindness and does it affect mentally retarded children?

A. Color blindness is usually defined as the inability to distinguish one or more colors. There are two basic forms: monochromatism and dichromatism. The former is the complete inability to discriminate different hues and saturations, although brightness perception remains normal. The latter is a condition in which the individual perceives only two of the three basic hues (red, green, or blue). It takes one of three forms: red blindness, green blindness, or blue-yellow blindness.

One out of every four or five mentally retarded children is color blind. Sex differences in color blindness, invariably found in intellectually normal children, do not appear. Consideration must be given to the possible need for a color vision test within the intellectual grasp of most retarded children. It is not known whether color blindness imposes a handicap.

Earlier in the century studies have shown many color blind persons in the general population overcome this disability when working in occupations dependent upon good color vision. But whether mentally retarded individuals can as readily overcome color blindness needs to be investigated.

If the rates for color blindness are as high as one in four, the problem is urgent. For even smaller proportions of children, the question needs to be reopened: Does the use of color dependent instructional techniques penalize the color blind, mentally retarded child? REF. Schein JD, Salvia JA.: Color Blindness in Mentally Retarded Children. Exceptional Children 35:8, 609-612, 1969.

396. Q. What are the characteristics of a so called rubella child?

A. Some of the characteristics of these children are:

(1) Thinness
(2) A low hairline with double cowlicks
(3) A bumpy nose with a deviated septum
(4) Delicate hands and feet
(5) An almost fanatical obsession with light
(6) A delay in physical progress
(7) Unusual pleasure in rocking
(8) Lack of recognition of human relationships
(9) Little interest in food
(10) Difficulties with toilet training
REF. Guldager L.: The Deaf Blind: Their Education and Their Needs. Exceptional Children 36:3, 203-206, 1969.

397. Q. What methods help prevent retardation in infants with Down's syndrome?

A. During 1967 and 1968, an eighteen-month study of the development of seven children with Down's syndrome was carried out. Its purpose was to establish guidelines for helping children with mongolism achieve greater developmental progress.

The children aged 4-17 months, were placed on wards with a home-like setting, toys and other items that would encourage tactile and visual stimulation. None of the children could be considered to be at their appropriate developmental age. Each child was provided with a "mother substitute" who cared for the child on a consistent basis in a consistent way.

Daily experiences such as shopping, being dressed and fed and playing with other children approximated the life of a normal child in a home setting. The children also attended nursery school, were provided special attention and stimulation, physical and occupational therapy.

At the end of the experimental period the children were functioning at their age level in gross motor activities and slightly below the norm in fine motor activities for their chronological age. For most of the children, adaptive behavior and language development were appropriate for their age. In addition, some had developed self-help skills and some were being toilet trained.

The experiment demonstrated that, with change, the hospital setting can meet and support the child's developmental needs.
REF. Kugel RB.: Combatting Retardation in Infants with Down's Syndrome. Children 17:188-192, Sept.-Oct. 1970.

398. Q. What is an exceptional child?

A. The term exceptional refers to that individual who has special needs which affect his or her development through the life cycle. It includes those who are physically handicapped and/or emotionally disturbed to the extent that part or all of their care and treatment occurs outside the family unit.
REF. Maddock J.: Sex Education for the Exceptional Person: A Rationale. Exceptional Children 40:4, 273, 1974.

399. Q. What are some attitudes toward the exceptional child?

A. A study was done using 132 men and 132 women college students to learn their attitudes toward the exceptional child. The categories were the following: blind, chronically ill, crippled, deaf, delinquent, emotionally disturbed, gifted, hard of hearing, mildly mentally retarded, nonexceptional, partially seeing, severely mentally retarded, and speech handicapped. The interpersonal situations were as follows:

(1) I would marry this person.
(2) I would accept this person as close kin by marriage.
(3) I would accept this person to membership in my fraternity (men), sorority (women), or club.
(4) I would invite this person to visit my home.
(5) I would accept this person as a co-worker in my occupation.
(6) I would accept this person as a playmate for my child.

A major finding was that there is a common set of attitudes toward the disabled which cuts across categories of disability and interpersonal situation. The general facts were differentiated into attitudes toward the physically disabled (with certain special emphases), attitudes toward the psychologically disabled, and attitudes toward the mildly retarded nonexceptional. The last named factor was particularly provocative, indicating that, except for the closest interpersonal relationships (marriage and acceptance as close kin by marriage), the mildly retarded shared in the same configuration of attitudes as are held toward the nonexceptional. Attitudes toward the gifted emerged as a separate factor, isolated in virtually all instances from those held toward the disabled.

REF. Jones R.: The Hierarchical Structure of Attitudes Toward the Exceptional. Exceptional Children 40:6, 430-435, 1974.

400. Q. How can one deal with the sexuality of the exceptional child/person?

A. Human sexuality has two basic dimensions: (1) how will one live out the implications of having been born a biological male or female, (2) sex refers to "genitalization" of one's personal identity. At what ages under what circumstances with whom, and in what forms is genital activity to take place in a person's life - and with what results, both for the individual and for society. Several guidelines are:

(1) Fostering the underlying personhood, the "human" in every person - that quality which transcends the inequalities of life. Striving to respect and appreciate the individuality of each person with whom we work.

(2) Recognizing the fundamental sexuality of every human being as a basic dimension of personality. Recognizing the meaning and significance of sexual expression distinct from reproductive functioning, composed of physical and symbolic aspects, both of which are important to the individual.

(3) Understanding the sexuality of the exceptional person in relation to his/her physical, mental, emotional, and social development so that appropriate channels of expression can be discovered. We should be willing to provide accurate information and sound guidance with the goal of enabling the exceptional person to become sexually active as his or her capacities, physical and emotional health, welfare of other persons and of society will allow.

(4) Fostering a morality which encourages personal autonomy and freedom within the limits of the individual's capacity for social and interpersonal responsibility.

Parents and institution personnel are those who most make the final decisions based on the above guidelines. The rewards and potential benefits are great: the unlocking of new capacities for self expression which in the exceptional individual which can lend to greater overall health and effective functioning.
REF. Maddock J.: Sex Education for the Exceptional Person: A Rationale. Exceptional Children 40:4, 273-278, 1974.

401. Q. Can exceptional foster children benefit from trained foster parents?

A. In this project it was shown that early educational intervention with handicapped children can be highly successful. The rapid mastery of assigned, specific skills through intensive parental and staff efforts also is supportive of intervention.

One of the keys to successful intervention is the training of foster parents to be attentive to the developmental process and its enhancement and to the subsequent intensive stimulation provided the child by them. The three primary objectives in the training are:

(1) To intervene early to attempt adequate remediation of handicapping conditions.
(2) To intervene sufficiently early to permit a more rapid acceptance of infants by prospective adopting parents.
(3) To establish prototypic techniques of early intervention through foster parent training procedures.
REF. Quick AD, et al.: Early Childhood Education for Exceptional Foster Children and Training of Foster Parents. Exceptional Children 40:3, 206-208, 1973.

402. Q. What science contributes to the study of cultural diversity and the education of exceptional children?

A. The science of linguistics. Language is a system of vocal sounds; it is systematic and symbolic; it is in a state of constant change. The ability to learn language (but not the specifics of any particular language) is innate in humans, and all languages and their variations are equally good.

The role of linguistics in the educational assessment of culturally different is emphasized. The linguistic and cultural bias of I.Q. tests, as well as the role of adaptive behavior and community acceptance are discussed. Identification of gifted children has never had a top priority in this country, especially those who are culturally different. When identified there is often resentment, feelings of hostility, apathy toward the gifted as a major problem.

Many youngsters in the U.S. grow up speaking languages other than English. Some would impose the same linguistic expectations on them in the early years as they would on native English speakers of the same age. We claim to live in a pluralistic society, there are those who would rob others of their native tongue or dialect, only to require its learning later as a prerequisite for graduation.

Though all languages and dialects have been shown to be appropriate for their time, place, and circumstance, there are those who would relegate speakers of language and dialects other than "standard" to an inferior or retarded status.
REF. Gonzalez G.: Language, Culture and Exceptional Children. Exceptional Children 40:8, 565-570, 1974.

403. Q. What is the definition of the term culturally different gifted child?

A. Various labels, some misnomers have been foisted on this child. Labels such as culturally disadvantaged, socially disadvantaged, culturally diverse, and culturally deprived.

The culturally different comprise one segment of a larger subpopulation called the educationally disadvantaged. This latter broader group includes not only the culturally different but also the economically deprived, female, handicapped, rural, and underachieving. Thus, the major qualification in the definition of the culturally different is membership in a culture other than the dominant one.

This article re-examines the identification procedure with an emphasis on environmental and sociological variables. The article points out what is being done to fulfill the special and different needs of the culturally different gifted child and offers information on the educational programs being instituted throughout the U.S. Some available resources which have generated new materials are provided.
REF. Sato IS.: The Culturally Different Gifted Child - The Dawning of His Day? Exceptional Children 40:8, 572-576, 1974.

404. Q. Are gifted children superior in the use of language?

A. The language of the gifted child has received little attention. This is perplexing when one considers the relationship between language and intellectual performance, as well as the demands placed by society on an individual's ability to express concepts symbolically through language.

The research investigated the relationship of language performance to intellectual factors only. The hypothesis to be tested: There is no difference between average and superior fifth grade boys and girls in casual and careful oral language fluency, grammatical control, and function.

The Lorge-Thorndike Intelligence Tests: Verbal and the Gates-MacGinitie Reading Tests were given to 80 fifth grade pupils. There were 20 each average boys and girls, and 20 each superior boys and girls.
REF. Jensen JM.: Do Gifted Children Speak an Intellectual Dialect? Exceptional Children 39:4, 337-338, 1973.

405. Q. What are some findings on testing gifted children versus average children on speech usage?

A. The conclusions are:

(1) All of the basic structural patterns of English occurred within the typescripts of both ability subgroups, with the usage pattern of the subjects closely paralleling that of adults.
(2) Standard English usage, characterizes the speech of both ability subgroups.
(3) The language differential between students who performed in the top and middle ranges on standardized tests of intelligence and achievement was not statistically significant on most comparisons.

Selected implications of the study relate to the formal teaching of grammar and usage, differential sex expectations in oral language performance, teacher preparation in individually diagnosed and prescribed language arts instruction, and the usefulness of the general label of gifted.
REF. Jensen JM.: Do Gifted Children Speak an Intellectual Dialect? Exceptional Children 39:4, 337-338, 1973.

406. Q. Are there ethnic differences in psycholinguistic abilities?

A. This article summarizes the results of several research studies on the psycholinguistic abilities, as measured by the Illinois Test of Psycholinguistic Abilities, of three ethnic groups, Blacks, Indians and Mexican Americans. The summary of studies reveals the following:

(1) The performance of Black children in auditory sequential memory appears to be superior to their performance in other areas and to the performance of other ethnic groups along this dimension as measured by a digit repetition test. This seems to occur in both middle class and lower class Black children.

(2) Indian children appear to have a superiority in visual sequential memory (visual short term memory), both with reference to their other abilities and with reference to Black and Anglo children.

(3) Mexican American children, similarly to bilingual Indian children, appear to be superior in visual sequential memory relative both to their other abilities and to both Blacks and Anglos.

Possible explanations for these results is that there may be hereditary ethnic differences.

The Indian hereditary difference which may be inherited is that in order to survive Indians had to have good visual abilities and particularly good visual sequential memory.

Among Black families learning occurs primarily through the auditory channel from the time the child is in the crib. The child begins to depend on what he hears and remembers for adaptation in a family situation. The author believes that there are major differences in early childhood training due to cultural differences among ethnic groups.
REF. Kirk SA.: Ethnic Differences in Psycholinguistics Abilities. Exceptional Children 39:2, 112-118, 1972.

407. Q. Who is a handicapped child?

A. He is a human being who deviates from capabilities we expect from any normal child. He may deviate a little, or a lot; he may have only a single learning disability, or combinations of learning disabilities. Many handicapped children are similar, but no two exactly alike. The children will vary in their needs for three definite reasons:

(1) All children are born with innate, inherited characteristics.
(2) Each child responds to his particular environment.
(3) The number of areas, the place, and the degree of brain damage will never be the same in any two cases.*

*Steps to Achievement for the Slow Learner. Ebersole, M., et al., Columbus, Ohio: Charles E. Merrill, 1968, p. 196.
REF. Book Review. Exceptional Children 35:5, 393-394, 1969.

408. Q. What is the educational process for developing skills in handicapped and normal children?

A. The right kind of auditory stimuli should surround the new-born baby. When the baby is mature enough he should be in the middle of family activities, and not left alone all day. The child enjoys participating in family activities and helping other family members. For instance, the child helps the mother in her household tasks, so everyday activities can be used as a learning medium.

Later when the child plays soccer, baseball, balances on the curb, climbs trees, swims, the child really is receiving training in motor coordination, eye-hand coordination, auditory localization, and figure-ground discrimination. The child is exploring the potential of the body, training the senses, and learning to judge distance and perspective and coordinate his body movements.

This development is basic for all children. If there has been a gap in the development for whatever reasons, the child is handicapped and needs special attention.

The earlier a deaf blind child can be identified and given direction in skill development, the better.
REF. Guldager L.: The Deaf Blind: Their Education and Their Needs. Exceptional Children 36:3, 203-206, 1969.

409. Q. Can college students contribute to the language development and general well being of severely handicapped children?

A. This article describes a program based on behavioral principles to develop verbal behavior in severely handicapped young children and designed to be conducted by college students. The results indicate that college students are able to apply their basic knowledge and technical skills obtained mainly from an increasing number of behaviorally oriented courses offered at the undergraduate level. The development of language repertoires in severely handicapped children initially requires an intensive one to one relationship between child and instructor. In most educational settings, especially where the population consists of low functioning children, sufficient professional staff is not available to perform this function.

The success of this project suggests that an expanded use of this resource, i.e., college students may ultimately contribute toward alleviating the shortage of technical personnel, especially in institutions and treatment centers serving severely handicapped children.
REF. Guralnick MJ.: A Language Development Program for Severely Handicapped Children. Exceptional Children 39:1, 45-49, 1972.

410. Q. Are siblings influenced by the handicapped child?

A. The advent of technological advances and knowledge has seen an increase in the number of salvagable handicapped infants and children. In the home, much attention is focused on them with a concomitant decrease in attention to siblings by the parents. Relationships with parents may become distorted because of the time, energy and care given to the handicapped child. Sometimes, parents may have negative feelings toward the handicapped child. Rather than expressing them toward him, they may be expressed toward another child in the family. The increased needs of the child with an impairment may cause the parents to be overprotective and overloving, thus creating a special relationship which, excludes healthy siblings. As siblings experience emotional neglect, psychiatric and behavioral problems may become manifest.

Health professionals are in a position to investigate whether or not the needs of other children in the family are being met. If they are not, parental counselling and perhaps child counseling may be necessary.
REF. Poznanski E.: Psychiatric Difficulties in Siblings of Handicapped Children. Clinical Pediatrics 8:232-234, April 1969.

411. Q. What are the role perceptions of parents of handicapped children?

A. Transition to any new role requires socialization - learning new ways of behaving and seeing oneself. Persons who have been socialized to the conception of parenthood through their previous children and those who are parents for the first time face a different socialization process when they meet the task as parents of a handicapped child. It has been said that "no parent is ever prepared to be the parent of a handicapped child. The identification of a mother and father in that role always comes as a complete surprise".

Socialization to the role of parent of a handicapped child is usually a traumatic and conflict producing experience. There are both instrumental (technical) and expressive (emotional) aspects of this role change which needs resolution. The agents of socialization, such as doctors, teachers, social workers, (nurses), and handicapped adults, play an important role in the socialization process. The transition in role perception is also influenced by the socioeconomic status, age, religion, and physical characteristics of the parents and by the sex and birth order of the child. An understanding of the

influence of these factors should assist the agents of socialization in helping parents and in turn be beneficial to the handicapped child in making an effective adjustment to his handicap.
REF. Meadow, KP, Meadow L.: Changing Role Perceptions for Parents of Handicapped Children. Exceptional Children 38:1, 21-27, 1971.

412. Q. What are the handicaps which may be found in children with congenital rubella?

A. The Developmental Evaluation Clinic of the Children's Hospital Medical Center in Boston studied 46 deaf children with congenital rubella. The 46 children exhibited the following handicaps:

(1) Mental retardation - moderate or severe in about 10% of the cases. Another 30% had low average intelligence ratings.
(2) Behavioral abnormalities in about 30% - in those not markedly retarded.
(3) Visual handicap - cataracts in 15% of the cases. Strabismus occurred in about 20% of the cases.
(4) Neurologic abnormalities and/or limitations in motor skills - excluding the group of retarded children, about 50% had faulty balance, coordination, and control of movement.
(5) Congenital heart disease - in about 25% of the children, with half of these having serious heart disease.
(6) Small size - 40% of the children were below the third percentile in height.
(7) Receptive language problems - this was difficult to evaluate.
REF. Guldager L.: The Deaf Blind: Their Education and Their Needs. Exceptional Children 36:3, 203-206, 1969.

413. Q. What are the steps in the child's development of the use of hearing?

A. Every child must first be a receiver of communication before he can express himself verbally. During the first few weeks of life a child will respond reflexively to sound. The infant responds to moods and emotional tones of voices rather than to words, for example the voice of the mother will evoke smiling and cooing behavior. By the age of 6 months, the child learns to move his eyes to locate the sound and begins to vocalize responses to the voices around him. In the second 6 months of life sounds of speech assume meaning and he may recognize words. By 9 months words such as "Mama" and "milk" will elicit specific responses. By the age of 1 year the child will recognize three or four word sentences such as "Get daddy's shoes". They respond to the context of the sentence rather than to each separate word.

Between 18 and 24 months, children enjoy the lilting auditory pattern of nursery rhymes even though they do not comprehend the meaning. By the third year of life the child can follow simple stories through hearing alone. By the age of four, however, the child can

carry on a conversation in a give and take manner. The child's use of audition as a mode of adaptation to his environment progresses somewhat ahead of his development of speech.
REF. McConnell F, Ph.D.: A New Approach to the Management of Childhood Deafness. Pediatric Clinics of North America 17:2, 347-362, 1970.

414. Q. What are some characteristics of the deaf child?

A. A child with perceptual handicaps is believed to be different from children without such impairment. Specifically, his perceptual environment is less complete, interaction with others will differ and the child's self-concept will be influenced by it.

Behavior disorders such as autism, mental retardation or compulsive-like traits often are manifest. If hearing loss can be corrected these behaviors often are reversed. Because of absence of a sensory modality, ego organization and emotional expression develop later than in hearing children.

Deaf children appear to have alternate periods of diffuse motor restlessness and periods of immobility. This appears to be due to lack of a hearing modality, necessary for diffuse scanning of the environment.
REF. Lesser SR, Easser BR.: Personality Differences in the Perceptually Handicapped. Journal of Child Psychiatry 11:458-466, 1972.

415. Q. What are some characteristic behavior patterns of children with hearing loss?

A. A hearing loss is often a subtle, undetected defect in children. It is not unusual for children with moderate auditory loss to be considered mentally retarded or minimally brain damaged because of their behavior and interest in the environment. Severe hearing losses can present fewer problems in diagnosis because of the child's lack of speech development, failure to respond to loud noises, and lack of response to verbal commands.

How can we detect children with some degree of hearing difficulty? Several authorities in the field of hearing have described the child's behavior, which can yield significant data.

(1) The child with a hearing loss is less interested in his environment than his peers, responding more to visual and tactile stimuli. He will respond more to one's facial expression than to one's verbal statements.

(2) He will appear to hear better at certain times, often leading people around him to doubt his defect. However, astute observation can help one distinguish when he hears better. For example, a quiet environment, the distance between the speaker and him, and quality of the speaker's voice will influence his hearing.

(3) If the hearing loss is sensorineural, certain words or letters will produce difficulty because of sound distortion. Speech problems usually accompany this type of defect. For example, high frequency sounds like "s", "sh", or "z" can be omitted, causing sentences like "I ee the un," for "I see the sun." Voice inflection may also be affected, so that all sentences are monotone.

(4) These children are usually shy, timid, and withdrawn. They do particularly poorly when in a group, especially if several people are talking at once.

(5) Frequent earaches should always herald suspicion of a possible defect.
REF. Payne P, Payne R.: Behavior Manifestations of Children with Hearing Loss. American Journal of Nursing 8:70, Aug. 1970.

416. Q. What are some developmental danger signals in detecting a hearing loss in young children?

A. Children with a mild or greater hearing loss can be detected during the first year of life by observing for these clues:

(1) lack of neonatal startle reflex in response to sharp clap within 3 to 6 inches,
(2) persistence of Moro reflex beyond 4 to 6 months as a sign of neurological impairment,
(3) failure to be awaken by loud environmental sounds during first 4 months,
(4) failure to localize a source of sound at 2 to 3 feet away anytime after 6 months,
(5) absence of babble sounds by 7 months,
(6) inability to understand words or short phrases by 12 months,
(7) use of gestures to establish needs.
REF. Gustafson S, Coursin D.: The Pediatric Patient. J. B. Lippincott Company, Philadelphia, 1966, pp. 154-179

417. Q. What types of hearing loss are common among children?

A. The major types of hearing loss are conductive, sensorineural, and central impairment. Conductive loss results when there is dysfunction of the outer or middle ear. The primary effect of this dysfunction is loss of loudness. As loudness is restored, so is perception of sound. Sensorineural loss results from a dysfunction of the inner ear or damage to the auditory nerve. This loss results in acoustic distortion and problems of tone discrimination. Unlike conductive loss, hearing aids may afford little help. Central impairment results from dysfunction along the pathways of the brain from the brainstem to the cerebral cortex. This usually results in problems in terms of receptive and expressive language.

Hearing loss is based on audiometric measurements of hearing level. Sound is measured in decibels from 0 to 120. Zero represents the faintest sound the normal ear can hear; ten decibels is about as loud as a heartbeat. The range from 30 to 40 db. represents normal speech, 70 to 80 range street noises. A slight hearing loss is defined as a loss of 24 to 27 db. This child usually has little difficulty in school, has no speech problem and has difficulty hearing faint sounds. A child with a mild loss between 41 to 55 db. is able to understand conversational speech at a distance of 3 to 5 feet when facing the speaker, but he will probably miss half the conversation if he is farther away or not facing the speaker. He probably has a limited vocabulary and speech defects with higher sounds. A child with a greater loss requires amplified sound to hear normal confersation and needs special education in voice, speech and language development.

REF. Chinn P.: Child Health Maintenance. C. V. Mosby Company, St. Louis, 1974, p. 472

418. Q. How does deafness affect a child's development of language?

A. Deaf children will develop physically the same as normal children and up until the age of 6 months will smile, laugh and vocalize completely normally. At about 6 months vocalization begins to diminish and by 1 year he is usually mute other than for reflexive sounds of distress or crying. Because he cannot hear, he does not receive the reinforcement of hearing his own voice. Visual alertness increases and vision becomes the primary sensory input. The hearing child by the age of 18 months can use some words to express ideas, the deaf child has continually failed in getting something he wants without words. He may display negative behavior in the form of tantrums. Feet stomping, for example, could express rage, as well as be a call for attention. By the age of 6 or 7 the hearing child has mastered all the essential components of his native language. The deaf child however, may not even begin to learn language until this age and by this time is very retarded in his verbal abilities. It is recommended the very early training in the first year of life be instituted to overcome some aspects of the problem.

REF. McConnell F, Ph.D.: A New Approach to the Management of Childhood Deafness. Pediatric Clinics of North America 17:2, 347-362, 1970.

419. Q. What measures can aid in the early detectionof hearing loss in children?

A. The diagnosis of children who are deaf or hard of hearing is often not made early enough for medical, audiological and educational intervention to be instituted at the optimum time. These children may be thought to be mentally retarded, emotionally disturbed or brain damaged if not diagnosed early. Early identification of the deaf or hard of hearing child will be assisted by the following guidelines:

(1) recognition of conditions in infancy which put a child at high risk for developing hearing impairment,

(2) listening to and regarding seriously parents concerns about their child's language development,

(3) be alert to language development in the 2 year old using the Denver Developmental Screening Test as a guide,
(4) prolonged jargoning, poor enunciation and excessive use of gestures may be symptomatic of hearing loss,
(5) be aware that informal screening tests for hearing may fail to identify partial hearing loss,
(6) if hearing loss is suspected the child should be referred to an audiologist, regardless of age, developmental level or behavior.
REF. Holm V, M.D., Thompson G, Ph.D.: Selective Hearing Loss: Clues to Early Identification. Pediatrics 47:2, 447-451, 1971.

420. Q. Is there a verbal deficit in children with hearing loss?

A. This study was designed to explore the relation between language and/or verbal ability and reduced auditory acuity at discrete frequencies and various frequency bands in children with high frequency impairment.

Results showed significant relationships between hearing levels, particularly at 1,000, 1,500, 2,000 and 3,000 cps, and verbal deficit as measured by the Wechsler Intelligence Scale for Children. When impairment at these frequencies occurs before or during the language learning years (0-5) and is of sufficient severity to interfere with the reception of speech, there are several considerations:

(1) A school group I.Q. test that is highly verbal-vocabulary dependent may result in low I.Q. score. Then teacher judgment and teaching procedures are affected.
(2) Reduced verbal skill can adversely affect academic achievement.
(3) Misunderstanding of content or oral communication and frustrations from such failures may negatively influence social and emotional development. The child will fail to profit from peer interaction.
(4) Early identification of impairment so remedial procedure may be instituted. Their failure to hear consonants adequately may yield an impression that they are merely slow and inattentive.
REF. Roach RE, Rosecrans CJ.: Verbal Deficit in Children with Hearing Loss. Exceptional Children 38:5, 395-399, 1972.

421. Q. Is immaturity in deaf children a consequence of auditory deprivation?

A. Research findings reporting teacher-counselor ratings of deaf children from differing home and school settings show significant differences in assessments for maturity.

An analysis of various developmental crises for which deafness has a definite impact is presented, based on Erikson's theory of epigenetic development.

The authors contend that the research findings and independent observations which characterize deaf individuals as "immature" are not a necessary consequence of auditory deprivation.

The research findings presented earlier, which show differential levels of maturity in deaf children from varying environmental conditions, and the applications of a developmental theory to the impact of deafness at varying stages of the life cycle both point to the reversible nature of this characterization.

REF. Schlesinger HS, Meadow KP.: Development of Maturity in Deaf Children. Exceptional Children 38:6, 461-467, 1972.

422. Q. Are there differences in academic learning ability among deaf children?

A. This study attempts to identify perceptual-motor characteristics which might account for, or attribute to, the differences in academic learning ability in deaf populations of comparable age and I.Q.

This investigation included the following: sensory avenues of kinestheses and vision, tasks of hand-eye coordination, gross body coordination, motor speed and planning, physical and motor fitness, and the balancing mechanisms.

The findings of the study indicated that significant differences existed between the groups on tasks involving muscular strength, motor speed, and motor planning, and also on tasks which involved greater integration of neuromuscular control. No significant differences were found between groups on tasks involving the balancing mechanism or sensory utilization.

By means of progressive-resistive training motor movements involving neuromuscular integration, gross strength, and ability to endure would improve. Sequential activity programs are feasible to enhance deficient developments of physical and perceptual-motor characteristics.

REF. Auxter D.: Learning Disabilities Among Deaf Populations. Exceptional Children 37:8, 573-577, 1971.

423. Q. How do deaf children develop communication skills?

A. In this study 74 children in 7 preschool programs for the deaf were assessed in a measure of receptive communication. Subjects ranged from 48 to 72 months with a mean chronological age of 61.96 months. Hearing losses ranged from 71 to 100 decibels with a mean loss of 95.49 decibels. Subjects were tested across five modes of communication:

(1) Sound alone
(2) Sound plus speech reading (lipreading)
(3) Sound plus speech reading plus finger spelling
(4) Sound and speech reading plus signs
(5) The printed word

Four levels of difficulty were assessed for each mode:

(1) number concepts
(2) adjective-noun phrases
(3) noun-conjunction-noun phrases
(4) noun-verb-prepositional phrase constructions

Results suggest that the most efficient means of receptive communication was simultaneous use of sound and speech reading plus signs. Children using this system receive information at least as efficiently as other deaf children when manual components are removed.
REF. Moores DF, et al.: Receptive Abilities of Deaf Children Across Five Modes of Communication. Exceptional Children 40:1, 22-28, 1973.

424. Q. What is the social status of hearing impaired children in regular classrooms?

A. This study examined the peer status and the self perceived peer status of 15 first and second grade hearing impaired children enrolled in regular classrooms.

Subjects included four children with mild to moderate hearing losses and 11 children with severe to profound hearing losses who were full time hearing aid users.

Three sociometric tests were used to assess the peer acceptance as well as the self perceived peer status for both normally hearing and hearing impaired students.

Results indicated that the hearing impaired children received a higher degree of social acceptance from normally hearing peers than reported in previous studies. They were also as perceptive of their own social status as normally hearing children.
REF. Kennedy P, Bruininks RH.: Social Status of Hearing Impaired Children in Regular Classrooms. Exceptional Children 40:5, 336-342, 1974.

425. Q. What are the etiological factors that can cause deafness among cerebral palsied children?

A. This study shows complications of the RH factor and indicates it to be the leading cause of the combined conditions of deafness and cerebral palsy. This is now preventable. Another cause of the conditions is rubella. The results of the 1963-1965 epidemic will remain a major habilitative responsibility for many years.

Meningitis, used to tesult in high mortality rates among infants, especially those born prematurely, and severe deafness, unaccompanied by other defects in children and adults, now generally does not deafen those older than 4 years of age. Because of medical advances many of the meningitic infants and prematures survive that would have formerly died, but those surviving are left with deafness and severe spasticity. Prematurity, the second most common condition associated with combined deafness and cerebral palsy, also contributes to the number of deaf cerebral palsied. The improved survival rate among children of low birth weight has probably increased the rate of combined deafness and cerebral palsy.

The findings of the collaborative perinatal project (Hardy, 1967; Masland, 1967) have revealed some new and preventable prenatal causes of the problem.

Some of the antibiotics used to treat meningitis (such as streptomycin, karomycin, neomycin, gramycetin, vancomycin, viomycin, gentamycin, and colistin) and some of the conditions associated with prematurity are atotoxic. Their removal from therapeutic regimes will prevent a small amount of the auditory component of the deaf cerebral palsy syndrome.
REF. Vernon M.: Clinical Phenomenon of Cerebral Palsy and Deafness. Exceptional Children 36:10, 743-751, 1970.

426. Q. What are the steps taken in the (Re)habilitation of the deaf cerebral palsied child?

A. Regular, thorough medical, audiological, and psychological examination beginning in infancy. Not only is diagnoses necessary but recommendation for prostheses and training for the correction or modification of the visual, hearing, perceptual, and other prevalent problems are necessary. The child will not only be able to utilize his capacities in the crucial early years, but throughout his life.

Another step in rehabilitation involves educational programming. Education of these children should involve the use of the readily visible and the understandable language of signs, fingerspelling, and reading which, in addition to being easier to perceive visually, also involve far less motoric skill than the movements required for speech. Some deaf cerebral palsied children with aphasia who are almost totally unable to communicate orally or with printed symbols can carry on meaningful conversations in the language of signs.

Vocational placement for the deaf cerebral palsied is low. Many with college degrees have no jobs, primarily due to poor or nonexistent counseling, public attitudes, and a lack of knowledge about appropriate areas of work for persons with this multiple handicap.
REF. Vernon M.: Clinical Phenomenon of Cerebral Palsy and Deafness. Exceptional Children 36:10, 743-751, 1970.

427. Q. How should the parents of deaf cerebral palsied children be treated?

A. It is crucial that valid available information about these children be communicated frankly to parents and that extensive counseling to help parents understand and accept these facts be available.

The psychological integration and acceptance of a deaf cerebral palsied child is a complex process involving parental emotional reactions to the trauma of having a multiple handicapped child.

Counseling of these parents may be long and somewhat expensive, but failure to provide it often adds an even more crippling emotional overlay to the child's physical handicaps.
REF. Vernon M.: Clinical Phenomenon of Cerebral Palsy and Deafness. Exceptional Children 36:10, 743-751, 1970.

428. Q. What is the intelligence rating of the deaf child with cerebral palsy?

A. This study suggests that almost half of deaf cerebral palsied children have average or better intelligence. Only about 20% are retarded. Particular care should be taken in obtaining and reporting data on intelligence, the crucial variable in determining prognosis for habilitation. It is easy for psychologists unknowledgeable about the behavioral implications of deafness to make gross errors based primarily on a confusion of the language lag due to deafness with a lack of intelligence.

There is much mental retardation among deaf cerebral palsied children, however, diagnoses should not be accepted unless confirmed by a psychologist with extensive knowledge of this specific problem.

When psychometric diagnoses stand in sharp contrast to the clinical judgment of people experienced in work with children, additional opinions should be obtained.
REF. Vernon M.: Clinical Phenomenon of Cerebral Palsy and Deafness. Exceptional Children 36:10, 743-751, 1970.

429. Q. What is the effect of "rock music" upon hearing?

A. The general attitude of adolescents who listen to rock and roll music is "the louder the better". This philosophy and practice is exposing the teenager to possible permanent hearing loss. Over the years, many wernings and evidence of hearing loss due to excessive noise have been issued.

Studies indicate that "exposures to noise intensities in the order of 100 db $cm^2$ can cause deafness. Noise levels in excess of 130 decibel may do permanent damage to the ears of normal persons, even after a relatively short exposure".

The greatest danger to the adolescent exposed to loud rock music seems to be at dances and discotheques when they are exposed to loud music for three to four hours. Noise levels in these environments have been measured at 120-140 db. Progressive, permanent ear damage is likely with frequent exposure to such noise.
REF. Rupp R, Koch C.: Effects of too-Loud Music on Human Ears. Clinical Pediatrics 8:60-62, Feb. 1969.

430. Q. How can nurses detect visual disorders in children?

   A. Visual acuity is measured by eye charts such as the Snellen scale. Visually impaired children are usually placed into one of two categories based on symptom severity. Type one is blind as defined by a corrected vision of 20/200 or less in the better eye or peripheral vision where the visual field extends and angular distance of less than 20 degrees in the better eye. Partially seeing is defined as corrected vision between 20/200 and 20/70.

Although all children should have their sight tested for visual acuity, refractory errors can be detected by observing for:

(1) retarded motor development in the infant, who may hitch on his buttocks rather than crawl to prevent banging his head,
(2) rocking for sensory stimulation,
(3) holding a book too close, or coloring with the head on the table,
(4) squinting and rubbing the eyes,
(5) clumsiness, and frequent accidents such as falling or bumping into objects,
(6) poor performance in school especially in subjects where blackboard demonstration is important, such as arithmetic.
REF. Marlow D.: Textbook of Pediatric Nursing. W. B. Saunders Company, Philadelphia, 1973

431. Q. What is the normal development of visual acuity in the young child?

   A. At birth, the pupils reach to light, the blink reflex and corneal reflex are present, and the infant can follow a light to midline. From one to three months, binocular fixation is established and the infant can follow a light or brightly colored objects to the periphery (180°). Tear glands function in response to emotion. Visual acuity is 20/200 by about five months. Between five and seven months, the color of the iris is established and hand-eye coordination is developing. By one year, depth perception has developed and visual acuity is about 20/100. At this time amblyopia may develop from lack of binocularity (strabismus). By two years, visual acuity is 20/40, he is able to scribble on paper, to identify forms and to maintain interest in pictures. By three years, visual acuity is 20/30, and toward the fourth year, reading readiness is present. After four years, there is minimal potential for amblyopia to develop. By six years, visual acuity approaches 20/20, depth perception is fully developed, and astigmatism may begin to develop.
REF. Chinn PL, Leitch CJ.: Child Health Maintenance: A Guide to Clinical Assessment. C. V. Mosby Company, St. Louis, 1974, p. 67

432. Q. What is the approach to visual performance deficits?

A. When a child has difficulty learning or behaving normally in spite of average or above average intelligence, normal visual acuity and hearing, the problem may be visual performance deficits. Children with such perceptual problems can have poor spatial judgment orientation and depth perception. In addition, deficits in hand-eye coordination negatively influence the child's ability to learn to read and write.

The child's poor performance in school and the resultant poor self-image and frustration often leads to behavior problems. They may be manifested by sullenness, arrogance and non-productiveness in school.

Early screening programs can detect visual dysfunction that is both common and correctable. Special optometric training, family support and school support can help the child become a school achiever with socially acceptable behavior.
REF. Kahn H.: Visual Dysfunctions. Nursing '74 26-27, Oct. 1974.

433. Q. How does a blind child differ in learning from a sighted child?

A. A comparative study of blind and sighted children in the 5 to 7 year age range was made, based on the responses to the Kephart Scale. It was found that blind children have misinformation, fragmented concepts, and a limited use of differentiation of information. Deprived of the visual process, they are deprived of a wide range of information gathering that is available to sighted children. This deprivation does not seem to be sufficiently compensated for by giving them auditory and tactile information. A Gestalt type of information coding, using a more nearly life-like situation, appears necessary in the coding process.

The results indicate that there are areas of research available which should be influential in offering broader curricula.
REF. Kephart JG, et al.: A Journey into the World of the Blind Child. Exceptional Children 40:6, 421-427, 1974.

434. Q. What is the significance of eye rubbing in blind children?

A. Eye rubbing, body rocking, head rolling, pacing, and other repetitive motor behaviors are loosely classified as blind mannerisms, or blindisms. Eye rubbing is one of the stereotyped behaviors occurring in blind children and is of concern to those who work toward the acceptance and adjustment of the blind in the sighted world. It is relevant to other issues, such as child development, sensory deprivation, and "critical periods". A critical period is that period when certain biologically based needs are most salient during specific periods of development. The need and response capability for certain experiences or sensory inputs upon which specific maturational events are dependent may be met only during limited segments of an organism's developmental time table. If not potentiated during

the preprogrammed critical period, the appropriate stimuli later
become ineffective and the specific behavior or response system is
lost to the organism's repertoire.

Confirmatory evidence for hypotheses was found from sensory and
social deprivation studies; children with capacity for only minimal,
unpatterned visual input were rated significantly higher in eye rubbing than either the totally blind or those with more usable, pattern-
ed vision. An additional finding, that similar significant differences
persisted but in diminished degree in older children compared to
younger, was related to both training effects and "critical period"
concepts. Given sensory social deprivation as critical ingredient,
plentiful substitute stimulation within an appropriate social context
appears to diminish, if not eliminate the blind mannerisms.
REF. Thurrell RJ, Rice DG.: Eye Rubbing in Blind Children: Application of a Sensory Deprivation Model. Exceptional Children
36:5, 325-330, 1970.

435. Q. What tests can nurses use to detect strabismus in young
children?

A. Strabismus is an ocular disturbance of malalignment of the
eyes. The earliest symptom associated with this disorder is double
vision or diplopia, where an object falls on different areas of the
retina of each eye. To overcome this, the brain supplies a functional blind spot or suppression scotoma. If the malalignment becomes
constant, the scotoma may become permanent, resulting in a visual
loss called amblyopia or "lazy eye".

This type of blindness is easily prevented by detecting and treating
strabismus. Several tests can be done to identify the disorder:

(1) In the "cover-uncover" test, fusion (the process of merging the
images from each eye into binocular vision) is disrupted by covering and then uncovering one eye at a time and observing its movement. If the eye does not move, the eyes are orthophoric (straight
or aligned). If the recently uncovered eye diverges to regain fusion
and normal alignment, an esophoric strabismus is present.

(2) The Maddox Rod test disrupts fusion by converting a bright fixation light source into a line in front of one eye. If the eyes are
aligned, the patient reports the centering of the line on the light.
If the line deviates from the light, the eyes are malaligned.

(3) The "cover" test requires useful vision in each eye. Test targets
used for visual acuity such as Snellen charts or the illiterate E's are
used. The eye is tested at 13 inches and 20 feet ranges. One eye
is covered, and the movement of the uncovered eye is observed. If
the uncovered eye remains fixated, there is no strabismus. The
same is done to the other eye. A patient's eyes can be orthophoric
at distant ranges of visions, but esotropic at near ranges.

(4) The corneal light reflex or Hirshberg test is performed by having the patient fixate on a bright light held 16 inches away. Normally, the light will be reflected slightly nasally as pinpoints in the pupil. In the presence of a deviation, the light reflex is decentered. This test is useful when the patient has poor vision or in infants.
REF. Hiles D.: Strabismus. American Journal of Nursing 74:6, 1082-1089, June 1974.

436. Q. Can visual acuity be assessed?

A. The phenomenon of optokinetic fixation may be used as the stimulus and end-point for minimal visual perception and fixation. The eyes of a normal subject fix and follow the movement of any object to the periphery of the field of fixation, and then jerk quickly back to take up fixation on the next object - such as in "railway nystagmus". It has been found that targets of decreasing size may be presented until they become too small to be fixed and nystagmus is no longer elicited.

A hand-held electrically operated instrument has been devised to assess visual acuity by means of the phenomenon of optokinetic fixation of nystagmus. An accurate determination of visual acuity has been obtained from an early age, and a graph of the normal visual development produced. It has been confirmed that adult acuity is reached by 3 years of age.
REF. Catford GV, Oliver A.: Development of Visual Acuity. Archives of Disease in Childhood 48:1, 47-50, 1973.

437. Q. What is the rationale for measuring visual perception?

A. By using a test of visual-motor integration: "The motor behavior of the small child...adapts itself to resemble the stimulus perceived in the optic field" (Bender 1938). This implies that the child's perception of a stimulus is reflected in his ability to copy it.

Opinion and research also exist which stress the value of measuring visual perception independently of motor activity. The rationale for this premise is that visual perception and motor development are to a considerable extent autonomous (i.e., separate) systems. Depressed performance on tests of visual-motor integration may represent problems in either one or both areas with the respective degrees of deficiency being undeterminable. Statements pertaining to visual perception based on these tests alone may not be valid. There is a need to measure visual perception of motor handicapped children with a motor-free and a motor-involved test in order to answer the following questions:

(1) Do motorically handicapped children as a group have serious deficiencies in visual perception?
(2) Are visual perception and motor development relatively independent systems?

REF. Newcomer P, Hammill D.: Visual Perception of Motor Impaired Children: Implications for Assessment. Exceptional Children 39:4, 335-337, 1973.

438. Q. Does childhood chronic illness lead to a visual motor perceptual deficit?

A. The visual motor perceptual development of 47 second grade children having a history of chronic illness was investigated. Confinement, poor attendance and frequent school transfers may have a subtle disruptive effect on the development of abilities prerequisite to early school success. The normal development of visual motor perception seems to be dependent upon one's opportunity to interact freely with one's environment and to perform visual motor experiments during the developmental period. Children who are confined with chronic conditions are unable to interact normally with their environment. Deficits may be global or specific and may be associated with comprehensive or specific development factors. The most significant results are:

(1) Visual motor perceptual ability is positively improved by training.
(2) Visual motor perceptual training positively improves reading achievement.
(3) Visual motor perceptual training given as soon as feasible after an illness to prevent developmental deficit suggests an affirmative answer.

Training programs routinely administered might serve to facilitate development and consequently facilitate early school success.
REF. Shepherd Jr., CW.: Childhood Chronic Illness and Visual Motor Perceptual Development. Exceptional Children 36:1, 39-42, 1969.

439. Q. What is the visual perception of motor impaired children?

A. Two arguments used to support the observation that children with motor handicaps have serious disabilities in visual perception are:

(1) As cerebral dysfunction is often the suspected cause of both motor impairment and visual misperception, the likelihood of a visual perceptual deficit is enhanced in any sample of children with motor disability.

(2) Many theorists postulate a direct relationship between motor development and perception; significant defects in one skill should produce some impairment of function in another.

The high incidence of perceptual disorder in motor handicapped children may be a function of the tests used to measure visual perception. Most of these tests require considerable motor ability. The devices are:

(1) Bender Visual Motor Gestalt Test for Children (Bender, 1938)
(2) Memory-For-Designs Test (Graham & Kendall, 1960)
(3) Marianne Frostig Developmental Test of Visual Perception
(Frostig, Maslow, Lefever, & Whittlesey, 1964).

These devices measure visual-motor integration since they include tracing or copying tasks. If perception is measured than the results may reflect a child's motor deficiencies rather than his perceptual inadequacies.
REF. Newcomer P, Hammill D.: Visual Perception of Motor Impaired Children: Implications for Assessment. Exceptional Children 39:4, 335-337, 1973.

440. Q. What were the findings when children were measured for visual motor-integration and on a motor-free test of visual perception?

A. Children perform progressively poorer on a test of visual-motor integration as the severity of their motor handicap increases. Conversely, they tend to function appropriately for chronological age on a motor-free test of visual perception regardless of level of motor disability. They do not have the difficulties with visual perception which are commonly attributed to them. Also, children's visual perception should be measured independently of motor development, especially when the children evidence motor problems.

The extreme influence of motor handicaps on the Bender performance test, and other tests of visual-motor integration, will likely result in a significant number of false positive diagnoses regarding visual perceptual deficiencies if they are interpreted as measures of visual perception.
REF. Newcomer P, Hammill D.: Visual Perception of Motor Impaired Children: Implications for Assessment. Exceptional Children 39:4, 335-337, 1973.

441. Q. How can visually handicapped/sensory handicapped children learn modality for motor orientation and spatial perception?

A. The relationships of motor involvement, perceptual-motor theories and neurophysiological evidence are examined for support of a motoric engramming approach to learning. Particularly noted is the necessity for motor involvement of the blind or sensory disabled child. The four motor generalizations postulated as basic to the establishment of body image and spatial perception in the education of sensory handicapped children are:

(1) Balance and posture: gravity is the one force in the constant direction. It must be established as a line of gravity through the observer's body in a direction noted by the observer. Then he can proceed to the development of coordinates of the space around him.

(2) Contact: with contact skills the child investigates the relationships within objects. There are three aspects of contact activities:
reach, grasp, and release.

(3) Locomotion: the child investigates the relationships between objects in space. Spatial directions and spatial orientations are developed through his own position and then... in relation to the position of another object. All objects occupy a position on a spatial
matrix with the three Euclidean coordinates as the principal axes.

(4) Receipt and propulsion: receipt relates to an object moving toward the child and propulsion involves activities with which the child
related to an object moving away from him.

The rationale presented explicates the use of motor engramming
for improvement and restoration of mobility and spatial orientation
for those who have experienced sensory deprivation or disability.
REF. Whitcraft CJ.: Motoric Engramming for Sensory Deprivation
or Disability. Exceptional Children 38:6, 475-478, 1972.

442. Q. What is the incidence of color blindness among deaf children?

A. There is a biological adage that when one physical defect
appears in a child there will likely be other defects present. This
study is a result of an investigation indicating a significantly greater defective color perception among mentally retarded children than
that found in nonretarded children.

The 308 deaf children were in primary through advanced grade level.
The tests were "Dvorine Pseudo-Isochromatic Color Vision Test",
a revision of the "Archer Word List" in an attempt to establish the
actual adjustment the subjects had made to the use of color in their
environment. Those found with defective vision by means of the
Belts Tele-binocular Vision Test were brought to a maximum point
of correction by ophthalmological treatment. The findings of this
study showed that:

(1) 3.806% had borderline degree of color blindness. Dvorine test
     shows 3% would fall in general population range.
(2) 5.844% had moderate degree of color blindness. Dvorine's test
     shows 2% in the general population.
(3) 0.974% showed severe color blindness.

The three degrees of color blindness indicates 10.714% of the children show some degree of color discrimination deficiency. Non
color blindness was found in 89.286% of the deaf children. The
typical incidence is reported as 4% among males and .4% among
females in the general population.

The incidence of color blindness among the deaf children tested is
greater than twice that of the general population, thus, adding a
further handicap to the deaf child's learning potential.

Implications drawn from this study are:

(1) Altering teaching aids used.
(2) Architectural decorations employed in classes.
(3) The concept of mass media usage in attempting to employ color for clarity with deaf students.
REF. Frey RM, Krause IB.: The Incidence of Color Blindness Among Deaf Children. Exceptional Children 37:5, 393-394, 1971.

443. Q. Are there vision deficiencies in deaf children?

A. Man has two primary distance senses, hearing and vision. By nature, perhaps to foster survival, vision is unidirectional while audition scans all directions simultaneously. Persons who have profound deafness are remarkably dependent on vision, their remaining distance sense. To maintain contact with the environment, they must use this modality for both foreground and background purposes. Only on this basis can adjustment be effective.

In deaf children the eyes provide the primary avenue of learning. The ophthalmological status of this group of handicapped children essentially remains to be investigated.

This study also kept in mind the interrelationships of hearing and seeing - an area of interest not only to the ophthalmologist, but to the educator, psychologist, and even the biologist.

The ophthalmological status of school aged deaf children was studied with control of age, sex, type of school, and success in learning. The incidence of eye defects was twice that found for hearing children. These deficiencies were equally distributed by age and school but were not directly related to success in learning. It appears that children with deafness also tend to have defects in vision. However, the precise nature of the association between visual deficiencies and deafness is not clear.
REF. Lawson Jr., LJ, et al.: Ophthalmological Deficiencies in Deaf Children. Exceptional Children 37:1, 17-20, 1970.

444. Q. What are the causes of deaf blind children?

A. A child may become deaf blind from the following causes:

(1) Congenital blindness, acquired deafness - meningitis.
(2) Congenital deafness, acquired blindness - retinitis pigmentosa.
(3) Congenital deaf blindness - congenital rubella.
(4) Acquired deaf blindness - accidents.
REF. Guldager L.: The Deaf Blind: Their Education and Their Needs. Exceptional Children 36:3, 203-206, 1969.

445. Q. What is the grouping used for the deaf blind child?

A. The deaf blind can be divided into the following groups:

(1) Congenital blindness, acquired deafness.
(2) Congenital deafness, acquired blindness.
(3) Acquired deaf blindness.
REF. Guldager L.: The Deaf Blind: Their Education and Their
Needs. Exceptional Children 36:3, 203-206, 1969.

446. Q. What does the deaf blind child do about the senses of sight
and hearing?

A. The deaf blind child/person has to substitute for these
senses - the near senses of touch, smell, and taste.

The senses of sight and hearing are normally used as the mediums
for communication. One hears an airplane come long before seeing
it but one does not know what kind it is before coordination sight
with hearing, "consulting" the brain, and comparing the stimuli with
what is there.

The deaf blind child in most instances, has some residual hearing
and vision to supplement the near senses. Most children labeled as
deaf blind do in fact have some usable sight and hearing.
REF. Guldager L.: The Deaf Blind: Their Education and Their
Needs. Exceptional Children 36:3, 203-206, 1969.

447. Q. Can preschool deaf-blind children benefit from a preschool
training program?

A. This study resulted because of the rubella epidemic from
1963 to 1965 which caused approximately 1,000 to 2,000 children in
the United States to be born with both severe hearing and vision impairments. With high social awareness at a time of greatly improved communication media, there was a forced major and immediate
changes.

After 4 years' experience with preschool deaf-blind children, the
following conclusions were reached:

(1) An organized program of training at the preschool level is beneficial for deaf-blind children. Emphasis was on total child development and parent support and counseling, rather than communication skills.
(2) A preschool habilitation program for deaf-blind children should
be inseparable from the testing and evaluation program.
(3) The close relationship of habilitation and evaluation, a hearing
and speech center is a reasonable place for a preschool program
providing:
   (a) A close relationship is maintained with the elementary
       school where the children will matriculate.

    (b) Emphasis is on total child development, different para-
        meters of progress, and smaller increments of progress
        than encountered with less involved hearing impaired chil-
        dren.
    (c) The program is expensive and the center should be pre-
        pared for a one-to-one teacher-child ratio, and staff visits
        to the home for training and evaluation.
(4) Operant conditioning procedures have limited value for testing
    and training severely involved deaf-blind children but holds prom-
    ise for those having good organization of the central nervous sys-
    tem.
(5) Procedures for realistic evaluation of the progress of the child
    and for evaluation of the program are an essential feature of an
    agency offering services to deaf-blind children.

The above was brought about because of new interest and activity of
many people from other areas of concern. As interest wanes the
care and education of these children will revert to a few specialized
institutions.

The responsibility for these children should remain broad, and hear-
ing and speech centers should have a place in this responsibility.
REF. Calvert DR, et al.: Experiences with Preschool Deaf-Blind
Children. Exceptional Children 38:5, 415-421, 1972.

448. Q. What are the factors in the teaching of speech to deaf blind
children?

    A. Before starting to educate a deaf blind child, one must be
sure that his needs have been properly evaluated. The child should
be seen, if possible, by a pediatrician, otologist, ophthalmologist,
neurologist, audiologist, dentist, and psychiatrist. The child should
have been fitted with the proper hearing aids if needed. The important factors in the teaching of speech to deaf blind children are:

(1) Start as early as possible with prespeech work.
(2) Make the child pay attention to the mouth with touch.
(3) Use the methods which adapt to both teacher and child.
(4) Be sure to use the child's residual hearing and sight.
(5) Be sure the child receives maximal help with his individual hear-
    ing aid.
(6) Teach parents or house mothers what they must learn to help the
    child.
(7) Use visual speech apparatus.
(8) Use good amplifiers in individual lessons.
(9) Make the child love speech.
REF. Guldager L.: The Deaf Blind: Their Education and Their
Needs. Exceptional Children 36:3, 203-206, 1969.

449. Q. What are the communication systems used with deaf blind
children?

A. The following systems are used with the deaf blind:

(1) Speech and vibration
(2) Fingerspelling
(3) Gestures
(4) Sign language
(5) Communication using a machine

Internationally, in most deaf blind departments, speech and vibration are stressed as the main form for communication. There are many children who never will learn to speak and, therefore, must use one of the other systems.
REF. Guldager L.: The Deaf Blind: Their Education and Their Needs. Exceptional Children 36:3, 203-206, 1969.

450. Q. Can the communication systems used with deaf blind children be described?

A. The communication systems used with the deaf blind are as follows:

(1) Vibration: (Tadoma Method) the sense of touch is used for receptive language. The child puts his hand on the face of the person to whom he is talking. The thumb covers the mouth and feels the movement of the lips, jaws, and tongue. The four other fingers are spread over the cheek and jaw to pick up vibrations.

(2) Fingerspelling: each letter in the alphabet has a specific finger position. The letters are spelled into the hand of the deaf blind person and the deaf blind person spells out his ideas to the person with whom he is talking.

(3) Gesture: the normal young child finds movement and language inseparable. Spontaneous gesturing is rare in the congenitally deaf blind child and he must be taught to use gestures as one of the first steps in learning language. Natural gestures are necessary, but not as the final goal.

(4) Sign Language: each word has as its symbol a movement of hands and arms. Movements are combined to form a language used mainly by deaf students. Deaf blind children can use this system, but speech and fingerspelling are more often preferred. The movements of sign language are difficult for the deaf blind child to pick up through touch or residual sight.

(5) Communication using a machine: one machine translates sound into vibration patterns in a number of keys. Not fully evaluated. Another machine consists of a typewriter keyboard and a braille cell. The deaf person puts his finger on the braille cell, the person talking to him uses the keyboard. For example, pressing "A" on the keyboard makes the braille "A" appear.
REF. Guldager L.: The Deaf Blind: Their Education and Their Needs. Exceptional Children 36:3, 203-206, 1969.

451. Q. What can be done to demonstrate behavioral change in a
deaf-blind child?

A. Use of videotaping behavior for the purpose of recording
and comparing behavior appears to be a unique and useful method
for illustration.

The child selected for this study showed a lack of improvement in
comparison with her peers. She showed a positive change in behavior in the situation most vital to the development of her learning
potential. When presented with sensory stimuli in the stimulus
orientation she showed improvement. This would indicate that she
is attempting to make use of sensory avenues available to her. Even
though labeled deaf and blind, she does make use of her residual
hearing and vision, as well as processing tactile, kinesthetic, and
olfactory information.

The video taping procedure may be a method whereby favorable behavioral change can be displayed to show the validity of special education programs and procedures.
REF. Tweedie D.: Demonstrating Behavioral Change of Deaf-Blind
Children. Exceptional Children 40:7, 510-512, 1974.

452. Q. What are the difficulties in helping the deaf-blind child
achieve his full potential?

A. The typical picture of a young deaf-blind child referred to
a facility for training and therapy is that of a youngster who is severely visually impaired, but usually possessing some perception of light
and shape; is unresponsive to any form of sound stimulation; lacks
toilet training; is not walking; displays many blindisms and self
gratifying mannerisms such as hand twiddling, head banging. Medical specialists have done as much as they can for the child. Normal
development never emerges in these youngsters without specific,
intensive teaching of the use of these systems.

Separation of early medical treatment from psycho-educational
management results in delays and partially met needs. Day care
programs should have a representative medical and psychoeducational consultative staff plus trained full time therapists. A team concept is essential for early intervention which is critical to ensure a
unified approach for the multifaceted problem. Four types of programs may be required:

(1) An early management program emphasizing psychoeducational
management conjointly with medical care should be designed to
identify and train the child who is nonambulatory, delayed in self
care skills, and whose potential for learning has not been determined.

(2) Day programs should be established for ambulatory deaf-blind
children with basic self care skills and a determined potential for
learning.

(3) Residential programs for children who are ambulatory, possess some self care skills, and show signs of learning potential that can best be developed through concentrated residential teaching.

(4) Custodial programs to be established for severely involved children who have not demonstrated any learning potential.

The realization of these goals is dependent on the interdisciplinary cooperation of the medical and health related professions, special education systems, and state level agencies.

REF. Stein LK, Green MB.: Problems in Managing the Young Deaf-Blind Child. Exceptional Children 38:6, 481-484, 1972.

## IV. EMOTIONAL AND PSYCHOLOGICAL PROBLEMS IN CHILDREN

453. Q. What is childhood psychosis?

A. Childhood psychosis can be defined as a heterogeneous group of clinical syndromes which have their onset any time from birth to eleven years of age. They present severe disturbances in the following areas:

(1) Relationship with social environment
(2) Sense of personal identity
(3) Affect and its expression
(4) Use of speech for social communication
(5) Total integration and organization of personality.

Such terms as Schizophrenic child, Autistic child, Symbiotic child, Borderline Psychotic child and Psuedoschizophrenic child are used to describe the particular variety of psychosis and its underlying psychopathology.
REF. Aug R, Ables B.: A Clinician's Guide to Childhood Psychosis. Pediatrics 47:2, 327-338, 1971.

454. Q. How common is childhood psychosis?

A. In general psychosis in children is much less common than in adults. The incidence reported varies from 2.1 to 9 per 10,000 population. The incidence of psychosis in children referred for either outpatient or inpatient treatment ranges from 4 to 75 per 10,000. Childhood psychosis is definitely more common in boys than in girls. The boy girl ratio ranges from 2:1 to 4:1.
REF. Aug R, Ables B.: A Clinician's Guide to Childhood Psychosis. Pediatrics 47:2, 327-338, 1971.

455. Q. Is the etiology of autism in children known?

A. It was felt in the 1960's that early infantile autism was the result of maternal factors alone. Parents, especially mothers, were described as cold, rejecting, aloof and unable to give love. More recent research has shown autistic children suffer from a number of cognitive and perceptual handicaps. Many organic abnormalities have also been found in autistic children as a group. It is now questionable whether environmental causes alone play a primary role in the development of infantile autism.

A number of tentative hypotheses as to the etiology of autism have been advanced. Dr. Lauretta Bender holds that autistic children suffer from a deviance of CNS maturation associated with disorganization and disintegration of normal developmental patterns. Another hypotheses is that autistic children suffer from CNS defect which involves the homeostatic regulation of sensory and motor functions. As a result of the defect the child fails to gain stable inner representation of his environment and hence cannot learn to interact normally

233

with others. A third hypothesis suggests that autistic children suffer from a deficit which prevents integrating and processing of the information which they have perceived. These hypotheses are not mutually exclusive and each may fulfill a role in any one case. Infantile autism is not childhood schizophrenia and it is felt that this term should be reserved for those cases of childhood psychosis which begin after 3 or 4 years of age. The onset of infantile autism is invariably within the first 2-3 years of life.

REF. Tanguay P, M.D.: A Pediatrician's Guide to the Recognition and Initial Management of Early Infantile Autism. Pediatrics 51:5, 903-910, 1973.

456. Q. What are the clinical characteristics of infantile autism?

A. The fundamental clinical sign of early infantile autism is an "aloneness" manifested in a variety of ways. Autistic children may appear placid and undemanding. They fail to develop a smiling response or to assume anticipatory posture prior to being picked up. Parents may note the child's blank stare and lack of response to verbal and nonverbal stimulation. These factors may lead parents to suspect deafness.

Autistic children achieve the appropriate motor development for their age and may even be extremely graceful and agile in their movements. Their facial expression may be alert and they may show skill at visual-motor tasks such as jigsaw puzzles. Speech development is characteristically non-communicative. Phonation and articulation are clear, but speech consists of unrelated words or fragments of speech. Speech may be echolalic or parrot-like and inappropriate. Later in childhood some autistic children do develop speech, but it remains stilted and stereotyped as compared to normal children.

Abnormal motor and perceptual behavior may be noted in infantile autism. Infants may show intolerance to solid foods with gagging, refusal to chew and swallow. They may under-react or over-react to stimuli and sometimes to the same stimuli at different times. Exploration of the environment is predominately through mouthing and smelling objects, running fingers over surfaces and listening to the sound produced. Texture and the feel of objects may fascinate them. Such self-stimulatory behaviors as rocking, whirling, flapping of arms or flicking their hands and fingers before their eyes while staring at bright lights may be noted.

REF. Tanguay P, M.D.: A Pediatrician's Guide to the Recognition and Initial Management of Early Infantile Autism. Pediatrics 51:5, 903-910, 1973.

457. Q. What is symptomatic autism?

A. Symptomatic autism occurs in children who have severe preceptual handicaps from birth or early infancy. The more his perceptive ability is different, the more likely he is to appear bizarre

and have distorted emotional and intellectual growth. Children who are deaf, blind and moderately to severely retarded may develop symptomatic autism. Because these children have handicaps in their perception, they may develop autistic tendencies. These symptoms of autism will eventually be the same as for children who are autistic from other causes e.g., infantile autism. This syndrome can be anticipated in perceptually deprived children and diagnosed early in order that effective treatment can be instituted.
REF. Easson W, M.D.: Symptomatic Autism in Childhood and Adolescence. Pediatrics 47:4, 717-722, 1971.

458. Q. Would autistic children benefit from reduced auditory input?

A. This study investigated attention and performance on simple tasks as well as classroom attention of seriously disturbed, communication impaired, "autistic" children under conditions of reduced auditory input (using ear protectors) and under conditions of normal auditory input (using a placebo device).

Under ear protector conditions, there was a significant increase in the amount of attention given to most of the tasks. Also, teacher ratings indicated a significant improvement in classroom attention under ear protector conditions. A decrease was noted in sudden noisy outbursts or in destructive or aggressive acts under ear protector conditions. One autistic child who was previously agitated and highly distressed became so much quieter under ear protection conditions that she resorted to withdrawal and regressive behavior, e.g., cradling her head in her arms, sighing, and thumbsucking.

An increase in calmness was reported under ear protector conditions, with emphasis on the possible value of such a potentially calming effect in psychotherapeutic and other situations as well as in the classroom appears to be indicated.
The authors suggest consideration of possible beneficial effects on seriously disturbed children resulting from sound reduction in their classrooms by means of carpeting, drapes, furniture placement and selection, and even the positioning of the children in the classroom.
REF. Fassler J, Bryant ND.: Disturbed Children Under Reduced Auditory Input: A Pilot Study. Exceptional Children 38:3, 197-204, 1971.

459. Q. Can the use of small groups help severely psychotic children?

A. Autistic children with gross, lifelong, deficit and surplus behavior can significantly improve. They can learn complex, cooperative, social behavior, academic achievement, self control, and can be taught to use language.

In under 4 years of this study the children no longer displayed the major autistic characteristics of aloneness and preservation of sameness or severely aggressive and destructive behavior. Also,

objective, behavioral concepts and techniques can be effectively developed and applied to groups of severely psychotic children. A behavior modification group program, organized and supervised by a professional but carried out by initially naive non professionals was arrived at.
REF. Graziano M.: A Group Treatment Approach to Multiple Problem Behaviors of Autistic Children. Exceptional Children 36:10, 765-770, 1970.

460. Q. How can lay persons be used in a group treatment approach to help the autistic children?

A. The author feels that highly selected nonprofessionals with a high school education but without previous experience with disturbed children can be trained in behavioral approaches and can function competently as therapists for children. Training of personnel for children's services would take one year.

The author states that the parents of the children must be closely involved. Direct training of the parents within the program would be included. There would be maximum involvement, and responsibility of the parent. In addition, the parents would be involved in specific planning and training for parallel home programs.
REF. Graziano AM.: A Group Treatment Approach to Multiple Problem Behaviors of Autistic Children. Exceptional Children 36:10, 765-770, 1970.

461. Q. What are the long-term effects of "failure-to-thrive"?

A. A follow-up study was done of 15 patients who had been hospitalized for failure to thrive during infancy. At the time of the study the children's age range was three to eleven years.

Of the fifteen children, nine were below normal in physical development, ten were below normal in intellectual development and seven below normal in acceptable behavior. Evidence of health problems in the mother and other siblings and growth failure among siblings was a common finding.

On interview, many of the parents were unconcerned about their children's intellectual and behavioral problems. Most mothers also exhibited emotional detachment from their children. Most did not take their children for further evaluation of problems when it was offered to them.
REF. Elmer E, et al.: Late Results of Failure-to-Thrive Syndrome. Clinical Pediatrics 8:584-589, Oct. 1969.

462. Q. When should a child be referred for psychological evaluation?

A. The most common reasons for referring a child for evaluation are:

(1) Delayed or uneven development.
(2) School failure or erratic performance in school.
(3) Following a head injury.
(4) Developmental, behavioral and/or emotional problems in a child younger than six years of age.

Once the evaluation process has been completed and a psychologic report submitted, appropriate action to help the child should be instituted. In addition, family counseling should be carried so that the child's problem can be understood by the parents in order to better support and treat him.

REF. Berry KK.: Effectively Using the Psychologic Evaluation with Children. Clinical Pediatrics 12:174-177, March 1973.

463. Q. What are some causes of childhood depression?

A. Because children and adolescents are dependent upon adults and are still in the process of identity establishment, their emotions are influenced by depressed adults. The child's response to adult depression is feelings of despondency and depression.

Death or separation of a significant person can cause lethargy, loss of appetite, affect and other problems in the infant and young child. A baby or young child suffering from depression may be diagnosed as retarded.

Over-strict child-rearing can also cause depression. If the child's behavior is frequently criticized and praise is rarely given, the child will have a poor self-concept. If the child has not been permitted to express rage and anger, these feelings are repressed. Both the smothering of feelings and failure to gain approval can cause depression in the child. This may manifest itself in the form of somatic complaints such as abdominal pain, headaches and rashes.

Among adolescents guilt feelings and depression may develop in response to rebellious acts against parents. Mourning for the less complicated days of childhood is common and normal.

Children and adolescents who feel they must excel at school and home often become depressed. To relieve this feeling, self-destruction is sometimes considered. Both the child who is a high achiever and the child that underachieves feel they are failures.

Children or adolescents who become depressed and consider suicide should be evaluated and treated by a therapist.

REF. Brandes N.: A Discussion of Depression in Children and Adolescents. Clinical Pediatrics 10:470-475, Aug. 1971.

464. Q. How can psychosomatic problems be treated?

A. In children, many emotional disturbances manifest themselves as physical problems. Many symptoms such as anorexia,
obesity, headaches, hysterical reactions and behavior changes should
point to the need for exploration of the child's emotional background.
The difficulty lies in the fact that these symptoms may also be caused by an organic disease.

With each history-taking the child's personality traits, child-family
relationships, drastic changes at home (such as death or new sibling)
and school progress should be explored. During the interview interaction between child and parent should be observed, especially parental discipline and the emotional responses to the child. The child
should be talked to directly and his feelings explored.
REF. Goodall JJ.: Clinical Clues to Emotional Disturbances in
Children. Clinical Pediatrics 12:178-181, March 1973.

465. Q. Can pupillary reactions be studied to determine the presence of psychosomatic and emotional disorders?

A. Recurrent abdominal pains affect 1 child in 10 and so is one
of the common disorders of childhood. Though an organic cause is
occasionally found, there is a great deal of clinical evidence to indicate that this symptom is commonly a somatic expression of emotional disturbance. As in other psychogenic disorders, one pathway by
which the disturbance is expressed in physical terms appears to be
the autonomic functions. Pupillometry is a method whereby the
reactions of the pupil are measured under controlled conditions.
Normal pupillary reactions are modified in children with psychosomatic disorder (recurrent abdominal pain with no physical cause)
or with emotional disorder.

A change in autonomic activity is shown by the occurrence of unstable pupil recovery after stress in patients with these conditions,
as compared to controls. The control group showed a significant
difference in pupil size between rest and stress. There was a trend
for pupil size to be smallest in the emotional group. Pupillometry
can be used as a method of diagnosis in disturbances of autonomic
function.
REF. Apley J, et al.: Pupillary Reaction in Children with Recurrent
Abdominal Pain. Archives of Disease in Childhood 46:247, 337-340,
1971.

466. Q. How does chronic illness of a child influence the family?

A. When a child in a family has a chronic disorder the entire
functioning of the family is affected. Initially parents may display
a typical grief reaction with a later resolution to act positively on
the child's behalf. Medical management and continuous follow-up becomes a part of the family's usual activities. In addition, guilt feelings may be experienced by the parents because of the genetic origin
of the child's illness. A decision may be made not to produce more

more children. Parental reaction to the diagnosis may also be related to the age of the child. The younger the child, the more pronounced the response of shock and bewilderment.

Siblings within the family may resent the increased attention given to the child with a chronic disorder. Parents may tend to care for the ill child and overlook the others even though the sibling must often help care for that child. The responsibility for the sibling's care may be a great burden for the other children.

Parental counseling may be necessary since all family members are affected by the chronic disease of one of its members. Guidance should be supportive during the crisis of diagnosis and focus upon present and future-oriented goals for the child. Parents should also be provided with the opportunity to discuss the child's problem and their feelings regarding future childbearing.
REF. Schild S.: Parents of Children with PKU. Children Today 1:20-22, July-August 1972.

467. Q. What are some of the psychological aspects of long-term illness on children and their families?

A. Long-term or chronic illnesses may cause significant interference with the normal emotional and physical growth and development of the child. The common causes for emotional stress associated with long-term illness are:

(1) Pain, physical symptoms and etiology of the illness: pain can cause psychic stress in anyone. In the young child it is often perceived as punishment for some real or imagined transgression. Children may feel they became ill because their parents failed to protect them. Diseases transmitted by hereditary factors may cause strain in the parent-child relationship when children discover the etiology of their illness.

(2) Hospitalization, nursing and treatment procedures: frequent and lengthy hospitalizations which result in separations from family, school and friends can be stressful for the child. Anger, humiliation and anxiety regarding needed nursing care may be evident. Children may resent the need to be helped with bathing, feeding and toileting. Painful procedures such as injections and surgery reactivate fears of bodily mutilation and fantasies of punishment.

(3) Stress related to special chronic syndromes: the causation and symptomatology of many long-term illnesses can pose special problems. For the diabetic child, this may be worry about hypoglycemic or acidotic episodes. A child with a convulsive disorder may fear having a seizure at school or among his peers. Children with chronic respiratory problems such as asthma or cystic fibrosis may fear suffocation. Children with hemophilia, congenital heart disease and chronic renal disease may find it difficult to live with restrictions on their activity and continual medical work ups.

Successful management of the child with a long-term illness and his family depends on several factors. The child and his family should receive continuous personalized support from the medical and nursing team. Allowance for verbalization of feelings should be made. The parents' acceptance of the child and the disease with its uncertain course implies mastery of conflicting feelings aroused by the illness. The goal of raising a handicapped child as normally as possible may be achieved by promoting reasonable activities with other children and regular schooling modified by the needs of the individual child.
REF. Mattsson A, M.D.: Long-Term Physical Illness in Childhood: A Challenge to Psychological Adaptation. Pediatrics 50:5, 801-819. 1971.

468. Q. How do children and families adjust after a catastrophic illness?

A. The authors of this study attempted to evaluate the impact of long-term rehabilitation on the psychosocial attributes of child and family following a kidney transplantation. The subjects were 35 children, ages 1 1/2 to 20 years who had received a transplant 1 to 5 years prior to the study. Interviews, questionnaires, and personality tests were used to gather data. Some of the results were:

(1) Most of the children were functioning as expected for their age groups. Activities, annoyances, and plans for the future were typical and appropriate for their age group. Concerns were rarely illness related, except in terms of body image, for example obesity from steroids. Overprotectiveness was a major complaint of most of the children.

(2) By the time of the follow-up most of the parents stated that their family life was back to normal. Fourteen mothers reported depression, irritability and fatigue. Others also mentioned a temporary increase in disagreements between marital partners. Most of the siblings reported that family life was normal again, their own resentment and feelings of neglect resolved except for three families.

(3) Major concerns of both patients and families centered around fear of rejection of the kidney and fear of change in body image. In terms of body image, the side effect of steroids caused the greatest concern: obesity, short stature, cosmetic problems, and bone changes. Obesity seemed to be of greatest concern to the adolescent females, while short stature worried the adolescent males.

(4) Personality problems were diagnosed in eight of the patients. It is interesting to note that noncompliance with immunosuppressive drugs was a frequent occurrence among this group as compared with the rest of the patients.
REF. Korsch B, et al.: Kidney Transplantation in Children: Psychosocial follow-up study on child and family. Journal of Pediatrics 83:3, 399-408, Sept. 1973.

469. Q. How is pain a contributing factor in the psychological re-action of the burned child?

A. Pain experienced by a child is thought to be related to the degree to which the pain is charged with psychic meaning. While anxiety is the predominant affect, anger, rage, submission, guilt, and depression may also be observed, depending on the child's conscious and unconscious interpretations of the traumatic event and his subsequent care.

Bodily pain occurs when the real boundary between the self and the outside world is breached by certain noxious stimuli. In mild burns, pain may assume a positive function by aiding the child in active mastery of the trauma and in adaptation to the hospital environment. With excessive pain this positive function of pain probably diminishes or disappears as the anxiety level attendant on the pain increases. Pain, augmented by anxiety, represents a major event in the child's life and is long remembered, the memory often being accompanied by phobic defenses against its return.

The sensitivity to pain would appear to be a function of the degree to which the pain is psychically charged.

The protective stimulus barrier has important preservation functions for the individual in holding back stimuli from the outer world. Pain associated with intense anxiety or so severe as to overwhelm the protective stimulus barrier loses its adaptive function for the child.

REF. Nover RA.: Pain and the Burned Child. The American Academy Journal of Child Psychiatry 12:3, 499-505, 1973.

470. Q. What are the causes of recurrent abdominal pain in children?

A. One hundred and two children with recurrent abdominal pain were hospitalized and studied. In addition to abdominal pain and tenderness over the colon, symptoms such as headache, pallor and dizziness were described. Workups performed revealed non-specific findings. A clinical definition of this complex of symptoms was termed "irritable bowel syndrome of childhood". The diagnosis of this symptom complex in children can be based on the following points: (1) a varied and erratic history of recurring abdominal pain, (2) additional symptoms of pallor, dizziness, headache and pellet stools, (3) precipitation of pain with stress, (4) tenderness over the colon on deep palpation, (5) improvement of pain on hospitalization, (6) negative lab and x-ray findings. The treatment should be aimed at emotional support.

REF. Stone R, M.D., Barbero G, M.D.: Recurrent Abdominal Pain in Childhood. Pediatrics 45:5, 732-738, 1970.

471. Q. Do stresses in a child's life serve as contributing factors in the development of diseases?

A. According to these authors social psychological events preceding the onset of illness do have an effect upon children. They developed a scale of life events, scoring each category for four different age groups. For example, the birth of a sibling was given a
score of 50 for all four groups (pre-school, elementary, junior high,
and senior high). Life events such as changing schools, loss of a
parent, divorce or parents were weighted differently for each age
group. Five patient populations were studied: juvenile rhematoid
arthritics, hemophiliacs, general pediatric patients, surgical patients, and psychiatric patients.

Results showed that two to three times as many patients in the above
groups had experienced more frequent and/or more severe life events
prior to the onset of their illnesses than did their healthy peers.
Thirty-four percent of these children developed illness following a
year in which they were faced with major psychophysiological adjust-
ments.

This association of life events with illness has implications for care
givers. Possibly, if we could screen for children with high scores
early, we could prevent illness from occurring, and be better able
to evaluate the total child.
REF. Heisel J, et al.: The Significance of Life Events as Contributing Factors in the Diseases of Children. Journal of Pediatrics 83:1,
119-123, July 1973.

472. Q. What are childrens' reactions to injections?

A. Children at different ages and developmental stages view
their world differently, and experiencing pain is no exception. An
infant during the first month reacts to painful stimuli as he would
to a loud noise or startle. He cries immediately, reflexly withdraws his legs, and then relaxes. As he matures, his response to
stimuli may be delayed. He may cry after the injection is given.
Somewhere between five and eight months, he begins to associate
the object that caused the pain with the painful experience, and
cries at the sight of the needle. This association process continues
to develop until about 14 months, when he can specifically locate
the site of pain, and tries to push the needle away. At this time,
he needs much restraint during the injection, and cuddling, rocking and speaking to him after the painful event. This is essential
if he is to develop trust in others, especially his parents.

The toddler does not have an intrinsic fear of needles, but has usually formed an association about them from past experience. This
mental image, now distorted by fantasy, can be especially frightening. How to support the child becomes a question of whether or not
the parents should stay. Two arguments exist: if the parents leave,
the child is subject to the stress and anxiety of separation; if the
parents stay, the child finds his protectors subjecting him to this
pain. A compromise is to have the mother remain in the background,
and comfort him immediately after the shot.

The preschool child is beginning to become aware of his body and its capacity. Through dramatic play, he is able to cope with threatening experiences. It is at this age that letting the child hold the syringe and giving a needle to the doll or nurse becomes his way of handling the painful event. If he plays with the equipment before the shot, he should do so just before to diminish the time he has to fantasize about the procedure. Because he fears intrusive experiences, privacy should be maintained. It is also at this age that a child knows he is punished for wrong doings, and may see an injection as punishment. An explanation should always be given about the reason for the needle.

The school aged child is becoming independent and is busy accomplishing projects. He thrives on praise, and wants to be cooperative and helpful, but he still fears the unknown. He needs an explanation of why the injection is given, and an opportunity to use the equipment.

The adolescent is striving for identity and acceptance. He may bear the pain in order to act like an adult, although he needs to also be reassured that crying or yelling are acceptable. He is very concerned about his body, and wants to understand about the medication. He wants to be treated as an individual and allowed privacy.
REF. Brandt P, et al.: IM Injections in Children. American Journal of Nursing 72:8, 1402-1402, Aug. 1972.

473. Q. What are the major categories of sleep?

A. Sleep is divided into two major categories, rapid-eye-movement (REM) sleep and nonrapid-eye-movement (NREM) sleep. NREM sleep is composed of sleep states 1, 2, 3 and 4.

As a person falls asleep stage 1 appears and is characterized by the absence of REMS and a low-amplitude, fast-frequency electroencephalographic pattern.

In stage 2, sleep spindles of 12 to 16 cps are present. Stages 3 and 4 sleep follow and are characterized by general slowing of the frequency and an increase in the amplitude of the electroencephalographic waves so that high-amplitude, slow waves dominate the record.

In all age groups, REM sleep constitutes about 20 to 25% of the total sleep time. Children have high levels of stages 3 and 4 sleep. There is a progressive decrease in stages 3 and 4 throughout life and the elderly have virtually no stage 4 sleep.
REF. Kales A, M.D., Kales JD, M.D.: Sleep Disorders - Recent Findings in the Diagnosis and Treatment of Disturbed Sleep. The New England Journal of Medicine 290:9, 487-499, 1974.

474. Q. What are the sleep patterns of children?

A. During infancy lapse into sleep is easy. Rocking or sucking a bottle is usually adequate. During the first eight months the child may develop "falling asleep methods": rocking and thumb-sucking, for example. Babies may wake during the night but usually go back to sleep without assistance. The two-year-old will make many demands at bedtime. This seems to be a normal aspect of sleep behavior. At two-and-a-half, rituals become part of bedtime. Rituals can be patiently accepted and handled by parents. Three-year-olds can fall asleep easily but may awaken several times during the night. Most children remain in bed and fall asleep again.

Bedtime behaviors and demands vary according to the child's age and individual character. Head-banging and rocking are usually observed between one and four years of age. The demand for mother's presence at bedtime most commonly occurs form 2 1/2 to 3 1/2 years. It appears to be a mild form of separation anxiety. Bedtime fears, nightmares and dreams are exhibited in most children. They vary with age.

Sleep needs and development patterns are individualized. Many varied behaviors and sleep changes are believed to be a developmental feature of the child's life.
REF. Battle CA.: Sleep and Sleep Disturbances in Young Children. Clinical Pediatrics 9:675-682, Nov. 1970.

475. Q. Can sleep problems be psychological in nature?

A. Psychological sleep disturbances, associated with normal sleep polygraph patterns, are more common and are often reflections of specific developmental stages. These may be referred to as insomnia and nightmares. During the first year of life the greatest concern is that of sleeping through the night. Seventy percent of babies achieve this by age 3 months and 13% by 6 months. Thus, during the first year, if physiological needs are met and excessive parental anxiety is allayed, sleep problems can be rapidly resolved. In the second year of life the major problem may reflect itself in the child's reluctance to go to sleep. This is often due to the child's anxiety regarding separation from the parent. Rituals such as bedtime stories and substitute objects such as toys or blankets may be a way of reducing the child's pre-sleep anxiety. Many children between 3 and 5 years experience some sleep disturbance such as difficulty falling asleep, night wakening, nightmares, fear of the dark or ghosts or some presleep ritualistic behavior. Most of these disturbances are transient and respond well to minimal environmental manipulation, e.g., leaving a night light on. Most often patience and support are sufficient to overcome these problems. If problems related to sleep persist or become severe, family counseling or psychotherapy may be indicated.
REF. Anders T, M.D., Weinstein P, M.D.: Sleep and Its Disorders in Infants and Children: A Review. Pediatrics 50:2, 1972.

476. Q. What are some of the common sleep disorders of children?

A. Nocturnal enuresis, somnambulism, somniloquy, night terrors and narcolepsy are considered to be the most common physiologic disorders of sleep in childhood. All but narcolepsy have been described as disorders of arousal, since they are associated with emergent sleep stage transitions from Stage 4 to Stage 1 NREM (non-rapid eye movement) sleep. Narcolepsy has been associated with abnormal transition from wakefulness directly into REM (rapid eye movement) sleep and is thus termed a disorder of sleep. Though these sleep problems may be associated with psychological factors, psycho-physiologic factors have been demonstrated and various specific pharmocologic agents have proven effective in their treatment. REF. Anders T, M.D., Weinstein P, M.D.: Sleep and its Disorders in Infants and Children: A Review. Pediatrics 50:2, 1972.

477. Q. Why are night terrors and nightmares often seen in children?

A. The night terror (pavor nocturnus in children and incubus in adults) is characterized by intense anxiety, extreme levels of autonomic discharge, motility and vocalization and little recall. Night terrors occur more frequently in children than in adults, and it is not uncommon for somnambulism and night terrors to occur in the same person, often simultaneously.

The nightmare that represents the ordinary, frightening dream is much more frequent than the night terror and occurs in all ages. There is much less anxiety, autonomic changes if present are slight, the sleeper is more easily aroused, and the content recalled is more lengthy and developed.
REF.Kales A, M.D., Kales JD.: Sleep Disorders - Recent Findings in the Diagnosis and Treatment of Disturbed Sleep. The New England Journal of Medicine 290:9, 487-499, 1974.

478. Q. What is somnambulism?

A. Somnambulism is sleepwalking. It is not a rare nocturnal disturbance. Its prevalence is estimated from 1-6%. It occurs predominantly in males, more commonly in children than in adults, and often there is a positive family history.

There is wide disagreement in descriptions of the actual somnambulistic incident, particularly regarding the general degree of motor performance and dexterity of the sleepwalker, and his ability and inability to carry out complex tasks. There is agreement that the episodes generally last for several minutes, with total amnesia for the incident.

A number of organic or functional conditions have been proposed as etiologic factors in somnambulism such as epilepsy and dissociative hysterical neurosis. A popular notion was that the sleepwalker is acting out a dream.
REF. Kales A, M.D., Kales JD, M.D.: Sleep Disorders- Recent Findings in the Diagnosis and Treatment of Disturbed Sleep. The New England Journal of Medicine 209:9, 487-499, 1974.

479. Q. What is the psychological evaluation in somnambulism?

A. Those favoring a psychological explanation most commonly regard sleepwalking as a dissociative hysterical state, similar to fugue. Psychiatric interviews of the parents of the child somnambulists studied in the sleep laboratory revealed considerable parental concern that the sleepwalking was a manifestation of psychopathology. Psychological testing did not demonstrate any consistent psychopathology, indicating that psychologic disturbances are not primary factors in child and adolescent somnambulism.
REF. Kales A, M.D., Kales JD, M.D.: Sleep Disorders - Recent Findings in the Diagnosis and Treatment of Disturbed Sleep. The New England Journal of Medicine 290:9, 487-499, 1974.

480. Q. What are some findings of the somnambulist in sleep-laboratory studies?

A. Studies of child and adolescent somnambulists have shown that sleepwalking incidents occur exclusively during nonrapid-eye-movement (NREM) sleep, especially stages 3 and 4 sleep, when dreaming is least likely to occur. Sleepwalking in the laboratory lasted for 30 seconds to several minutes. During the incidents, subjects exhibited low levels of awakeness, reactivity and motor skill. They were totally amnesic for the events.

Somnambulistic episodes (induced sleepwalking) could not be induced in normal children.

Follow up studies showed that most of the somnambulists had "outgrown" the disorder after several years, suggesting a delayed central-nervous-system maturation in these children and adolescents.
REF. Kales A, M.D., Kales JD, M.D.: Sleep Disorders - Recent Findings in the Diagnosis and Treatment of Disturbed Sleep. The New England Journal of Medicine 290:9, 487-499, 1974.

481. Q. What is the management and treatment of the child somnambulist?

A. The most important consideration in managing the child sleepwalker is to protect him from injury. Prophylactic measures such as locking doors and windows, removing potentially dangerous objects and having him sleep on the first floor, if possible, are essential to the safety of the sleepwalker.

Psychologic tests and psychiatric interviews of child somnambulists did not indicate serious psychologic disturbances. Child sleepwalkers usually "outgrow" the disorders within several years; extensive psychiatric evaluation and treatment is not indicated. It is important to communicate this information to the child's parents so that they do not treat the child as if he has psychologic disturbances and, by so doing, compound the problem.

When sleepwalking is frequent and severe and does not diminish over a period of years, the use of stage 4 suppressant drugs is under investigation. The benzodiazepines, such as diazepam and flurazepam have been found to suppress stages 3 and 4 very effectively. Use of these drugs with somnambulists has not resulted in a clear-cut decrease in the incidence of sleepwalking episodes.
REF. Kales A, M.D., Kales JD, M.D.: Sleep Disorders - Recent Findings in the Diagnosis and Treatment of Disturbed Sleep. The New England Journal of Medicine 290:9, 487-499, 1974.

482. Q. Does the positioning of an infant have a psychophysiological effect?

A. According to the author of this study, the supine or prone positioning of an infant does have certain benefits or disadvantages. Their experiment included 30 fullterm normal newborns, who were positioned on their back or on their abdomen for a two-hour uninterrupted session in the nursery. The dependent variables studied were heart rate, respiration, motor activity, and behavioral state. The first three variables were monitored by electrical equipment and behavioral state was rated by an experimenter on a 6-point scale ranging from quiet sleep to crying awake.

Results indicated that when the infants were prone, they slept more, cried less, and moved less. They also tended to have slower heart rates and more regular respiration, although these differences were not statistically significant. Infants in the supine positioned cried about five times as much, and slept about 26% less. The "lost sleep" time was supplemented primarily by increased crying and drowsiness.

An important consideration besides the physical benefits of prone positioning is the possible effect it may have upon the mother-child relationship. Accumulating evidence shows that neonatal arousal level is an important factor in the initial mothering process. Cranky, fatigued and drowsy infants seem to elicit different maternal responses than, happy, well-rested and alert infants.
REF. Brackbill Y.: Psychophysiologic Effects in the Neonate of Prone versus Supine Placement. Journal of Pediatrics 82:1, 82-84, Jan. 1973.

483. Q. Does curtailment of physical activity influence the child?

A. In the inner city setting, residents tend to view the street and stranger as personally threatening. Most adults are extremely fearful for their children's safety and well-being. Consequently, children are kept indoors thus restricting their physical activity and no provision for expending physical energy.

The primary alternative to outdoor activity is watching a great quantity of television daily. Many children seen in an inner-city hospital responded to curtailed physical activity with "hyperactivity" in school,

listlessness and inattentiveness. However no physical abnormality was present. The remedy for this problem is social in nature. Adequate, safe settings for physical activity must be provided.
REF. McNamara JJ.: Hyperactivity in the Apartment Bound Child. Clinical Pediatrics 11:371-373, July 1972.

484. Q. What are some important facts about suicide?

A. Suicide is one of the leading causes of death among adolescents. Several studies have been done to try and characterize the dynamics of suicide in young people. A composite review of these studies reveals several pertinent aspects:

(1) Frequently, these people are "social isolates," living under stress.
(2) They may come from disorganized homes, where they felt unloved and unwanted.
(3) They may be impulsive, restless, depressed, and have a sense of failure.
(4) If they are angry, their anger and guilt are turned inward toward the ultimate punishment, death.

Some important facts to remember about suicide include:

(1) people who talk about suicide frequently do it,
(2) the more detailed the plan for killing oneself, the more likely the act will occur,
(3) there is frequently a triggering event, such as a tragedy or argument, before the suicide,
(4) attempted suicide may be a call for help,
(5) "improvement" during a period of depression may really signal a person's decision to commit suicide,
(6) individuals who are suicidal at one time in their lives are not necessarily suicidal forever.
REF. Shneidman E, Mandelkorn P.: How to Prevent Suicide. Public Affairs Pamphlet No. 406.

485. Q. What is the "replacement child" syndrome?

A. The "replacement child" syndrome refers to a child, either conceived for this purpose or another sibling, who is used by the parents as a substitute for a sibling who has died. It is a sign of unresolved parental grieving, and may occur with an "anniversary reaction".

Several factors easily identify this replacement child syndrome. The parents never fully grieve for the loss of their child, and soon after the death replace this child either by conceiving a new one or by choosing a younger child. This new child is prescribed a set of behaviors and expectations previously held for the dead child, but tremendously exaggerated because of the idealization of the lost child. The replacement child usually finds it difficult, if not impossible, to become a living version of the idolized dead child. She is never allowed an identity of her own.

The parents attempt to preserve this child by over-protection and domination. They usually have an exaggerated concern for illness or accidents, a fear which may be incorporated into the child's personality. One of the hazards of the "replacement child" is the fear that a similar fate awaits them.

People working with parents who have recently lost a child need to be aware of this phenomenon, and need to anticipate its occurrence if parents want another child before grieving has taken place. Replacing a child with another acts as a barrier which protects the parents from the full acknowledgment of their loss and prematurely arrests the mourning process. Completed bereavement involves acceptance of the loss through a lessening of emotional attachment and an increase of reality towards remembering the deceased.
REF. Poznanski E.: The "Replacement Child": A Saga of Unresolved Parental Grief. Journal of Pediatrics 81:6, 1190-1193, Dec. 1972.

486. Q. How can nurses help young children handle their aggression?

A. Toddlers are in an age of newly developing motor and social skills. They are feeling an independence that is reinforced by ritualistic activities in the home. They are beginning to have feelings of aggression in the "NO" stage, and are learning ways of coping with them. Hospitalization erases these routines, imposes dependency and often separation from loved ones, and takes away any individuality of the newly found "ME".

Nurses can help make this traumatic ordeal more pleasant by establishing routines learned at home and letting the child feel important by helping in activities he has mastered, such as dressing himself or eating with a spoon. Besides finding out what these rituals are, nurses must ask parents how the child normally shows aggression or frustration at home. One child may become quiet and withdrawn when angry while another screams and acts out. For one child, intervention might be talking, while for the other, it might be banging on a drum.

We also need to help parents understand what hospitalization means to a child. Besides his loss of familiar routines, loss of autonomy, and fear of pain, he feels that his parents have caused the illness and are punishing him for some wrong-doing. He may lash out at them, or at the staff. Nurses must realize that it is healthier for a child to be angry with them and continue to see his parents as his source of security.
REF. Penalver M.: Helping the Child Handle His Aggression. American Journal of Nursing 73:9, 1554-1555, Sept. 1973.

487. Q. Do childhood problems continue or become worse if left untreated?

A. The major objective of this study was to investigate spontaneous improvement in public school children who had been identified as behavior problems but who had not had the help of any special educational or psychiatric care.

Two-thirds of the children in the study exhibited spontaneous improvement but it was not clear which children and under what circumstances. Major reason for spontaneous improvement was the child's progress in academics and adjustment to school. The child adjusted and learned that basically there is one set of outside norms (the schools) and one job (academic success). If a disorder persists to indicate a prognosis of continuing disturbance then the limited mental health resources could be directed to those children or family circumstances which suggests that spontaneous improvement is not likely to occur.

Schools should play an increasingly prominent role in modifying disturbing behavior in specific ways both in the classroom and in the child's other social contexts.

The higher incidence rate for emotional disturbances was among boys. One speculation for recovery without intervention being that the child improved in school. Persistent disturbances were found in 30% of the children. It should be remembered that most emotionally disturbed children continue to remain in regular public school classrooms.
REF. Glavin JP.: Persistence of Behavior Disorders in Children. Exceptional Children 38:5, 367-376, 1972.

488. Q. What family dynamics characterize a child's development when one parent is an alcholic?

A. A child learns social behavior and norms through relationships in his family. Communication, compromise, sharing, attitudes and feelings are learned by watching other significant people interact. However, this learning can have particular impact on a child when one parent is an alcoholic.

One dominating characteristic of the alcoholic family is inconsistency. Children, who need rules and regulations, suffer from inconsistency and lack of structure. Communication is half-truths and white lies, because the non alcoholic parent tries to protect the children from the truth. Empty promises lead them to place little importance on verbal communication, so they learn to act out their impulses, usually following the behavior of the alcoholic parent. They often learn to rely on themselves, rather than placing trust in others.

Roles that are ordinarily learned by imitating a parent are distorted or absent in these homes. The father may be passive, unreliable, even violent and impulsive. Instead of supporting the family, he is a burden. The wife and mother assumes all responsibility. Because of her priority of helping and protecting her husband, the children's problems and minor refractions go unnoticed. It is not unusual that when the alcoholic parent improves, the parents become concerned about problems that have actually existed for a long time.

When the mother is the alcoholic, other problems arise. Often her drinking problem is gradual and more readily concealed. Often, to allow herself time to be alone to drink, she permits the children an excess of freedom. During sober periods, she feels guilty about such behavior and becomes overly demanding and protective. In an attempt to run the household, she delegates household chores and sibling care to the oldest daughter. It is not unusual for this older daughter to marry early in order to escape such responsibilities.

Children want to love their parents, and they want affection from them. But the broken promises, the financial crisis, the arguments, all cause the children to be angry, resentful, and rebellious. Yet, the children feel guilty, and turn the anger inwards. One result of this is self-punishment, achieved through provoking authority figures to punish oneself (ex. school officials or police). Besides the self-punishment, the feelings of shame and disgust, and the lack of a model to identify with, the child lives in fear that his home won't remain intact, and what little he has will be lost. Studies show that these children are especially prone to delinquency, depression, hostility, and sexual confusion.

Health professionals, such as nurses, need to understand these family dynamics and need to realize that as a system, one "element" always affects the other. Improvement of one person in the family necessitates the inclusion of all family members in treatment or therapy so that healthy relationships can be fostered.
REF. Hecht M.: Children of Alcoholics are Children at Risk. American Journal of Nursing 73:10, 1764-1767, Oct. 1973.

489. Q. Does special class intervention help emotionally disturbed children?

A. The school, as an instrument of society, attempts to provide the opportunity for all children to be educated to their fullest extent. This study was designed to investigate long term changes in achievement, overt behavior, and social position of children identified as emotionally disturbed.

The findings suggest that special classes do not result in long term changes for emotionally disturbed children as compared to emotionally disturbed children placed in regular classes. The salient points are:

| In Special Class | In Regular Class |
| --- | --- |
| 1. Achievement gains did not exceed those in regular class. | 1. Greater degree of achievement growth. |
| 2. Overt behavior - no significant difference. | 2. Overt behavior - no significant difference. |

3. Did not receive more positive or negative choices.
4. No significant differences
when compared to normal
children.

3. Did not receive more positive or negative choices.
4. No significant differences
when compared to normal
children.

In conclusion the data support the notion that emotionally disturbed
children who did not receive special class intervention are accomplishing the objectives of academic achievement, overt behavior, and
social position at the same level as children who did have the advantage of a special class. Thus, the concept of placing emotionally
disturbed children in special classes for rehabilitation is called into
question.
REF. Vacc NA.: Long Term Effects of Special Class Intervention
for Emotionally Disturbed Children. Exceptional Children 39:1,
15-22, 1972.

490. Q. Should the ecological conditions be changed to help the
emotionally disturbed child?

A. The disturbed child can be viewed as a collective object of
a micro-community who becomes both a generator and receptacle of
reverberating emotions and behavior. Introducing a "strange"or
"peculiar" child into any microcommunity (a classroom, group cot-
tage, family home) he then becomes the locus of collective dynamics
which flow and ebb around him. It is like a reverberating circuit of
disturbed mood-behavior exchanges. This is an ecological exchange,
a reciprocity between the child and his living environment, which
is disquieting and uneasy.

By placing him in a specially constituted setting (a therapeutic
milieu, for instance) something happens. He is no longer strange
or generates constant currents of mood-behavior excitation. He
seems different - more "normal". He is more a part of his micro-
community, more in harmony with his setting.

Intervention into the emotional disturbance of the child should take
into consideration the reciprocal nature of the phenomenon and
should not treat the child as the sole possessor of the disturbance.
A child is helpless to resist our intrusion. The rest of the community resists reciprocal change. The child is more malleable
and adaptable to change. The effort made should not only be one of
shaping a particular child to fit a static culture in a community,
but also one of constant revision in the community's accomodation
to wide ranges of differences in individuals. Such capacity to accomodate should make for fewer intense, disruptive convulsions in
the total community.

Consultation is favored over psychotherapy as an intervention process.
The totality of the problem is realized when one enters into the ecological context of the condition and attempts to influence the quality
and nature of the exchange between the child and his microcommunity.

Also the ecological conditions under which children have to live and grow has to be changed. The number of occasions of disturbance and the number of children who are extruded or alienated from their living units has to be reduced. This is the only way in which our society can hope to come to terms with the magnitude of the problem called emotional disturbance.

REF. Rhodes WC.: A Community Participation Analysis of Emotional Disturbance. Exceptional Children 36:5, 309-314, 1970.

491. Q. What can be done to integrate emotionally disturbed children into regular classes?

A. For a great number of emotionally disturbed children, special education should be regarded as a temporary intervention which can prepare students for their return to regular classes. If a special class is provided which helps the child develop acceptable behavior patterns while maintaining academic skills, it is likely that some students will be able to be integrated into regular classes. But a child considered ready for integration faces a major impediment, not created by the child's deficits but rather by the apprehension and lack of knowledge felt by the regular school staff toward the child.

A questionnaire was developed to help delineate current problems in the communication which exists between directors of special education and regular school staff and to establish guidelines which might facilitate the effective integration of emotionally disturbed children.

A need exists, it was demonstrated,for the development of more positive channels of communication. These channels have to be continually fluid to assure the most positive growth of all exceptional children in the public school, integrated or not. The importance of this level of communication cannot be minimized.

REF. Schultz JJ.: Integration of Emotionally Disturbed Students: The Role of the Director of Special Education. Exceptional Children 40:1, 39-41, 1973.

492. Q. What happens to the personality of a child from a sociocultural deprived environment?

A. This article presents some of the evidence indicating the importance of noncognitive variables in determining how well the socioculturally retarded child will achieve in structured testing and scholastic situations. Intellectual and experiential restrictions appear to influence the personality structures of these children. They approach formal testing and scholastic situations with poor achievement motivation, with little expectation for success and high expectation of failure, with heightened anxiety, with poor self concepts, and with a need for emotional nurturing. These noncognitive variables influence learning so that consideration must be given these factors along with the consideration given to cognitive variables in formal academic programs.

An effort should be made to change the environmental conditions from which these children may derive their personality structures. An emphasis should be on the child's attempting tasks and trying new solutions, on exploration, on creativity, and on socialization, along with an emphasis on attending to and completing tasks and utilizing appropriate language in school.

As the teacher (nurse) should give adequate and consistent emotional support, the parents also should give emotional support, since some degree of failure tolerance may ensue.
REF. Tymchuk AJ.: Personality and Sociocultural Retardation. Exceptional Children 38:9, 721-728, 1972.

493. Q. How does the emotionally disturbed teacher influence students?

A. The influence of a teacher upon a child can be powerful. As humans, teachers are liable to emotional problems and emotional illness.

Teacher-pupil relationships may be greatly influenced by displacement of hostility and anger upon the school child or a teacher with a poor self-concept may force his class to excel in order to demonstrate to others his superior abilities. These behaviors and others are not pathologic in themselves. It is the degree of response that is the important variable.

The emotionally disturbed teacher can cause great damage to students. Children may experience anxiety, hostility, poor learning ability and physical problems that arise from adverse interaction with such a leader.
REF. Brandes NS.: Influence of the Emotionally Disturbed Teacher of School Children. Mental Hygiene 53:606-610, Oct. 1969.

494. Q. What traits characterize the speech of disturbed children?

A. Disturbed children often exhibit speech deviations such as complete silence or silence except for non-speech sounds. Deviations in pitch, stress, inflection and voice quality are also common. Irrelevant and disordered meaning and pronoun reversals are frequently observed. Children who usually speak infrequently, in single words or short sentences will sometimes suddenly verbalize long, complex sentences. Indefinite echolalia occurs in some children as well as poor comprehension of yes-no questions.
REF. Millman IK, Canter SM.: Language Disturbances in Normal and Pathological Development. Journal of Child Psychiatry 11:243-254, 1972.

495. Q. How does the emotionally disturbed mother influence the mother-child interaction?

A. Because the child is totally dependent upon his mother for care, mother-child interaction will greatly influence the child's development. As ego development, sexual identification and other differentiations develop, so does thought. Through parents, children learn what constitutes reality. This enables him to organize his life and set objectives.

Severely disturbed mothers have an intensely close relationship with the infant. When the infant begins to work toward independence, the mother threatens to reject the child if he is separate from her. In order to survive, the child complies with his mother's demands. This type of negative interaction and negative fantasies are responded to by the child. They can be destructive and have a deleterious effect upon mother-child interaction.
REF. Newman MB, San Martino MR.: The Child and the Seriously Disturbed Parent. Journal of Child Psychiatry 10:358-373, 1971.

496. Q. What is the impact of foster home placement on the child?

A. When a child is removed from his home, the impact is great. At the same time, parental rejection is experienced and a new foster family is introduced. The child may feel lost and helpless, insecure with lost identity in such a crisis.

Because of his past experiences and present emotional turmoil, the child is expected to have difficulties as he adjusts to a foster home. Behavioral reactions may be hostile and belligerent. At other times detachment and emotional isolation from the foster family may be exhibited. Foster parents are often frustrated by this behavior as they seek to gratify and receive gratification from the child.

Because of parental rejection, foster children feel unworthy and inadequate. When children are moved from one foster home to the other, the feelings are reinforced.

If the child forms any attachment to his foster parents, he feels guilty because of the loyal feelings still held for his own parents. This attempt to relate to two sets of parents keeps the child in a state of constant emotional confusion.

The foster home experience can have many positive dimensions. However, this is contingent upon a carefully planned and carefully handled foster home placement.
REF. Maluccio AN.: School Problems of the Emotionally Disturbed Foster Children. Mental Hygiene 53:611-619, Oct. 1969.

497. Q. Does foster care influence school functioning?

A. Since the foster child is vulnerable to stress, the pressures of school will evoke problems. Many foster children have learning difficulties. These learning problems lead to further anxiety, emotional and social problems.

The child's problems in school are factor-related. He must prove his own worth and respond to school demands even though he feels worthless. His anxiety intensifies the feeling.

Because much of his energy is used to cope with his emotional problems, little energy remains for learning. In addition, he is unable to relate to others and has poor interaction with teachers and peers.

The fact that he is a foster child, rather than living with his parents, is a painful reality for the child to accept. Most tend to deny their status.

Sometimes, aggressive behavior is acted out in school but not in the foster home. School demands and peer group pressure may be the precipitating factors. Although the foster child has many difficulties, the school can serve as a therapeutic setting as it helps the child and offers many opportunities for positive growth.
REF. Maluccio AN.: School Problems of the Emotionally Disturbed Foster Children. Mental Hygiene 53:611-619, Oct. 1969.

498. Q. In what ways can divorce affect children?

A. The divorce rate in the U.S. continues to rise and the children affected are numerous. The reaction of children to divorce and its effect on their future growth and development may in many ways be similar to the death of a parent. There may be confusion on the part of the child and the parents, projections and compensation for guilt, retaliation by use of the children and relocations of geography and economy, all of which can produce problems. The initial response of the child is similar to separation anxiety initially and is later followed by a mourning reaction. How these reactions are manifested depend on the child's age, sex and psychosexual development. In spite of the emotional upheaval of the parents, they can be helpful in allaying anxiety and meeting the child's needs. Some parents may find this difficult without professional help.
REF. Sugar M, M.D.: Children of Divorce. Pediatrics 46:4, 588-595, 1970.

499. Q. What are some of the factors influencing identity development in the adopted child?

A. Some children because of their adoptive status may experience a degree of emotional stress that does not occur in children living with natural parents. The waiting period before adoption is finalized may be an anxious one for adoptive parents and may inhibit to a degree their emotional closeness to the child. In many adoptions there is the unavoidable factor of the presence of more than one mother figure, depending on the length of time a child is in foster care prior to adoption. Many adoptive parents are older and may be less flexible and more anxious in caring for the child. Also, the value of the adopted child may lead parents to react in overprotective, inconsistent ways in their childrearing practices.

If an adopted child remains an only child he is subjected to the stresses inherent in the single-child home. When at some point the child
learns that he is adopted, he may begin to seek out the meaning of
this fact. This may complicate the resolution of normal parental
relationships. Every opportunity should be used to help the adopted
child develop a sense of worth, importance and a true sense of identity.

REF. Committee on Adoptions: Identity Development in Adopted
Children. Pediatrics 47:5, 948-949, 1971.

500. Q. What are some origins of homosexuality?

A. Homosexuality is believed to be learned behavior that is
the consequence of disturbed development. It is the most common
adult sexual deviation.

During pre-school period children experience sexual pleasure, primarily through self-stimulation. Also, the child becomes attached
to the parent of the opposite sex, an analog to future heterosexual
behavior. Identification with the parent of the same sex is a major
developmental task. The degree to which parents perceive their
sexual role in a positive light will be a strong determinant of the
child's acceptance of sexual role.

During the latency period the child identifies with his parents and
mimics their sexual role behavior. A child of latency age prefers
peers of the same sex. By contrast, the potentially homosexual
male prefers to play with girls and avoids male type activities.

Puberty dramatically brings with it biologic, physical, sexual and
emotional changes. Since psychosexual development continues
through adolescence, a diagnosis of homosexuality is most appropriate at this time.

The male who is developing homosexual characteristics often appears to be pale and clumsy. They are overdependent upon their
mothers and are very fearful. He will shy away from age-appropriate, aggressive activities. In addition, excessive closeness
with the parent of the same sex stimulates the child to reject his
own sexuality as a defense against close contact with that parent.
If a boy is repeatedly approached by older peers and adults with
homosexual behavior, further investigation regarding sexual identification should be done.

Homosexuality is best managed by recognition of early signs and
counselling of the parents and child. Direct, private consultation
with the adolescent concerning his self-concept and sex role identification is vital. For more fixed homosexual behavior, psychotherapy is indicated.

REF. Davenport CW.: Homosexuality - Its Origins, Early Recognition and Prevention. Clinical Pediatrics 11:7-10, Jan. 1972.

501. Q. What are some patterns of illicit drug and alcohol use among high school students?

A. The present study was undertaken to determine patterns of drug and alcohol use and its correlation with demographic, social and personal factors of users. The study group was representative of a private school population, rather than a public high-school population. Some of the results were:

(1) Alcohol was the most commonly used drug (52%). Tobacco was smoked by 18%, and illicit drugs had been used by about 14%. Marihuana was the most commonly used illicit drug (12%). Multiple drug use was the rule with 59% using two or more drugs, and 7% using as many as seven. A most important finding was the parallel increase in the use of tobacco, alcohol and illicit drugs in relation to factors which have a correlation with high rates of drug usage. One can conclude that drug seeking behavior is a characteristic of personality type rather than a response to a particular effect elicited from the substance.

(2) Boys (20%) outnumbered girls (6.6%) in the use of alcohol and illicit drugs. Increasing age also correlated with increasing drug usage. Significant differences were found in religious backgrounds: Jewish students had the lowest usage of drugs and alcohol, Protestants the highest for illicit drugs, and Catholics and Protestants for alcohol use.

(3) Poor academic achievement, negative moods, anti-social behavior, rebellious attitudes, and social and sexual precocity were positively correlated with higher drug use, as well as psychiatric difficulties.

(4) There was a high correlation between the percentage of friends or classmates using drugs or alcohol, emphasizing the importance of peer influence and the tendency of users to limit their contact to other users.
REF. Milman D, Su W.: Patterns of Illicity Drug and Alcohol Use Among Secondary School Students. Journal of Pediatrics 83:2, 314-320, Aug. 1973.

502. Q. What are some physical effects of heroin addiction?

A. Data collected at Samaritan Halfway Society, a therapeutic community treatment program, indicate that frequently there is a physical basis for the addict's complaints of pain or discomfort. Some of these findings include:

(1) The first and most obvious physical problem is often severely carious or absent teeth. Because of its high incidence among heroin abusers, it has been called the "heroin longevity sign". This "sewer mouth" may be the result of poor nutrition, altered metabolism, or a direct action of the drug itself.

(2) The next most obvious sign is dermatitis, both fungal and bacterial. These lesions are present as pustular acne on the back, chest, or face, and infection of the nailbeds, particularly the toenails. Systemic fungal infections occur in the neurological system.

(3) Bone infarction, possibly from emboli elsewhere, can occur, and osteomyelitis from septic areas under the skin can cause bone destruction. Addicts are especially prone to tetanus from poor injection technique.

(4) Gastrointestinal complaints are common. Autopsies revealed a transverse myelitis, possibly from a vascular clot or inflammation. Complaints suggestive of peptic esophagitis, gastritis, and cardiospasm are frequent. Generalized lymphadenopathy is also common.

(5) Hepatomegaly with or without clinical hepatitis is seen frequently. The asymptomatic patient, under stress or ill from another disease, can present with acute hepatitis.

(6) Effects on the reproductive system include gynecomastia in the pubertal or just postpubertal male. Females often have vaginitis, secondary amenorrhea, and verrucae venerium (veneral warts). There is a high incidence of false positive serological tests.

(7) Complaints such as fatigue, faintness, dizziness and anxiety might be due to a low blood sugar, which may be related to liver damage.
REF. Pillari G, Narus J.: Physical Effects of Heroin Addiction. American Journal of Nursing 73:12, 2105-2108, Dec. 1973.

503. Q. What is one pattern of drug use among youth?

A. Three hundred adolescent and young adult patients were interviewed in a Youth Clinic program. The primary purpose was to investigate personal drug use.

A consistend finding was that the objective of taking any drug was to erase the present. There was no fixed drug usage. Rather, intake was dictated by drug availability and peer group customs. In addition, more than one type of drug was often ingested at the same time. Marijuana and hashish were most commonly used. An equal number of youths used "uppers" and "downers". Probably because of the declined interest in their use, there were few "speed freaks" (users of injected amphetamines) and "acid heads" (users of LSD).

Alcohol was used more frequently than drugs by more young people. The trend toward greater alcohol or marijuana use indicated a move toward indulgence in more socially accepted ways of altering one's mood.
REF. Minowski WL, et al.: A View of the Drug Problem. Clinical Pediatrics 11:376-381, July 1972.

504. Q. What is the use of drug education?

A. Many adolescents who experiment with drugs need an understanding, trusted non-judgmental person with whom thoughts, feelings and experiences can be shared. A supportive, respectful and tolerant attitude will motivate the teen-ager to openly discuss his experiences.

For the drug experimenter, drug education is the best preventative solution to drug abuse.

This approach coupled with opportunities to develop useful skills could specifically help the potential school drop-out who is at high risk for drug use. If their educational programs held their interest and they were active in their self-development they might begin mastery of school and not turn to drugs.
REF. Proskauer S, Rolland RS.: Youth Who Use Drugs. Journal of Child Psychiatry 12:32-47, Jan. 1973.

505. Q. Is there a relationship between ego structure and drug use?

A. Among young drug users, use of drugs is believed to be resorted to in order to decrease or avoid anxiety and to deal with personal and developmental problems. It has been hypothesized that many of these youths manifest early impairments of the capacity for object relations and impulse and affect control. In addition, they do not possess a positive or stable self-concept and perceive themselves as "freaks" or outcasts. As other stresses occur throughout their lives, cognitive function and ego functions become impaired.

The central detriment in their lives appear to be a relative absence of enduring ego structure to successfully handle stress. This is believed to occur because these young people have constantly been under stress or excessively stimulated throughout life. It is perhaps through drug use that the childlike stressful freedom of latency can be achieved.
REF. Pittel SM, et al.: Developmental Factors in Adolescent Drug Use. Journal of Child Psychiatry 10:640-660, 1971.

506. Q. What is the nurse's position as therapist of drug addicts?

A. These authors provide some excellent guidelines for the nurse therapist in helping her face the realities of this difficult therapeutic relationship. When first seeing a drug user, the nurse must make it absolutely clear that she will never supply him with drugs or money (even for a telephone call). She must keep all personal values and objects in her environment under lock and key. The therapist must inform the patient that she doesn't trust him because of her knowledge and experience with other drug users, but that she looks forward to the day when she can. She also has to put the responsibility of quitting with the patient by telling him that little can be done until he quits, but that she can listen to his plans to quit and then his plans for the future. At the same time, she should encourage him to socialize with people out of the drug culture, to find an easy job, to think about school, etc. If the patient is on probation while under treatment, the nurse should get to know the probation officer, so that the patient can't play one against the other.

This author also suggests looking at the patient's history for clues to his prognosis. For example, the earlier the addiction started, the lower the educational level, the shorter the job record all add up to a harder climb in society.
REF. Morgan A, Moreno J.: Attitudes Toward Addiction. American Journal of Nursing 73:3, 497-501, March 1973.

507. Q. What is the lethal dose of methadone?

A. The lethal dose of methadone is unknown, however 10-20 mg/kg will kill a rhesus monkey. The average dose for patients in a methadone program is 80-120 mg/day taken by mouth in 2-4 oz. of Tang or fruit juice. When taken by these patients, who have developed a tolerance for the drug, no adverse side effects occur. However, the same dose if taken by a non tolerant person will cause severe respiratory depression and in children this dose is likely to be fatal. A child aged 2-6 years who takes a full dose of methadone will become increasingly comatosed over a period of 1 1/2 to 3 hours, and if untreated, can die of respiratory failure.
REF. Arena J, M.D.: Two Current Poisonings: Tricyclic Drugs and Methadone. Pediatrics 51:5, 919-922, 1972.

508. Q. What is the current therapy for methadone intoxication?

A. Methadone has become a prominent aspect of treatment of heroin addiction. This therapy has been accompanied by childhood addiction, poisoning and death. Methadone intoxication should be suspected in any child with unexplained respiratory depression or drowsiness. If the child is alert, emesis should be induced with Ipecac. In other patients, gastric lavage is indicated.

The antidote of choice is Naloxone (Narcan) IV 0.01 mg/kg/dose every three to four hours. Nalorphine (Nalline) 0.1 mg/kg/dose or Levallo-orphan (Lovfan) 0.02 mg/kg/dose may also be used.

The child should be given supportive care and observed for 48 hours following methadone ingestion. The parents should be informed of the dangers of methadone ingestion in children. All cases of methadone intoxication should be investigated by the appropriate agencies.
REF. Lee KD, et al.: Childhood Methadone Intoxication. Clinical Pediatrics 13:66-68, Jan. 1974.

509. Q. What are the manifestations of neonatal withdrawal in an infant born to a drug addicted mother?

A. Drug withdrawal represents the final insult to the newborn who has been exposed to pharmacologic agents in utero. Infants born to heroin addicts are notoriously small and there is evidence that heroin may be a factor in growth retardation, although the mechanism for growth inhibition is not known. Intrauterine exposure to heroin can affect the course of maturation of fetal liver and lungs.

Onset of withdrawal in the newborn is determined by the time and amount of the mother's last dose of drug, metabolism of the drug by the infant and the presence of other drugs which would modify withdrawal symptoms. Most newborns who withdraw from heroin start within the first 24-48 hours after birth. All infants showing withdrawal symptoms are irritable, jittery and tremulous. They may sneeze, appear hungry, taking formula vigorously and vomit soon after feeding. As withdrawal progresses, diarrhea starts. These infants will suck ferociously on their fists, drop off to sleep, awaken in a short time, sucking their fists and thrashing about. Their pattern of sleep and wakefulness, as well as quiet and active sleep are disturbed. Other signs are high-pitched cry, hyperreflexia, hypertonicity, sweating, tachypnea and nasal congestion. Not all infants born to addicts suffer withdrawal symptoms and symptoms may range from mild to severe. There is increasing evidence that methadone withdrawal may be more severe than heroin withdrawal. The signs of withdrawal are the same, however there may be more signs for a longer period with methadone withdrawal. Treatment is aimed at reducing irritability, allowing sleep and reducing vomiting and diarrhea. This is accomplished by the use of opiates, barbiturates or other depressant drugs such as chlorpromazine or diazipam.
REF. Rothstein P, M.D., Gould J, M.D.: Born With A Habit: Infants of Drug Addicted Mothers. Pediatrics 51:5, 1972.

510. Q. What signs and symptoms should alert the nurse to narcotic withdrawal syndrome in neonates?

A. Several investigators have reported that between 60 to 90% of infants born to drug dependent mothers show symptoms of withdrawal. Infants can become addicted to heroin or methadone; different investigators report varying degrees of severity among each group. The larger the dose of heroin, the longer the addiction, and the closer to delivery that heroin was taken are factors affecting the severity of the infant's withdrawal. Withdrawal symptoms become most pronounced between 48 and 72 hours after birth. The majority develop clinical signs after 4 to 24 hours, if the mother has been on heroin alone. Methadone addicted babies may not show withdrawal signs until the first or second week.

The most common symptoms of withdrawal are those of the central nervous system: hyperirritability, tremors, restlessness, and increased muscle tone. Gastrointestinal disturbance such as vomiting, diarrhea and an exaggerated, but ineffectual and uncoordinated sucking and swallowing reflex are common. About a third of these infants exhibit a shrill, piercing high-pitched cry. The respiratory system is also affected, characterized by excessive nasal secretion, stuffy nose, and rapid respirations sometimes accompanied by retractions, intermittent cyanosis, and apnea. One interesting finding in relation to these infants and the respiratory system is a lower incidence of respiratory distress syndrome than among non-addicted infants. One possible reason is accelerated lung maturation in the addicted infant.

To summarize, nurses should be alert to the following infant behaviors: tremors, confulsions, hypertonicity, hypersensitive Moro reflex, tachypnea with mottling of the skin, regurgitation or vomiting after feeding, followed by loose stools, poor feeding in general, sneezing, yawning and nasal stuffiness, frantic sucking of thumb and fist despite poor sucking of the nipple, inability to sleep, and a persistent high-pitched cry.
REF. Finnegan L, Macnew B.: Care of the Addicted Infant. American Journal of Nursing 74:4, 685-693, April 1974.

511. Q. What problem areas are involved in the nursing care of addicted infants?

A. The nursing care of the addicted infant can be classified into three major areas:

(1) the physical care of the infant, based on the signs and symptoms present,
(2) the treatment of the addiction and withdrawal, and,
(3) the mother-child relationship existing between the drug-addicted mother and baby.

Because the physical care of this infant is based upon the presence of certain symptoms, one of the first nursing responsibilities is observation of the infant's behavior. These observations must be specific: duration, onset, frequency, severity. Also, what events precipitate symptoms such as tremors, and what actions decrease these behaviors? Generally, the signs of withdrawal fall into three categories, those involving the central nervous system, the gastrointestinal system and the respiratory system. The infants need a quiet subdued environment, with infrequent handling, swaddling, and feeding on a demand schedule. They need small, frequent feedings to maintain fluid and caloric requirements, or an intravenous feeding may be warranted. Daily weights are essential to monitor the effectiveness of oral or parenteral fluids. They need good skin care, but an organized schedule that allows for as much rest and quiet as possible. Frequent suctioning of the oropharynx is often necessary, as well as positioning to assure patent airway. Seizure precautions are also essential because of the possibility of generalized convulsions.

Often, supportive care is insufficient and drug therapy must be initiated. The pharmacological agents frequently used include paregoric, phenobarbital, chlorpromazine (Thorazine), or diazepam (Valium). The nurse must be familiar with the action and side effects of each. For example, paregoric must be used in large doses to treat severe withdrawal and infants often dislike its taste and refuse to swallow it. Duration of therapy often is longer than with other drugs. Advantages, however, are its oral administration and its inhibition of bowel motility which helps diminish the diarrhea. Phenobarbital, although especially effective in controlling irritability and insomnia, can cause respiratory depression. Chlorpromazine reduces withdrawal symptoms, and has few side effects. Diazepam seems safe and effective, and needs a shorter time of therapy, although some authors found it caused a depressed sucking reflex.

A very important aspect of the care revolves around fostering a positive mother-child relationship. Some authors advocate placing the child in a foster home, while others believe the mother can be supported in her effort to care for this child. To stimulate maternal attachment, the mother needs to be encouraged to enter the nursery to see and touch her baby. The mother needs a great deal of attention and consideration because of her own problems and fears. She needs continual communication about the infant's progress and management. Family members should be encouraged to visit, especially if the father is present, because the mother will need emotional support from these people after discharge.

The authors of this article feel that with strong support from a team of the nursery nurse, pediatrician, social worker, obstetrician, and public health nurse and with intensive psychosocial services during pregnancy and after delivery, this woman can more realistically cope with motherhood.
REF. Finnegan L, Macnew B.: Care of the Addicted Infant. American Journal of Nursing 74:4, 685-693, April 1974.

512. Q. Which drugs can be present in mother's milk and can they effect the newborn?

A. The mammary gland is a relatively unimportant route for total drug excretion, however any drug in the maternal organism must traverse the endothelium of capillaries into the alveolar cells and then be secreted into the lumen with the milk. The mere presence of drugs in milk does not imply adverse effects on the infant, as the drug may be pharmacologically inactive, destroyed in the G.I. tract, or not absorbed at all.

It has become apparent that a number of drugs should not be given to the mother while she is nursing. Included in this group are atropine, anticoagulants, antithyroid drugs, antimetabolites, cathartics, dihydrotachysterol, iodides, narcotics, radioactive preparations, bromides, ergot, tetracyclines and metronidazole (Flagyl). Some drugs may be noxious to the infant if taken continuously and although not specifically contraindicated, require close observation of the infant. These include steroids, diuretics, oral contraceptives, nalidixic acid, sulfonamides, lithium carbonate, reserpine, diphenylhydantoin and barbiturates.

Drugs not contraindicated include insulin, epinephrine and occasional aspirin. Other compounds, which used in moderation do not seem to be harmful to the infant include alcohol, nicotine (cigarette smoking) and caffeine.

Adverse effects of drugs can produce alterations in the homeostasis of the infant by their cumulative effect, interference with normal physiological functions, causing hypersentivity reactions or affecting normal developmental pattern.
REF. Catz C, M.D., Giacoia G, M.D.: Drugs and Breast Milk. Pediatric Clinics of North America 19:1, 151-165, 1972.

513. Q. What are the clinical features of congenital morphinism?

A. The diagnosis is not difficult if the mother is known to be an addict. The clinical features are fever, irritability, and fits. The cry is peculiarly high-pitched and persistent. The vomiting and diarrhea may lead to dehydration, electrolyte loss, and collapse. The mortality in untreated cases is as high as 90%.

A differential diagnoses includes causes of convulsions, especially hypoglycemia, hypocalcemia, and meningitis and the causes of diarrhea and vomiting.

Offspring of addicted mothers are usually small for dates and tend to suffer from dysmaturity complications. Pneumonia is a frequent finding at necropsy.

It is important to remember that symptoms of withdrawal are rarely present at birth and may begin as late as 96 hours.
REF. McMullin GP, Mobarak AN.: Congenital Narcotic Addiction. Archives of Disease in Childhood 45:239, 140-141, 1970.

514. Q. What is the treatment for congenital morphinism?

A. Treatment is essentially maintenance of nutrition and fluid and electrolyte balance combined with small doses of morphine analogues.

There have been discussions regarding the relative merits of paregoric, methadone, and morphine, but not one seems to have exclusive merit.

Some authors have used paregoric or methadone in doses equivalent to morphine 0.13-0.5 mg. 6 to 8 hours apart. Sedative such as phenobarbital, chloral, and chlorpromazine have generally been used in addition to a narcotic.

Chlorpromazine seems to have a morphine-sparing effect and improves the infant's general condition and enables the complete withdrawal of narcotics.
REF. McMullin GP, Mobarak AN.: Congenital Narcotic Addiction. Archives of Disease in Childhood 45:239, 140-141, 1970.

515. Q. Do salicylates have teratogenic properties?

A. Eight cases were reported in which pregnant women medicated themselves with 650 milligrams or more of salicylates or salicylates and another medication. In every case, the neonate was born with a congenital anomaly. The defects included cleft lip and palate, dextrocardia, abnormal extremities and anencephaly. The most severe anomalies occurred in infants whose mothers had taken salicylates and another medication.
REF. McNeil JR.: The Possible Teratogenic Effect of Salicylates on the Developing Fetus. Clinical Pediatrics 12:347-349, June 1973.

# V. SOME ASPECTS OF THE NURSE'S ROLE IN PEDIATRICS

516. Q. How can the nurse help prepare the pediatric patient for procedures and surgery?

A. At all ages, the hospitalized infant or child needs to be provided with some means of dealing with his anxiety in the form of a familiar person, a calm person or a familiar object from home. In order to provide the child with ego support, comfort and assurance, the nurse must understand the child's feelings. Concomitantly, she must be able to respond appropriately to the verbal and non-verbal cues given by the child.

During the initial period of hospitalization, the child should be introduced to the new hospital environment by familiarizing him with positive aspects of the setting and the personnel. In addition, early care chould be provided by one person. The first few days of the hospital stay the nurse should help the child cope with the reality of his situation, help meet the child's dependency needs and assist him towards independence.

Preparation for surgery is of utmost importance. It should be provided prior to hospitalization by parents and, following admission, continued by the nurse and doctor. The child should be given the opportunity to express his perception of the surgery and provided with information appropriate for his age level of comprehension.

With the nurse's support and guidance, care of the hospitalized child by the family should be fostered.
REF. Scahill M.: Preparing Children for Procedures and Operations. Nursing Outlook. 17:36-38, June 1969.

517. Q. How can a nurse use play therapy with a child?

A. "Play is the child's natural medium of expression." Because a child's defenses are not as fully developed as an adult's and because his verbalization skills are still rudimentary, expressive nonverbal communication is the key that unlocks the door to his inner thoughts and fears. In play the child's ego can be supported and encouraged to become wholly integrated. He can learn more socially adaptive and personally satisfying ways of coping with his environment. But all of this does not just happen because he plays. Rather, for play to be therapeutic, he must know that he is genuinely accepted, that his freedom of expression is without boundaries, and that his actions and behaviors are accepted, rather than judged.

Allowing play to be creative means that the therapist must have a working knowledge of children. She must be able to look beyond a hint or a clue and see meaning. Frequently, she merely listens, acknowledges and supports the child's own use of play. If this sounds simple then it is deceiving because merely listening necessitates objectivity, a skill most difficult to learn. For example,

267

freedom doesn't imply limitless permissiveness, but appropriate limit setting. One principle to follow is to see that the child cannot harm himself, the therapist, or the playroom.

The tools of play therapy are as varied as the child's use of them. What is important is how they are used. For example, a checker game can become an emotional full scale war in which the child is trying to win in order to gain control. Puppets might easily become parents and siblings. Aggressive toys such as guns can become instruments through which the child can feel powerful and let out angry, hostile feelings, paving the way for healing to take place.
REF. Hyde N.: Play Therapy: The Troubled Child's Self-Encounter. American Journal of Nursing 71:7, 1366-1370, July 1971.

518. Q. How do therapeutic play and play therapy differ?

A. Play therapy is a psychiatric practice which must be conducted by a psychiatrist, psychologist or psychiatric nurse clinician. By contrast, therapeutic play can be utilized without special training.

Play therapy is used in one-to-one treatment of emotionally disturbed, psychotic or neurotic children in a controlled environment. Its objective is to help the child gain insight into his behavior and feelings. The technique requires frequent reflection and interpretation of the child's expressive behavior over long periods of time.

On the other hand, therapeutic play can be conducted with a hospitalized child by a professional nurse. Verbal cues provide the nurse with insight into the child's needs and feelings. Sessions are short and only one may occur while the child is in the hospital.
REF. Green CS.: Understanding Children's Needs Through Therapeutic Play. Nursing '74 31-32, Oct. 1974.

519. Q. How can nurses use "puppets" to help prepare children for procedures for surgery?

A. Nursing students at the University of South Carolina are using hand puppets to prepare children and their families for expected procedures. Their guidelines are essential for any nurse who wants to relate to children through a "child's mind".

The pupped family consists of figures representing the patient, the father, the mother, the nurse and the doctor, in outfits that characterize their role and their culture (for example--black puppets to characterize a black family). Construction paper toys represent any of the equipment that will be used during the "show".

Each show is preceded by preparation by the nurse who must assess several factors:

(1) What is the child's age and his level of development and understanding?
(2) What is the actual procedure to be done? (Specific details are necessary because each hospital can have different routines).
(3) What do the parents and the child already know? (The nurse might need a conference with the physician in order to insure consistency of information).
(4) What is the scheduled time and length of the procedure?
(5) What preoperative preparation will be required, for example, any shaving, medication and route, respiratory therapy for post-operative recovery?
(6) Will the parents be able to accompany the child to the procedure, where will they wait for him, will the parents both be present?
(7) What method of anesthesia will be used, for example, local anesthesia while the child is awake or general anesthesia?
(8) What post-operative changes will there be, such as casts, bandages, drainage tubes, etc.?

Such an assessment by the nurse allows for individuality in the care of each child. The nurse arranges a time for the show when child and parents are present. The child wears the "patient" puppets, while the nurse acts out the other characters. Generally, the information conveyed is concrete, rather than abstract and limited to only what the child will hear, feel, or see. When the puppet show is finished, the child is asked to play back the events, in order to help the nurse evaluate and if necessary clarify or reinforce any aspects of her teaching.
REF. Whitson BJ.: The Puppet Treatment in Pediatrics. American Journal of Nursing 72:9, 1612-1614, Sept. 1972.

520. Q. How can the nurse help foster healthy mother-child interaction?

Because there is absence of observable physical pathology, the nurse needs independent and sophisticated assessment tools. Data collection must include parental attitudes and values related to family life and motherhood. In addition samplings of family interaction and discussions may reveal other aspects of the family's life style.

The nurse-family relationship is the critical factor in any nursing intervention. The mother is recognized to be inadequate for carrying out the mothering role. Also, since she probably has not resolved her dependency needs, she may be minimally dependent upon the nurse during periods of stress. With help, the mother may be able to identify her difficulty in interacting her child.

In addition to focusing upon the mother, mother-child interaction should be encouraged. Realistic goals should be planned for the child with the mother.

Family planning is an integral part of maintenance of family stability. Nursing intervention may consist of information-giving, various contraceptive methods and resources for obtaining them.
REF. Stewart RF.: The Family That Fails to Thrive. Family Health Care D. Hymonich, M. Barnard (ed.) N.Y., McGraw-Hill Book Co., 1973.

521. Q. What is the role of the nurse when a defective child is born?

A. The birth of a defective child constitutes a family crisis. The professional nurse can utilize the tools of nursing assessment and intervention to provide the child and family with comprehensive and effective nursing care.

Case-finding as a means of identifying potentially defective offspring is the ideal means of preventing birth defects. However, since this is not always possible, instruction and counseling of the public may be utilized as an additional preventive measure.

When a child is born with an anomaly, normal post partum care should be followed as closely as possible. Mother and child should have emotional and physical contact with one another. Whenever feasible, the mother should be permitted to care for the child. The anxiety, doubt, guilt and questions of the parents can be responded to. When the parents express readiness, they should be instructed in child care and comprehensive child care. Equally as important, the abilities of the child should be emphasized.

The nurse must consider the family as a unit. Thus, communication will remain open and the child will have a strong, coping mechanism through the family. Developmental assessment, appropriate instruction and reinforcement, anticipatory guidance and prevention are all facets of the nurse's role in dealing with the defective child and his family. In addition, referrals to other facilities by the nurse help provide comprehensive care and continuity of care.

Public health is of utmost importance since the family's environment is the community. In such a setting, the nurse's primary concerns are to meet the child's needs to sustain health and life and promote development. The nurse may help foster development by identifying child and family strengths.

Since the needs and problems of the exceptional child and family exist for a lifetime, anticipatory guidance is ongoing. If the question of institutionalization of the child is explored, the final decision must rest with the parents.
REF. Tudor MJ.: Family Habitation: A Child With a Birth Defect. Family Health Care. D. Hymonich and M. Barnard (ed.) N.Y., McGraw-Hill Book Co., 1973, pp. 284-299.

522. Q. What is the professional nurse's role in a pediatric multiphasic program?

A. The Kaiser-Permanente Medical Center in San Francisco is a pre-paid health care system. One of its goals is to detect physical or psychological problems in otherwise symptomless children. This project has three phases: (1) actual testing, (2) computer processing or results, and (3) examination by a physician six weeks after the tests. The actual testing involves psychological screening of various types (Rutgers Drawing Test, Peabody Picture Vocabulary, Columbia Mental Maturity Scale, Draw a Person Test, and others) and physical tests (body measurements, vital signs, blood pressure, hearing and visual acuity). Laboratory tests include urine and blood samples. These tests are administered by specially trained aides or technicians.

The role of the nurse in charge of this multiphasic unit is primarily in four areas: supervision of testing, evaluation of procedures, coordination with other departments, and health teaching. Test results and questionnaire data are not only used to evaluate the child's condition but also as data base for research. She is responsible for the initial training of all nursing personnel who work with the children. She constantly evaluates the procedures to insure precision and uniformity in performance. She evaluates the performance of individual nursing staff members. A large part of her job is working with other departments, helping them maintain a high level of performance. A large part of her responsibility is health teaching for parents, children, and staff. She uses booklets, visual aids, and eventually closed-circuit T. V. as educational media. REF. Galli P.: Nursing in a Pediatric Multiphasic Program. American Journal of Nursing 74:5, 892-894, May 1974.

523. Q. What services should be provided in a comprehensive health program?

A. At present, few comprehensive programs for children exist in the United States. However, comprehensive planning is needed so that all children and youth will have access to quality health care. If a plan is to be national in scope geographical, and economic restrictions would have to be eliminated so that services would be inter-related and available to every child irrespective of other factors.

In general, comprehensive health services consist of: primary care at the point of entry; intermediate care for seriously ill children and advanced specialty care for children with complicated problems. At each level the following services should be provided:

a) Level one:
    (1) Social casework.
    (2) Nutrition education.
    (3) Basic laboratory and diagnostic tests.
    (4) Health screening.
    (5) Treatment services for minor illnesses.

b) Level two:
   (1) More sophisticated diagnostic and treatment services.
   (2) Association with a medical or teaching hospital.
   (3) Referral service.
c) Level three:
   (1) Provision of highly sophisticated diagnostic and treatment
       centers.

In the future, the concept of family care should become an integral
part of comprehensive care. Thus, any individual receiving health
care would have all family members cared for. As these goals are
carried out quality health care must always be a priority.
REF. Wallace HM.: Some Thoughts on Planning Health Care for
Children and Youth. Children May-June 1971.

524. Q. What are the skills of the school nurse practitioner?

A. The school nurse practitioner, as opposed to a school nurse
can increase and improve the health care given to children. Because
of her special preparation, she is able to utilize interviewing techniques. In addition, she can take a health history, carry out physical
examinations and perform laboratory tests and procedures. She
has also learned how to assess and identify many childhood problems.
In her capacity, the practitioner can also assess over-all health
status of the child, do health screening, provide emergency care and
counsel children and parents. Problems which require other modes
of management are referred by her.

Thus, specially prepared school nurse practitioners can increase
the quality of school health care for children.
REF. McAtee P.: Nurse Practitioners in our Public Schools. An
Assessment of the Expanded Role as compared with School Nurses.
Clinical Pediatrics 13:360-362, April 1974.

525. Q. How can the nurse do effective suctioning of the newborn?

A. Clearing the upper and lower airways immediately during
and after birth is vital to the survival of infants. During the first
10 to 30 minutes of life, the infant is experiencing a neurological
stimulation called the first reactive phase, during which time mucus
secretions are abundant. The second reactive phase occurs two to
four hours after birth, when again mucus is abundant. Besides these
factors, an infant's anatomy of the air passages enhances the danger
of obstruction: he is a nose breather only, nasal passages are
small, he has relatively large tongue while the glottis and trachea
are small, and the ciliated columnar epithelium is especially susceptible to edema.

A newborn needs suctioning even before his entire body has passed
through the birth canal. As his head is born, a rubber bulb syringe
is used to suction the mouth, then the nose. The bulb is compressed
before insertions to prevent forcing material into the bronchi. After

birth suctioning is done while the baby in a position which facilitates drainage. A hand or rolled towel under the shoulders not only lowers the head but also separates the tongue from the posterior pharyngeal wall. In order to suction the oro-nasopharynx, the nurse can use a DeLee mucus trap or mechanic suction. With a DeLee mucus trap, she places one end of the tubing in the area to be suctioned and the other end in her mouth. She creates suction by sucking as she withdraws the catheter. With mechanical suction and the proper size catheter, she applys suction while withdrawing and rotating the tubing to prevent mucosal damage. Suctioning should be done for 10 seconds or less since prolonged and deep suction can produce laryngospasm or bradycardia and cardiac arrhythmias from vagal stimulation.

REF. Roberts J.: Suctioning the Newborn. American Journal of Nursing 73:1, 63-65, Jan. 1973.

526. Q. How can a nurse effectively do postural drainage on an infant or child?

A. Percussion along with proper positioning helps loosen trapped secretions in different lobes of the lungs. Tapping over the rib cage, never over the stomach, sternum or kidney, with a cupped hand produces a hollow sound which causes vibrations throughout the lungs to loosen material lodged in the bronchial tubes. Postural drainage should not be done after meals, but preferably first thing in the morning and just before bedtime.

Psitioning the child in a head-down position frequently causes crying, which is beneficial in causing diaphragmatic movement that stimulates coughing. Frequently, the child will swallow these secretions instead of coughing them up. Positioning is best done by placing the child in your lap, either lying prone or supine with head and knees supported by one hand, and clapping with the other.

REF. Pinney M.: Postural Drainage for Infants. Nursing '72 2:10, 45-48, Oct. 1972.

527. Q. What are nursing implications when phototherapy is used for hyperbilirubinemia?

A. An abnormally high serum bilirubin can cause severe brain damage by passing the normally protective blood-brain barrier. An increased bilirubin occurs in newborns from blood group incompatibility, large doses of vitamin K, certain drugs such as sulfisoxazole (Gantrisin) given to the mother, and prolonged neonatal cyanosis. Bilirubin is a pigment formed from the breakdown of hemoglobin. Hemoglobin is broken down into globin and heme, which is further catabolized into bilirubin. In its free state, bilirubin enters the bloodstream causing the skin, sclera, and mucous membranes to turn yellow or jaundiced.

Until recently, the only known method to lower bilirubin quickly was exchange blood transfusions. However, this carries several risks, such as allergic reaction. Recently, the use of sunlight has been shown to increase destruction of bilirubin. Since sunlight is not always available, a fluorescent light is used. The baby is placed under the light for several days, or until the bilirubin is at its normal concentration of 1.0 mg/100 ml. of blood. Several nursing precautions are necessary:

(1) the baby should have as little covering as possible to increase skin exposure to the light,
(2) the infant's eyes should be shielded with patches, making sure the eyelids are closed to prevent corneal abrasions,
(3) the infant's temperature should be checked because the lamp can overheat the baby,
(4) loose stools are a common side effect as bilirubin is more rapidly excreted; dehydration is a potential risk,
(5) priapism, a painful, continued erection of the penis can occur from sensory irritation of light; diapering or placing the infant prone will resolve the problem.

REF. Williams S.: Phototherapy in Hyperbilirubinemia. American Journal of Nursing 71:7, 1397-1399, July 1971.

528. Q. Why should a nurse have some knowledge of an infant's temperament?

A. One of the nurse's responsibilities in comprehensive care of an infant is advice, counseling, and guidance of the parents. However, often factors such as the infant's behavior pattern affect that astute offering of such counsel. The author of this study tried to correlate measurements of temperament with the incidence of colic, development at one year, and the frequency of injuries by use of a questionnaire. The nine categories of temperament in the questionnaire included: activity, rhythmicity, adaptability, approach, sensory threshold, intensity, mood, distractibility, and persistence. The nine categories were rated as difficult, intermediate (high or low), and easy. Results showed the following correlations:

(1) Of the 13 babies with colic, four were rated as difficult, four as intermediate high, and four as intermediate low, one as easy. Also 11 had low sensory thresholds. (Colic was defined as "paroxysms of crying lasting for a total of more than three hours a day and occurring on more than three days in any one week").

(2) The very active babies were walking more than babies who were very inactive. The very persistent babies were speaking two words with meaning more often than the nonpersistent ones. There was no difference in the walking or talking of difficult babies and easy babies.

(3) Although the difficult babies did not have more injuries, they needed more suturing for lacerations than any other group.

REF. Carey W.: Clinical Applications of Infant Temperament Measurements. Journal of Pediatrics 81:4, 823-828, Oct. 1972.

529. Q. What sites can be used for intramuscular injections in children?

A. The American Academy of Pediatrics recommends using the vastus lateralis in all children, but particularly in infants. The correct site is located by dividing the area between the trochanter of the femur and the knee into thirds, and injecting in the middle third, lateral to the midline. To give the injection, the skin should be pinched before and during the procedure, and the needle injected at a 90 degree angle to a depth of one inch or less. This site has several advantages: it is well developed at birth, relatively free of major blood vessel and nerves except the femoral artery, and relatively large in older children if several injections have to be given. If a hypersensitivity reaction occurs, a tourniquet can easily be applied above the injection site.

Another good site is the ventrogluteal, located by placing the index finger on the anterior superior iliac spine, the middle finger along the posterior iliac crest, and the webspace between these two fingers on the greater trochanter. Injections are made in the center of the triangle at about a 90 degree angle. It has several advantages including easy location by bony landmarks, accessibility in several positions, and absence of major vessels and nerves.

The gluteus maximus can be used only after the child has been walking, so that the muscle is well developed. As a general rule, it should be avoided because of the presence of the sciatic nerve and used only if the child is over two years old. It is located by drawing an imaginary line from the trochanter to the posterior iliac spine, and injecting above and outside this line at a 90 degree angle. The person should always be lying down when this site is used.

The deltoid is usually underdeveloped and small until the child grows considerably, and should be abandoned in favor of the vastus lateralis and ventrogluteal sites.
REF. Brandt P, et al.: IM Injections in Children. American Journal of Nursing 72:8, 1402-1406, Aug. 1972.

530. Q. How can the nurse function in a therapeutic role for the adolescent with VD?

A. The sixties witnessed the advent of an epidemic of veneral disease in the United States. It is estimated that approximately 300,000 teenagers contract VD annually.

In order for the nurse to act as a therapeutic force, she must examine her own attitudes about sex. Then, with insight, she will be better able to work with the adolescent in a non-judgmental manner. As a health professional, the nurse can improve sex education and treatment services for teenagers. Case finding and encouraging the adolescent to get treatment is a vital activity for the teenager's well being and that of others. The counseling role is of vital importance since the teenager often seeks out someone with knowledge in whom he has trust. Equally as important, the nurse can help the adolescent explore the meaning of adolescence, health care and their implications.

The nurse's use of self can be vital in helping adolescents become better-informed as they achieve maturity.

REF. Brown MA.: Adolescents and VD. Nursing Outlook 21:99-103, Feb. 1973.

# OTHER BOOKS OF INTEREST

## PEDIATRIC NEUROLOGY HANDBOOK
Edited by J. T. Jabbour, M.D., D.A. Duenas, M.D.
R.C. Gilmartin, Jr., M.D., and
M. I. Gottlieb, Ph.D., M.D.

**About 550 pages ● 2nd Edition ● Price: $15.00**
**1975 ● Illustrated**

A clear, concise reference source in the diagnosis
and treatment of neurological disorders in children, with a unique emphasis on genetics and
metabolism. Condenses and simplifies complex
material, utilizing many illustrations and tables
to supplement descriptive text. A valuable aid
for the neurologist, pediatrician, pediatric sur-
geon, and residents in these specialties.

## HANDBOOK OF PEDIATRIC SURGICAL EMERGENCIES

By Diller B. Groff, M.D.

**176 pages ● Illustrated ● 1975 ● Price: $10.00**

A practical handbook which describes the more
common pediatric surgical emergencies, designed
for the physician who is not specifically trained
in the discipline of pediatric surgery. Offers
basic techniques, helpful procedures, and step-
by-step course of patient management, as well
as photographs, x-rays, charts, diagrams, and
current references.

## CHILD PSYCHIATRY – Medical Outline Series
Edited by John C. Duffy, M.D.

**185 pages ● 1973 ● Price: $10.00**

This volume provides the reader with a concise
overview of child psychiatry. Among the topics
covered are: normal child development, genetics,
classification, psychotic disorders, adolescent
psychiatry, and drug treatment.

## PEDIATRIC NEUROLOGY
### A Practitioner's Guide

By *Lester L. Lansky, M.D.*

*About 270 pages* ● *1975* ● *Price: $12.00*
*Illustrated*

A clear and concise volume which covers all aspects of pediatric neurology, including developmental assessment in infancy and childhood, congenital malformations of the nervous system, convulsive disorders, vascular disease, brain tumors, genetic disorders, metabolic and neuromuscular diseases, and disorders of learning and communication in childhood.

## PRACTICAL POINTS IN PEDIATRICS

By *John E. Allen, M.D., Vymutt J. Gururaj, M.D., and Raymond M. Russo, M.D.*

*300 pages* ● *1973* ● *Price: $10.00*

A brief, concise and practical survey of pediatrics with emphasis on useful clinical information. Invaluable as a quick-reference guide, covering all aspects of child health and disease, from both the ambulatory and inpatient points of view.

## CHILD PSYCHIATRY CASE STUDIES

By *R. Dean Coddington, M.D.,*
    *L. Eugene Arnold, M.D.,*
    *David R. Leaverton, M.D., and*
    *Marjorie Rowe, Ph.D.*

*282 pages* ● *1973* ● *Price: $10.00*

64 case studies related to child psychiatry, psychology and development, with special emphasis on deductive clinical reasoning as applied to troubled children and adolescents, practicality and efficiency, and prevention. Written with educators, clergy, pediatricians, family physicians, and medical students in mind, as well as mental health professionals.

# Other Books Available

Prices subject to change.                                    P

# Other Books Available

Prices subject to change.